MW01089073

How to Think Like a Radiologist

Radiologic investigations can be confusing to clinicians and radiologists alike. Questions invariably arise as to which type of imaging study best answers the clinical question posed. Once a modality is determined, decisions must be made regarding the technical manner in which the study is performed and if IV contrast is required. Patient factors, risks, benefits, and other variables must also be considered.

This pocket guide is written for anyone who needs to understand enough about radiology to know which study to order in a patient workup. The book addresses imaging studies by modality, body region, and type of study in bulleted outline format for easy reference. General considerations for each modality – including advantages and disadvantages – are presented, followed by information on patient preparation and requirements for each type of examination. Dr. Tara Marie Catanzano explains how specific studies are performed, what information can be obtained, study indications, contraindications, and limitations. The book also includes two appendixes.

Educated at the Royal College of Surgeons in Ireland, Dr. Tara Marie Catanzano learned the value of appropriate medical indications for imaging. During her internship, residency, and fellowship in diagnostic radiology at Yale-New Haven Hospital, she performed a variety of research projects and was awarded the title of Fellow of the Year as well as the RSNA Resident/Fellow Research Award. Dr. Catanzano is formerly Assistant Professor of Diagnostic Radiology and Chief of Cardiac Imaging at Yale University School of Medicine.

How to Think Like a Radiologist

ORDERING IMAGING STUDIES

Tara Marie Catanzano

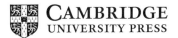
CAMBRIDGE
UNIVERSITY PRESS

CAMBRIDGE UNIVERSITY PRESS
Cambridge, New York, Melbourne, Madrid, Cape Town, Singapore, São Paulo, Delhi

Cambridge University Press
32 Avenue of the Americas, New York, NY 10013-2473, USA

www.cambridge.org
Information on this title: www.cambridge.org/9780521715232

First published 2009

Printed in the United States of America

A catalog record for this publication is available from the British Library.

Library of Congress Cataloging in Publication Data

Catanzano, Tara Marie, 1973–
How to think like a radiologist : ordering imaging studies / Tara
Marie Catanzano.
    p. ; cm.
Includes bibliographical references and index.
ISBN 978-0-521-71523-2 (pbk.)
1. Diagnosis, Radioscopic – Handbooks, manuals, etc.   2. Radiography, Medical –
Handbooks, manuals, etc.   I. Title.
[DNLM: 1. Diagnostic Imaging – Handbooks. WN 39 C357h 2009]
RC78.C39   2009
616.07′57–dc22   2008014183

ISBN   978-0-521-71523-2 paperback

In loving memory of my grandparents. Thank you for being my guiding light, my inspiration, my hope, and my future. Without your love and support, none of my achievements would have been possible. This book is a representation of your dedication to me . . . thus I dedicate it to you.
Forever love.

Contents

Preface

Diagnostic imaging is a constantly evolving specialty with new technology and new imaging methods constantly arising. It can be extremely challenging to navigate the ever-changing tide of medical imaging. Clinicians are continually plagued by a variety of questions when requesting imaging studies.

"What study is best to evaluate right upper quadrant pain?"
"Does the CT require IV contrast?"
"Can the patient eat before the upper GI?"
"What information will I get from the CT versus the ultrasound?"

These and other questions can make it difficult for the referring clinician to request the most appropriate investigation and to counsel the patient on the required preparation for the examination. It is the intention of this text to guide clinicians through the maze of medical imaging by providing information on different imaging modalities (e.g., x-ray, fluoroscopy, ultrasound, CT, MR, nuclear imaging, interventional procedure). Consideration will be given to general information about the technique, how the procedure is performed, patient preparation, contraindications to the examination, and limitations of the studies.

The text is divided into imaging by body region and technology (e.g., body MR imaging, neuroradiology, genitourinary imaging, and so on). Charts are provided for some of the more common imaging requests.

Clearly, given the scope of diagnostic imaging and the rapidity with which it changes, it is not possible to be exhaustive in the discussions of each type of study or modality. Some topics are beyond the scope of the text and are not included for discussion. What is provided is meant to act as a general guide to the available technologies. Its purpose is to determine patient suitability for an examination, study suitability for the question posed, and significant limitations and contraindications to the examination.

Tara Marie Catanzano

Radiation and Contrast Concerns

General Considerations

- The risks of iatrogenic injury from radiation exposure and contrast administration (in any route) should always be seriously considered prior to the request for an imaging study. Remember, *primum no nocere . . .* "first do no harm."
- Almost every imaging investigation carries with it risks, some of which are yet unknown for newer modalities.
- Risks include radiation-induced malignancy (a cumulative risk over the lifetime of a patient), contrast reaction, contrast-induced nephropathy (CIN), and nephrogenic systemic fibrosis (NSF). These entities are considered in this chapter.

Radiation Risks

- Every human is exposed to radiation on a daily basis, in the form of solar radiation. Individuals living in areas where there is loss of the protective ozone layer have increased exposure to this ionizing radiation. Individuals also receive increased exposure to background radiation when they fly in airplanes.
- The highest single exposure to ionizing radiation on record occurred in the fallout from the atomic bombs dropped on Hiroshima and Nagasaki. This fallout totaled a radiation dose of 5–200 mSv.
- Medical radiation is the highest exposure to ionizing radiation that most individuals receive, putting them at increased risk of radiation-induced malignancy.
- The following is a rough estimate of the amount of radiation involved with most imaging exposures; these and other values

are available online. The total effective radiation dose is dependent upon the equipment used and varies from center to center.

Background Radiation	0.3 mSv
Chest Radiograph	0.5 mSv
Abdominal Radiograph	1.2 mSv
Chest CT	5–8 mSv
Routine Abdominopelvic CT	10–20 mSv
Hematuria Protocol CT	30–40 mSv
Flank Pain Protocol CT	6–10
Head CT	2 mSv
Cervical Spine CT	2 mSv
Cardiac Nuclear SPECT	10–20 mSv
Coronary CT Angiography (CTA)	7–15 mSv
HIDA Scan	2–3 mSv
PET	14 mSv
Coronary Angiography	5–20 mSv (diagnostic catheter)

- The risk of malignancy is approximately 1 in 2,000 if a patient receives 10 mSv of radiation, according to FDA data.
- Many patients undergo repeated examinations that require ionizing radiation. The total radiation exposure can far exceed that received from the fallout in Hiroshima. For example, a patient may present with chest pain to the ER. A hypothetical (but plausible) evaluation of this patient may include the following:

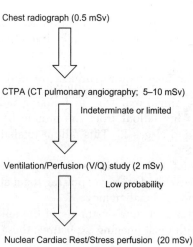

Chest radiograph (0.5 mSv)

CTPA (CT pulmonary angiography; 5–10 mSv)

Indeterminate or limited

Ventilation/Perfusion (V/Q) study (2 mSv)

Low probability

Nuclear Cardiac Rest/Stress perfusion (20 mSv)

Total radiation exposure: approximately 32.5 mSv

■ If alternative imaging modalities that do not involve radiation are available and they can provide adequate information to confirm a suspected diagnosis or direct appropriate treatment, they should be seriously and carefully considered. An example would be use of a retroperitoneal ultrasound to evaluate for hydronephrosis in a patient with known renal stones who is presenting with classic flank pain. Use of retroperitoneal ultrasound would obviate the need for a flank pain protocol CT (6–10 mSv) and would direct therapy because percutaneous or transureteral stenting would only be required if renal obstruction was present. The treatment, otherwise, would be medical with hydration and pain control.

Contrast Agents and Administration

■ *Oral contrast:* For studies in which bowel opacification is necessary (e.g. appendicitis) or useful (e.g. mesenteric metastases), oral contrast is administered. Oral contrast allows the bowel wall to be visualized, and it allows the presence and location of bowel obstruction, extrinsic compression, inflammation, and so on to be determined. Three main oral contrast agents are routinely used: barium, Hypaque, and water. Water is a "negative" contrast agent, which makes the bowel low in density (attenuation). Barium and Hypaque are "positive" contrast agents, which make the bowel dense (or white appearing). Barium is used for routine outpatient imaging and is an inert substance. Its drawback is that if it leaks from the bowel into the peritoneum (e.g. in bowel perforation), it becomes thickly adherent to the peritoneal surfaces, which can complicate surgery. Hypaque does not have this property, thus it is used for inpatient and ER patients who may require surgical treatment. Hypaque, however, can cause pulmonary edema if aspirated into the lung.
■ *IV contrast:* There are two main types still used in routine clinical practice: ionic and non-ionic. There are a variety of preparations of each, with various viscosities and different risks to the kidneys, particularly in the diabetic population. Non-ionic contrast is less nephrotoxic and has a reported lower risk of contrast reaction than ionic contrast; however, non-ionic contrast material is slightly more expensive than ionic.
  □ IV contrast can be nephrotoxic; therefore, it should not be administered to patients with chronic renal insufficiency or acute or chronic renal failure. The level of renal

dysfunction at which individuals still receive IV contrast varies by institution. At our institution, contrast is not administered if the creatinine (Cr) is >1.5 mg/dL. Patients with elevated Cr may be hydrated and given acetylcysteine (Mucormyst) prior to a study in an effort to be renoprotective. The radiologist should be consulted at the time of the study request for these patients in order to determine if IV contrast should be administered or if an alternative imaging study should be considered.

☐ Patients taking oral hypoglycemic agents (e.g. metformin) are at risk for lactic acidosis when IV contrast is administered. To decrease this risk, the patient is advised to discontinue the metformin on the day of and for 48 hours following the examination. They are also advised to have Cr redrawn 48 hours following the contrast administration to evaluate for CIN.

☐ Patients with IV contrast allergies should be premedicated where appropriate (see the following).

☐ IV contrast may be administered by hand injection; however, this technique has limitations. Although it may be the only manner in which IV contrast can be administered to small children or to patients with small caliber or tenuous IVs (in whom "power injection" with a machine is not safe), hand injection means that the bolus of contrast material is spread out over time. This leads to delayed scanning of the patient, often minutes after contrast administration, at which time contrast may have already left the arterial vascular bed and may be in later phases of organ enhancement (e.g. portal venous phase in the liver). This delay may significantly compromise an examination, particularly if the study must be timed to a specific vascular bed such as the pulmonary arteries for evaluation of pulmonary embolism. CT pulmonary angiography (CTPA) cannot be performed if the patient must be hand injected.

☐ Most studies are performed with the use of a power injector; this is a machine that holds contrast material to inject intravenously, which is controlled from the scanner console. These injectors have pressure safety monitoring devices such that if the pressure exceeds a certain amount, the injection is stopped. Because of this, large bore IVs are required for rapid contrast administration under pressure (usually required for vascular studies such as pulmonary embolism aortic dissection, and CT coronary angiography). If routine chest, abdomen, pelvis, or neuro CTs are performed, a slower rate of contrast administration is sufficient, which can be performed through a smaller IV. It is advisable to check with your department to determine the required IV size for study indication (e.g. 20-gauge IV is required for CTA and CTPA).

☐ PICC lines and central lines cannot be injected by power injector or by hand (unless a special "power PICC" specifically designed for this indication is used). The reasoning behind this is that there is a risk of shearing off the tip of the catheter with the pressure from the contrast injection or showering thromboemboli from around the catheter tip.

▪ *Angiography (intra-arterial contrast administration):* The risks of performing contrast tests are the same as for IV administration, although the risks surrounding contrast may be more severe and immediate.

☐ For enteric contrast (i.e. bowel), barium is the agent of choice over Hypaque unless there is concern about bowel perforation. Barium is an inert substance (a member of the periodic table), which is very dense and thus is well visualized on x-ray (fluoroscopic) studies. Barium has the advantage over Hypaque in that it is easily seen with fluoroscopy and thus outlines bowel pathology well.

• There are differences in the preparations/suspensions of barium for different imaging modalities. The barium used for fluoroscopic studies is an extremely dense suspension that is not appropriate for CT as it causes the CT x-ray beam to be deflected in various directions and causes so-called streak artifact, which can render the CT uninterpretable. Therefore, if a CT is considered for a patient already scheduled for a fluoroscopic barium study, the CT should be performed first. The x-rays in fluoroscopy can "see through" the CT barium, if necessary.

Premedication for Intravascular Contrast

▪ Experts differ in their opinions about what constitutes an increased risk of contrast reaction; it is best to discuss the local policies for premedication with your radiology department.

Radiation and Contrast Concerns

- There is a theoretic increased risk of contrast reaction in patients with multiple allergies, atopy, and shellfish allergy.
- Patients with previously documented contrast allergy should be premedicated for a contrast-enhanced examination unless an anaphylactic reaction to contrast was previously documented. In these patients, intravascular contrast SHOULD NOT be administered.
- Contrast reaction includes minor and major reactions and may present as any of the following:
  - ☐ Sneezing
  - ☐ Vomiting
  - ☐ Hypo/hypertension
  - ☐ Cutaneous reactions (e.g. itching or hives)
  - ☐ Throat tightness
  - ☐ Wheezing
  - ☐ Chest tightness/shortness of breath
  - ☐ Anaphylaxis
- The following are normal side effects of contrast administration that some patients experience and are not contrast reactions:
  - ☐ Metallic taste
  - ☐ Flushing
  - ☐ Nausea
  - ☐ Warm feeling
- Premedication regimens:
  - ☐ A variety of regimens are in clinical use for the premedication of patients with known or suspected contrast reaction.
  - ☐ The need for premedication must be communicated to the scheduler at the time of the imaging request so that the examination may be scheduled for a time when the premedication regimen has been completed. For inpatients requiring premedication, it is suggested that the housestaff stay in communication with the technologists/schedulers to ensure completion of the regimen.
  - ☐ The following regimens are suggested:
  - ☐ Regimen 1:
    - • Medication: Prednisone
    - • Route: Oral
    - • Dose: 50 mg
    - • Schedule: 13, 7, and 1 hour prior to contrast-enhanced CT (CECT)

- Diphenhydramine (Benadryl) 50 mg oral or IV is also administered 1 hour prior to CECT
- Cimetidine may also be administered for its H_2 antagonist effects
□ Regimen 2:
  - Medication: Methylprednisolone sodium succinate (Solu-Medrol)
  - Route: IV
  - Dose: 125 mg
  - Schedule: 4–6 and 1 hour prior to CECT
  - Benadryl 50 mg oral or IV is also administered 1 hour prior to CECT
  - IV cimetidine may also be administered for its H_2 antagonist effects

Nephrogenic Systemic Fibrosis

- NSF is a recently recognized disease that has been linked to the IV administration of gadolinium contrast agents for MR examinations.
- NSF is a scleroderma-like disease that progresses over the course of several years and may result in death.
- NSF is associated with the administration of gadolinium in patients with impaired renal function. Currently, there are no national guidelines as to the precise level of renal dysfunction at which it is safe to administer gadolinium. Institutional policies vary and are based on the estimated glomerular filtration rate (eGFR), which is more accurate than serum Cr for evaluation of nephron function.
- At our institution, patients at risk for or with known renal impairment must have an eGFR calculated within 1 month prior to the study. Patients with severe liver disease must have labs within 24 hours before the study. For patients with renal disease, gadolinium may be administered if the eGFR is > 30; it must be > 40 for patients with severe liver disease due to the partial hepatic excretion of gadolinium.
- It is recommended that the local policy be determined prior to request for a contrast-enhanced MR examination.

2

Chest Imaging

Conventional Radiographs

■ A CXR is the initial step in imaging acute cardiopulmonary disease.

■ A CXR may be performed using a stationary or portable radiography unit.

■ Indications for portable CXR include unstable patients in acute distress, intubated patients in ICUs, and intraoperative/recovery room radiographs.

■ Optimal CXR includes frontal and lateral projections. It may only be possible to obtain frontal views due to a patient's clinical status, body habitus, or pregnancy. Pregnant patients are required to give verbal consent after discussion of the risks of radiation to the fetus, and these patients are double or triple lead shielded for the study. The risk to the fetus is low, particularly in later pregnancy when the fetus has developed beyond the stage of organogenesis. The patient (mother) is "triple shielded," meaning that lead aprons are placed over the abdomen and pelvis to protect the fetus from the x-ray beam. The actual scatter radiation from a single x-ray is quite low and typically of no significant risk to the fetus.

■ CXR findings often lag behind clinical findings by up to 48 hours.

■ In certain disease processes, the CXR may be normal.

■ CXR findings may be non-specific and can be seen in a variety of diseases; for example, it may not be possible to differentiate pulmonary edema from multilobar pneumonia. The clinical history is often key to interpreting radiographic findings.

Decubitus Radiographs

- This is the radiographic imaging study of choice to evaluate layering versus loculated pleural effusions; however, ultrasound is becoming the overall study of choice. Ultrasound allows quantification and characterization of pleural fluid (e.g. loculations), which radiographs cannot.
- Bilateral decubitus images are obtained to evaluate right and left pleural abnormalities.
- Decubitus radiographs may allow for evaluation of underlying pulmonary parenchymal abnormalities.
- Decubitus radiographs may occasionally be useful to evaluate for subtle pneumothorax, particularly in premature infants.
- They may be used to evaluate for air-trapping in patients suspected of aspirating foreign bodies.
- CT should be performed to evaluate for loculated pleural effusions only if the patient is too unstable or immobile for decubitus positioning; ultrasound may be performed to evaluate for complicated pleural effusions or loculation and does not require a radiation exposure. Ultrasound has the added advantage of performance at the bedside if the patient is too unstable to be transported to the CT scanner.

INDICATIONS
- ☐ Assessment of layering pleural effusion
- ☐ Assessment of underlying pulmonary parenchymal abnormality
- ☐ Assessment of air trapping from aspirated foreign body (usually pediatric population)
- ☐ Assessment of pneumothorax (usually pediatric population)

CONTRAINDICATIONS: None

LIMITATIONS
- ☐ Patients may be difficult to position due to clinical condition, contractures, or body habitus.
- ☐ Obese patients may have suboptimal films due to the increased soft tissue penetration required in the decubitus position.
- ☐ Patients should be maintained in the decubitus position for several minutes before imaging to allow for changes in location of fluid or air that occur with change in position. If patients are imaged too quickly after repositioning, there may be insufficient time for relocation of fluid or air.

Inspiration/Expiration Radiography

- Expiratory CXR (i.e. taken with patient in full expiration) is useful to evaluate for subtle pneumothoraces. The change in intrathoracic pressure draws the lung away from the pleural space and accentuates the pneumothorax.
- Inspiratory CXR (i.e. taken with the patient in full inspiration) should always be attempted. This allows for full expansion of the lungs, thus allowing for the optimal evaluation of the lung parenchyma. Full inspiration also allows for optimal assessment of cardiac size.

INDICATIONS:

- ☐ Inspiratory films should be obtained in all patients to optimize evaluation of cardiopulmonary disease.
- ☐ Expiratory films should be obtained if there is clinical or radiographic suspicion of subtle pneumothorax.

CONTRAINDICATIONS

- ☐ If patients cannot comprehend or comply with verbal commands, the study cannot be performed adequately.

LIMITATIONS

- ☐ Poor patient cooperation may make it difficult or impossible to obtain inspiratory or expiratory images.

Apical Lordotic Imaging

- Apical lordotic imaging is obtained with the patient in the AP/PA projection. The x-ray beam is angled toward the patient's head.
- It is useful when evaluating the lung apices, particularly for suspected nodules or masses overlying the first costochondral articulations.
- This type of imaging should not be performed as routine practice but rather as a problem-solving tool.

INDICATIONS

- ☐ Evaluation of the lung apices in patients with abnormal AP/PA chest film in which there is a suspicion of mass or nodule overlying the first costochondral articulation

CONTRAINDICATIONS: None

LIMITATIONS

- ☐ Patient positioning may be difficult, particularly in older or immobile patients.

Shallow Oblique Radiographs

▨ Shallow oblique radiographs are obtained with the patient positioned in 15 degrees of obliquity. Both right and left oblique views are obtained.
▨ They are useful to evaluate suspected nodules in order to confirm the finding and to assess if the nodules are within the skin, within the pulmonary parenchyma, or within bone.

Nipple Markers

▨ These are stickers with a metallic marker that are placed on the nipples.
▨ They are particularly useful in males, cachectic patients, and small-breasted women in whom a nipple may mimic a nodule.
▨ They assist in differentiating a parenchymal nodule from nipple shadow.
▨ Although some institutions employ nipple markers for all patients imaged, markers increase the time required for the examination and the cost of imaging.

INDICATIONS
☐ Male patients or females with small breasts in whom the nipple overlies the thorax. This may simulate a lung nodule. Nipple markers allow the radiologist to identify the "nodule" as a nipple.

CONTRAINDICATIONS: None

LIMITATIONS
☐ Nipple markers increase the cost of the examination.
☐ The placement of nipple markers requires additional time for patient preparation and may slow patient throughput, particularly in busy imaging departments.

Rib Films

▨ Most rib series include a frontal view of the chest and bone algorithm views (i.e. higher radiation dose) of the ribs. Multiple projections are obtained.
▨ These films are often unnecessary as the main complication of rib fracture is pneumothorax, which is best assessed on frontal views of the chest. Displaced rib fractures are often seen on conventional chest radiographs. Non-displaced rib fractures are often NOT visible on CXR or rib films.

- CT is NOT an appropriate method to evaluate for rib fractures as the images are obtained in the axial planes, thus, fractures oriented in this plane are often not visible.

Indications for Repeat Chest X-Ray

- Suboptimal radiographs
- Acute change in clinical status, particularly if further imaging (e.g. for evaluation of pulmonary emboli) is contemplated
- Following placement of percutaneous catheters, endotracheal tubes, or feeding tubes
- Daily portable films for intubated patients to assess line positioning, change in pulmonary findings
- Follow-up radiographs in patients with infiltrates to ensure resolution, as neoplasms may mimic the CXR findings of pneumonia (performed approximately 6–8 weeks after completion of therapy to allow for radiographic findings of acute infection to resolve)

CT of the Thorax

There are four main categories of chest CT: routine non-contrast CT of the thorax; contrast-enhanced CT (CECT) of the thorax; CT angiography (CTA) for pulmonary embolism, and high-resolution CT of the thorax.

Non-Contrast CT of the Thorax

- This is the most common protocol.
- It images the thorax from the thoracic inlet through the upper abdomen to include the adrenal glands.
- No IV contrast is administered.
- It is most often employed to evaluate findings noted on conventional radiographs (e.g. pulmonary nodules).

  INDICATIONS
  - ☐ Evaluation or follow-up of pulmonary nodules and masses
  - ☐ Staging and restaging of lung carcinoma (unless vascular invasion/involvement is known or suspected or hilar adenopathy is known or suspected; CECT is required for these indications)
  - ☐ Staging/restaging of lymphoma (with the exception of hilar lymphadenopathy)

□ Evaluation of aortic size/follow-up of aneurysms

LIMITATIONS

□ Non-contrast CT has a low sensitivity for hilar lymphade-nopathy.

□ CT is of little use in patients with acute processes such as pneumonia. If a patient demonstrates clinical findings consistent with an infectious process and conventional radiographs demonstrate an infiltrate, there is little to be gained from CT in the acute setting (unless there is a question of lung abscess or necrosis; contrast is required for these indications). The parenchyma involved by the infectious process cannot be further evaluated. If, however, radiographic findings persist following appropriate therapy for an infectious process (with expected radiographic resolution lagging behind clinical findings by several weeks), a CT may be appropriate at that time to evaluate for occult malignancy.

Contrast-Enhanced CT of the Thorax

▪ CECT is used less commonly than non-contrast CT.

▪ The most common indications for CECT are central lesions with a question of hilar lymphadenopathy or vascular involvement.

▪ Average contrast dose: 100 cc non-ionic contrast

▪ CTA requires a 20-gauge IV line minimum; a smaller gauge IV line may be used if a slower rate of contrast is to be administered (e.g. as used in routine CECT). In general, PICC lines are not used unless they are specially made "power PICCs" capable of handling high flow rates from IV contrast power injectors.

▪ Renal function: There is variability amongst institutions with regard to renal function and the level of creatinine (Cr) above which contrast cannot be administered. At our institution, contrast is administered to patients with a Cr $\leq$ 1.5 mg/dL.

▪ Contrast allergies: For patients with a history of contrast allergy, premedication with steroids is required. There are a variety of protocols in use for premedication. The two most common are as follows:

□ 50 mg prednisone orally 13, 7, and 1 hour prior to the study + 50 mg diphenhydramine (Benadryl) IV 1 hour prior to the study

□ Stress dose 125 mg IV methylprednisolone sodium succinate (Solu-Medrol) every 4–6 hours

INDICATIONS

- Evaluation of central lesions to evaluate for hilar involvement of lymphadenopathy
- Evaluation of vascular structures, particularly SVC obstruction by tumor and aortic dissections (performed without and then with IV contrast)
- Evaluation for possible vascular abnormalities such as aortic aneurysm or pulmonary artery pseudoaneurysm (e.g. post Swan)
- Evaluation of empyema (IV contrast is required to evaluate for enhancement of the pleura, which allows for the diagnosis to be made)
- Evaluation of mediastinal abscess (e.g. mediastinitis)
- Evaluation of lung abscess or necrosis

CONTRAINDICATIONS

- IV contrast is not necessary for the identification or follow-up of pulmonary nodules.

LIMITATIONS

- Loculated or complex pleural effusions may not be identifiable on CT; ultrasound is more sensitive for the evaluation of septated pleural fluid.
- If the study is performed to evaluate for venous thrombosis (e.g. SVC obstruction/occlusion), timing of the contrast administration is crucial. If there is not enough time delay, a false-positive result can occur from mixing of opacified and unopacified blood. If too much time elapses after IV contrast administration, false negatives may occur due to washout of contrast from the vessel, thus making the thrombus inapparent.

CT Angiography for Pulmonary Embolism

- This study is performed for the sole indication of evaluation of suspected pulmonary thromboembolic disease. Images through the pulmonary vasculature are obtained at intervals of 1.3 mm with overlap.
- The study should not be performed in lieu of a CXR in a patient with an acute event as there are a variety of CXR findings that may provide an explanation for the patient's symptoms and circumvent the radiation dose and contrast load of a CTA.

■ The study is performed with IV contrast, which is administered at a rate of 4–5 mL/second through a power injector. In young patients, rates of contrast administration may be increased to up to 8 mL/second in order to provide an adequate contrast bolus in patients with fast circulation times. Due to the high rates of IV contrast injection, a well-functioning, large-gauge IV line is required (20 gauge).

■ Average contrast dose: 100 cc non-ionic contrast

■ Renal function: As in the section, Contrast-Enhanced CT of the Thorax, earlier

■ Contrast allergies: As in the section, Contrast-Enhanced CT of the Thorax, earlier

INDICATIONS

☐ Evaluation of acute or chronic thromboembolic events

CONTRAINDICATIONS

☐ Relative: Patients with radiographic findings that explain the clinical presentation and who are at low risk for thromboembolic disease may not require the additional radiation dose of a CTA. Careful consideration should be given to the pretest probability of pulmonary thromboembolic disease in these patients so that an unnecessary examination may be circumvented.

☐ Pregnancy: Women in the second and third trimester are at relatively lower risk of fetal injury from the examination as the fetal thyroid has already formed (there is a risk of congenital hypothyroidism in early pregnancy from fetal thyroid damage caused by IV contrast during thyroid development); radiation risk to the fetus is lower after organogenesis has been completed. A lower extremity venous Doppler to exclude DVT is generally recommended as a primary imaging investigation as the treatment for both entities is the same and the fetal risk of CT is eliminated.

LIMITATIONS

☐ Patients with rapid cardiac circulating times may have poor quality studies due to the rapid washout of the IV contrast or the mixing of unopacified (dark) blood returning in the inferior vena cava from the abdomen.

☐ Patients with poorly functioning IVs may have a poor contrast bolus, limiting evaluation of clots.

☐ Respiratory or cardiac motion artifacts can render studies uninterpretable.

Chest Imaging

□ Slower CT scanners (e.g. single-, 4-, or 8-slice) may not be able to scan quickly enough to catch the contrast bolus. This may produce false-negative or false-positive results.

High-Resolution CT of the Thorax

■ This study is performed as a non-contrast examination. Images are obtained with a slice thickness of 1 mm at intervals of 10 mm in both inspiration and expiration. Thus, only 10% of the pulmonary parenchyma is imaged. However, at our institution, a routine non-contrast CT of the thorax is obtained prior to the high-resolution images.

■ It is performed solely for the evaluation of interstitial lung disease.

■ It is NOT an appropriate study to evaluate for pulmonary nodules as only approximately 10% of the lungs are imaged (unless local protocol includes a routine CT of the chest).

■ Patients must be able to breath-hold for at least 20 seconds for the study, thus, it is suggested that the study not be performed on patients hospitalized with superimposed acute pulmonary processes. Rather, it is suggested that the study be performed electively following resolution of the acute illness.

INDICATIONS

□ Identification and evaluation of interstitial lung diseases such as usual interstitial pneumonia, interstitial pulmonary fibrosis, sarcoid, lymphangitic spread of tumor, amiodorone toxicity, and so on

□ Follow-up/surveillance of the activity of the disease (this often can be determined based on the amount of ground glass opacity that is present)

□ Differentiation of abnormal perfusion from air trapping

CONTRAINDICATIONS

□ Inability to lie flat for the examination

□ Inability to comply with breath-holding instructions

□ Presence of acute superimposed pulmonary process (e.g. pulmonary edema or pneumonia). These acute processes make it difficult or impossible for the patient to comply with breath-holding instructions and will often mask the underlying pulmonary abnormality on the CT images.

LIMITATIONS

□ Many interstitial lung disease processes have similar imaging appearances. This may make it difficult or impossible to make a definitive diagnosis of a specific interstitial lung disease. Tissue sample is often necessary for diagnosis.

☐ If patients cannot comply with breath-holding instructions, it may not be possible to differentiate between air trapping and vascular abnormality. This may make it difficult or impossible to determine which portion of the lung is abnormal and what pathology is present.

"Triple Rule Out": Contrast-Enhanced CT Angiography of the Thorax

▪ This is a trade name coined by GE Healthcare. It indicates a CECT angiogram of the thorax, which has the contrast bolus timed in such a way that it will allow visualization of the aorta, pulmonary arteries, and coronary arteries.

▪ The studies can only be performed on a 16-slice or higher multidetector CT scanner; single-, 4-, and 8-slice scanners are not fast enough to allow image acquisition during contrast bolus injection.

INDICATIONS

☐ Evaluation of patients with chest pain in whom differential diagnosis includes aortic dissection, pulmonary embolus, and acute coronary syndrome (coronary artery disease)

CONTRAINDICATIONS

☐ Patients with contraindications to IV contrast material, including patients with contrast allergies, impaired renal function (elevated Cr), and so on

LIMITATIONS

☐ Every effort should be made to clinically differentiate between aortic dissection, pulmonary embolism, and coronary disease. This will allow the study to be tailored for optimal detection of the disease process in question.

☐ Contrast bolus timing may be difficult due to patient factors (e.g. poor IV access requiring smaller gauge IV), technical factors (e.g. slow infusion rate, inaccurate triggering of scanner), or physiologic factors (e.g. mixing of unopacified blood and contrast material leading to appearance of filling defect, leading to a false positive).

☐ If patients' heart rates are elevated (e.g. >90 beats/minute), evaluation of the coronary arteries is compromised. Patients may receive an oral or IV beta blocker prior to the examination if appropriate to slow the heart rate.

- [ ] Patients with renal impairment are not candidates for the study.
- [ ] As with all examinations, obese patients may be difficult or impossible to image as the radiation beam may not penetrate the chest wall well.
- [ ] Patients with cardiac pacemakers may be difficult to image as the right ventricular lead in particular produces an artifact that can obscure the right coronary artery.

3

Musculoskeletal Imaging

Conventional Radiographs

▪ These are the first steps in evaluation of musculoskeletal abnormalities.

▪ The radiographs may be performed using a stationary x-ray unit in the radiology department or using a portable unit in the patient's hospital room or in the operating room.

▪ Indications for portable imaging:

□ There are few true indications for portable musculoskeletal radiographs. Portable radiographs tend to be limited by technique and the patient's clinical condition. They may be performed on unstable patients to evaluate suspected acute fractures.

□ Portable films may be obtained in the trauma room on patients in whom osseous trauma is suspected and who are unstable.

□ Intraoperative films are obtained portably to confirm equipment or internal fixation device positioning. Fracture fragment positioning also may be evaluated with portable radiography in the operating room. Films are often obtained in the recovery room as a baseline for hardware positioning (e.g. hip prosthesis), fracture alignment, and so on. Fluoroscopy is used in the operating room to assess bone positioning while the bone is being manipulated.

▪ Optimal radiographs include a minimum of two projections at 90 degrees to each other (i.e. frontal and lateral views). For most long bones (i.e. femur and humerus), two views are sufficient. Imaging of a joint often requires three projections: frontal, oblique, and lateral views. Additional views may be obtained as warranted for evaluation of specific clinical questions. If an unusual or additional view is required, it is advisable for the clinician to discuss the case with the radiologist or technologist so that the best imaging is performed with minimal radiation exposure.

INDICATIONS

☐ Evaluation of suspected fracture. In patients with long bone fractures, imaging of the joints above and below the fracture site should be considered to evaluate for dislocation or additional fractures.

☐ Evaluation of patients with known or suspected arthritis. These films are obtained with a different technique than films obtained for the evaluation of bony injury and thus should be specifically requested. Conventional radiographs may be used for the diagnosis and follow-up of the arthridities.

☐ Evaluation of bone tumors. Conventional radiographs are often the diagnostic modality of choice for characterization of bone lesions. CT is of limited value in evaluation of bone tumors with the exception of determination of the matrix of the bone, which may help to narrow the differential diagnosis. MR may be performed to evaluate the same bone (e.g. femur) for second (synchronous) lesions.

☐ Evaluation of bone destruction, e.g. in osteomyelitis, septic arthritis Charcot joints, that is, joint fragmentation and destruction in patients with sensory depravation such as diabetes, syringomyelia, and so on.

CONTRAINDICATIONS

☐ Direct radiographs to the pelvis in early pregnancy are relative contraindications due to radiation risks to the fetus. However, if the risks to the mother from trauma or acute bony abnormality outweigh the risks to the fetus, the films should be obtained. If the patient or a family member is able, verbal informed consent for the films should be obtained.

☐ If the question is soft tissue or cervical/thoracic/lumbar spine disc disease, plain films are of limited value. A more definitive study (often MR) should be obtained without the added radiation exposure of conventional radiographs, which are unlikely to provide additional information. For example, the radiation dose to the gonads from lumbar spine radiographs is high, with very little yield in patients in whom disc disease is likely as the etiology of the patient's pain.

LIMITATIONS

☐ Postreduction films with the patient in an external cast are of limited value due to the cast. The x-ray beam cannot penetrate the cast, thus the fracture alignment may be difficult to assess, as may healing.

☐ Radiographs are of little use in the evaluation of suspected muscle, cartilage, or ligament injury as these are not visible on conventional radiographs. MRI is the optimal modality for these indications.

☐ Radiographs are of little use in evaluation of suspected early osteomyelitis as there is often a 10–14 day lag in radiographic manifestations of osteomyelitis. Radiographs may be useful in the early stages of osteomyelitis to evaluate for the presence of a foreign body acting as a nidus of infection and for air in the soft tissues, which would suggest a gas-forming organism infection. In late stages (>14 days), bony erosion may be present, indicating infection.

☐ Some fractures, particularly if non-displaced, may not be visible on radiographs obtained immediately following the acute trauma. Follow-up films in 7–10 days should be obtained in patients with high clinical suspicion of fracture. This will allow for periosteal new bone formation (i.e. callus formation) to occur, signifying healing of an occult fracture. It will also allow time for fracture line bone resorption (osteoclastic activity), which may render the fracture line visible.

Arthrography

▪ Arthrography involves the instillation of a contrast agent into a joint.

▪ The contrast agent instilled into the joint is dependent upon the modality to be used to image the area; non-ionic or iodinated contrast material only is used for conventional fluoroscopic arthrography. A mixture of saline, non-ionic/iodinated contrast (for the purpose of confirmation of needle placement in a joint), and gadolinium are instilled if MR arthrography is to be performed.

Musculoskeletal Imaging

■ Generally, the needle is positioned in the joint under fluoro-scopic guidance. Once the needle is confirmed to be within the joint, the joint is injected with the contrast material and the patient is imaged on CT or MR (as indicated). The injection should be performed no longer than 1–3 hours before the scan is to occur so that the contrast material does not seep out of the joint with normal joint fluid.

■ Conventional arthrography can be performed on a fluoroscopy unit. The joint is localized and contrast injected while the radi-ologist watches with fluoroscopy and manipulates the joint to evaluate for ligamentous injury. This is often performed for joints such as the wrist, although MR is generally the preferred method.

INDICATIONS

□ Evaluation of ligamentous injury, particularly rotator cuff tears (shoulder), ACL/PCL tears (knee), wrist ligaments

□ Evaluation of unstable joints (ligamentous injury)

□ Evaluation of joint pathology in patients who are unable to undergo CT or MR arthrography (e.g. pacemakers may cause streak artifacts on CT, limiting evaluation of a joint; pacemakers are contraindications for MR)

CONTRAINDICATIONS

□ Allergy to non-ionic IV contrast; small amounts of the con-trast instilled in the joint are absorbed into the systemic circulation from the joint lining. Therefore, it is possible to experience a contrast reaction from the arthrogram even though there is no IV administration of contrast.

□ Active or suspected joint infection; there is a small risk of infecting a joint by needle placement, even if performed under sterile conditions. Contrast itself is bacteriostatic. If there is concern for a septic joint, IV contrast-enhanced MR may be performed or imaging-guided joint aspiration may be undertaken.

LIMITATIONS

□ Conventional arthrography is an indirect evaluation of lig-aments; it does not directly visualize the ligament or its attachments (unlike MR).

□ The bones of the joint cannot be adequately evaluated with this technique; MR is the imaging modality of choice to eval-uate for bone edema or occult fracture, which may suggest a more significant injury.

☐ Partial ligament injuries such as partial or incomplete rotator cuff tears may not be identified with this technique (i.e. false negative).

CT

■ The majority of CTs performed for the evaluation of musculoskeletal pathology are performed as non-contrast studies (i.e. without IV contrast).

■ Images are most commonly obtained directly in the axial plane. With multislice CT technology, the axial data can be reconstructed into images in the sagittal and coronal planes.

■ Imaging is confined to the specific region of clinical interest. CT is NOT an appropriate modality to screen for diffuse disease (e.g. diffuse osseous metastatic disease, for which a bone scan is a more appropriate investigation).

INDICATIONS

☐ Identification of occult fractures not demonstrated on conventional radiography

☐ Preoperative planning of documented fractures

☐ Evaluation of congenital anomalies (e.g. tarsal coalition)

☐ Characterization of the matrix of a bone lesion identified on conventional radiography

CONTRAINDICATIONS

☐ Evaluation of ligaments, tendons, menisci, and so on; MR is the study of choice for this indication.

☐ Evaluation of suspected abscesses as IV contrast is required to evaluate for enhancing collections

☐ Evaluation of osteomyelitis; bone destruction does not occur until late in the disease. If there is concern for osteomyelitis, nuclear medicine bone scan or MR is recommended.

LIMITATIONS

☐ Patient factors: If the patient cannot be properly positioned (e.g. in patients with contractures or fractures), it may be difficult to image the fracture in a useful plane.

☐ Images may be degraded by streak artifact if an external fixator or internal fixation is present.

☐ Collections such as hematomas can be identified without the administration of IV contrast. However, infected hematomas (unless they contain air) and abscesses cannot be identified without IV contrast.

Musculoskeletal Imaging

☐ Soft tissue masses such as liposarcomas and malignant fibrous histiocytomas cannot be characterized on non-contrast CT. MR with IV contrast is the optimal imaging modality for primary soft tissue tumors as it allows for localization, characterization, and extent of tumor involvement.

☐ Primary bone tumors may be characterized on non-contrast CT; however, if there is a soft tissue component to the tumor, this may not be recognized or characterized on a non-contrast CT examination. Contrast-enhanced CT (CECT) or, preferably, MR should be performed for the evaluation of a known or suspected soft tissue component.

Musculoskeletal Contrast-Enhanced CT

INDICATIONS

☐ Evaluation of suspected abscesses

☐ Evaluation of vascular compromise by the presence of a soft tissue or an osseous mass

CONTRAINDICATIONS

☐ Poor renal function or contrast allergy

LIMITATIONS

☐ Small abscess collections may be below the resolution of CT.

☐ Intraosseous abscesses (i.e. an abscess in the bone marrow or cortex) is not typically visualized on CT. Contrast-enhanced MR is the imaging study of choice for this indication.

☐ Infected joint prosthesis cannot be definitively determined on CT; nuclear medicine imaging or contrast-enhanced MR are the studies of choice.

☐ Streak artifact from metal prosthesis can mask collections, particularly if small.

☐ Obese patients may be difficult to image, particularly if the area of interest is small, if the patient is too large and touches the sides of the CT scanner gantry (causing artifact), or if the collection is small.

CT Arthrography

▪ CT arthrography is performed in the same manner as conventional arthrography and MR arthrography; the joint is accessed and contrast is instilled. The study may be performed under fluoroscopy or may be performed under CT guidance. Once contrast is placed into the joint, the CT scan is performed.

INDICATIONS

☐ Evaluation of internal joint derangement (i.e. rotator cuff injuries, ACL/PCL graft injury)
☐ Evaluation of the postoperative joint
☐ Evaluation of labral injuries (i.e. shoulder glenoid labrum), evaluation of postoperative rotator cuffs for reinjury, evaluation of loose bodies in the joint
☐ Evaluation of ACL/PCL graft repairs; evaluation of postoperative menisci, evaluation of loose joint bodies
☐ Evaluation of the hip labrum

CONTRAINDICATIONS

☐ Allergy to non-ionic/IV contrast; small amounts of the contrast instilled in the joint are absorbed into the systemic circulation from the joint lining. Therefore, it is possible to experience a contrast reaction from the arthrogram even though there is no IV administration of contrast.
☐ Active or suspected joint infection; there is a small risk of infecting a joint by needle placement, even if performed under sterile conditions. Contrast itself is bacteriostatic. If there is concern for a septic joint, IV contrast-enhanced MR may be performed or imaging-guided joint aspiration may be undertaken.

LIMITATIONS

☐ Bone pathology such as bone edema or non-displaced fractures are not demonstrated on CT; MR is the modality of choice for this indication.
☐ In obese patients, artifacts related to body habitus may render the study suboptimal for evaluation of subtle injury.
☐ MR is a more optimal imaging modality for loose bodies that are not ossified or calcified; nonossified or noncalcified loose bodies may not be visible on CT.
☐ Evaluation of the articular cartilage is inferior to MR.

Musculoskeletal MRI

▪ It is the study of choice to evaluate ligamentous, tendinous, and cartilaginous injuries.
▪ Three types of studies may be performed: non-contrast MR, IV contrast-enhanced imaging, and MR arthrography

■ Suitability of candidates for MRI should be assessed prior to a request for a study.

CONTRAINDICATIONS

☐ Presence of a pacer/automatic implantable cardioverter de-fibrillator

☐ Recent cardiac stent placement (relative contraindication); currently, MR may be performed within 24 hours of stent placement.

☐ Obese patients (>350 lbs)

☐ Claustrophobic patients (relative contraindication)

☐ Unstable patients

Non-Contrast Musculoskeletal MRI

■ It is the study of choice for the evaluation of sports injuries (particularly of the knee).

■ Non-contrast study is an efficacious way to evaluate for occult fracture without the additional radiation of CT.

■ Non-contrast studies are inadequate to evaluate for labral pathology of the glenoid and acetabulum; MR arthrography is the study of choice in these patients.

■ In the postoperative sports injury patient (e.g. rotator cuff repair, ACL/PCL repair), MR arthrography is the study of choice.

INDICATIONS

☐ Evaluation of ligament, cartilage, tendon injuries

☐ Evaluation of occult fracture

☐ Evaluation of avascular necrosis, particularly of the hip

☐ Evaluation of muscle injuries

CONTRAINDICATIONS

☐ Contractures: If patients cannot be appropriately positioned, the study may be suboptimal or false positives/negatives may occur.

☐ Inability to maintain positioning: If patients cannot remain still, the imaging will be suboptimal and may be of no diagnostic value.

☐ Unstable patients should not be placed in the MR magnet for routine, non-emergent imaging.

☐ Claustrophobia: This is relative; sedation may be given as the patients are not required to comply with instructions such as breath holding.

LIMITATIONS

☐ Partial thickness ligament or cartilage tears may not be identified on non-contrast examinations.

☐ Loose bodies may be difficult to recognize in the absence of joint fluid or intra-articular contrast.

☐ Labral injuries are difficult to diagnose without intra-articular contrast.

IV Contrast-Enhanced Musculoskeletal MRI

■ The study involves the administration of IV gadolinium, which is a water-based compound that is visible with MRI.

■ Non-contrast images are obtained first, followed by contrast-enhanced images.

■ Given the recent recognition of gadolinium-related nephrogenic systemic fibrosis (NSF), patients with known or suspected renal dysfunction should have a creatinine (Cr) level drawn prior to the examination, as per institutional guidelines. Gadolinium is less nephrotoxic than ionic and non-ionic CT contrast and is generally safe for use in patients with elevated Cr levels up to 5.0 mg/dL.

■ Although less common than in ionic/non-ionic contrast imaging, contrast reactions can occur and may occasionally be life threatening. Premedication protocols are the same as those for other contrast allergies.

INDICATIONS

☐ IV gadolinium is required for the evaluation of all suspected or documented musculoskeletal masses.

☐ Evaluation of osteomyelitis

☐ Gadolinium-enhanced MR is the study of choice for the evaluation of soft tissue tumors including location, extent, and neurovascular involvement.

☐ Preoperative planning for possible limb-sparing procedures for treatment of musculoskeletal malignancies

☐ Follow-up of resected neoplasms to evaluate for residual or recurrent disease

☐ Evaluation of known or suspected marrow replacing lesions such as lymphoma, metastatic disease, and infection

☐ Evaluation of presence and extent of osteomyelitis

☐ Evaluation of soft tissue vascular and lymphatic malformations (MR angiography may be needed for evaluation of vascular malformations)

CONTRAINDICATIONS

☐ Renal dysfunction due to the risks of NSF
☐ Lack of adequate IV access

LIMITATIONS

☐ It may be difficult to differentiate recurrent tumor from normal postoperative appearances in cases of soft tissue tumor resection.
☐ Metallic hardware (e.g. intramedullary rods, hip prostheses, surgical clips) cause artifacts, which may render study performance suboptimal or difficult.
☐ Some slow flow vascular malformations (e.g. venous malformations) may be difficult to differentiate from lymphatic malformations.
☐ Vessel occlusion may be difficult to differentiate from very slow flow.

MR Arthrography

■ It involves fluoroscopically guided instillation of a gadolinium-based solution into the joint of interest in order to evaluate for pathology.
■ As with the IV administration of contrast, there is a risk of contrast reaction. As with any percutaneous procedure, there is also a minimal risk of bleeding or infection related to the procedure.

INDICATIONS

☐ The majority of MR arthrograms are performed in the postoperative patient to evaluate for reinjury.
☐ Shoulder arthrography is often performed to evaluate for rotator cuff pathology as well as for labral injury.
☐ Hip arthrography is useful to evaluate for injury to the acetabular labrum.

CONTRAINDICATIONS

☐ Active joint infection
☐ Immediate postoperative state (relative)

LIMITATIONS

☐ Metallic hardware (e.g. bone anchors, prostheses) may make image acquisition and interpretation difficult.

☐ It may be difficult to differentiate postoperative appearances from reinjury in ligament/tendon repairs.

☐ It may be difficult to access a joint following surgery due to fibrous scar tissue; therefore, it may be difficult or impossible for an adequate amount of contrast to be instilled into the joint.

Musculoskeletal Imaging

4

Genitourinary Imaging

Conventional Radiographs

■ These are of limited value in the evaluation of genitourinary pathology.
■ They may be useful in the following settings:
  □ To evaluate the presence of renal/ureteral or bladder calculi; this is most useful as a follow-up examination in patients in whom a stone has been documented on CT. Typically, if a stone can be seen on the scout view of a flank pain protocol CT, it can be seen with conventional radiographs. Kidney, ureter, and bladder (KUB) views can then be used to evaluate for stone migration without the need for a follow-up, higher radiation CT.
  □ To grossly evaluate stone burden
  □ To evaluate for stone passage or changes in stone size or shape following nephroureteral stent placement or lithotripsy
  □ To detect air in cases of emphysematous pyelitis or cystitis
  CONTRAINDICATIONS
  □ Pregnancy is a relative contraindication for the examination due to the risk of direct fetal exposure to the x-ray beam.
  □ If patients are already scheduled to undergo a CT for the evaluation of nephroureterolithiasis, there is no indication for the additional radiation exposure of a KUB.
  □ Morbid obesity: If a KUB is being requested for the evaluation of the presence and location of a stone in an obese patient, there is little role for the film. The limitations of the film (due to underpenetration of the body by the x-ray

beam) will render it useless for identification of a stone; CT
or ultrasound should be performed in these patients.

LIMITATIONS

☐ Only approximately 80% of renal/ureteral calculi are radiopaque (i.e. appear dense and are thus visible on x-ray).

☐ Non-obstructing stones (which do not cause collecting
system dilation) cannot be differentiated from obstructing
stones (which are often the cause of acute flank pain/renal
colic). Non-contrast CT (i.e. the flank pain protocol CT) is
the study of choice to identify, localize, and characterize a
calculus. It also allows for evaluation of the presence and
degree of obstruction (hydronephrosis). If calculi are known
to be present in patients who have symptoms typical of
renal colic, an ultrasound may be the study of choice to
evaluate for obstructive uropathy (i.e. hydronephrosis) in
order to minimize radiation exposure from a CT.

☐ Small stones (even if radiopaque) may be below the resolution of the film.

IV Urogram/Pyelogram

▩ Conventional radiographs (KUBs) are obtained without and
with abdominal compression following the administration of an
IV contrast medium. IV access is acquired after an initial KUB is
obtained. The initial KUB allows for evaluation of bowel preparation (stool may prevent adequate evaluation of the kidneys)
and the presence of renal/ureteral calculi. After determining
that there are no contraindications to IV contrast administration, a bolus of contrast is administered by hand (typically 100
cc of non-ionic IV contrast). Additional films are then obtained
at 1, 3, and 10 minutes to allow for evaluation of the renal cortex
(1-minute nephrogram phase film), collecting system (3-minute
excretory film), and ureters (10-minute delayed films). Depending upon the institution, compression films (i.e. with a compression device applied to the abdomen) may be obtained to further
evaluate the collecting system and kidneys. The compression
allows for distension of the collecting system. In some institutions, compression is not applied and the patient is evaluated
with CT in addition to the IV pyelogram (IVP). The bladder is
also evaluated in the examination.

- Renal function: Serum creatinine must be ≤ 1.5 mg/dL for contrast administration.
- Study preparation: The patient should be fasting for at least 4 hours prior to the study. All IV fluids must be discontinued for at least 4 hours prior to the study to avoid dilution of the contrast medium. A bowel preparation is helpful but not an absolute requirement.
- IVPs have largely been replaced by non-contrast (flank pain protocol) CTs for the evaluation of renal abnormalities. IVPs, however, remain superior to CT for evaluation of the urothelium (the lining of the excretory tract), particularly within the intrarenal collecting system and ureters. (This is less frequently the case with the advent of the CT urogram, however; please refer to the body CT section). The two studies are often performed in conjunction with one another (i.e. CT-IVP). The most common indication in current practice is evaluation of hematuria. Depending upon the institution, either the kidneys only are scanned or the level of the kidneys to the bladder are scanned on CT. Consult the radiologist at your institution prior to requesting the examination to determine which protocol is utilized. The CT and IVP must both be ordered.
- IVP allows for evaluation of:
  - □ Renal: Function (ability to filter and excrete), obstruction, morphology/size, cortical loss (i.e. scarring), and positioning (e.g. ectopia)
  - □ Collecting system: Obstruction, infundibular stenosis, filling defects suggesting neoplasm, blood, course and caliber of the ureters, and ureteral strictures or obstruction
  - □ Bladder: Morphology and size, trabeculation (suggesting chronic outlet obstruction or infection), masses, extrinsic impressions from masses, postvoid residual urine volume

INDICATIONS
  - □ Evaluation of hematuria
  - □ Evaluation of renal function. The rate of renal enhancement and excretion can be assessed in a relative manner. If quantitation of renal function is required, nuclear medicine studies should be performed as these studies allow for measurements of renal flow, function, and excretion (see Chapter 11).
  - □ Evaluation of renal obstruction. This is less commonly performed currently due to the superiority of CT and ultrasound

for this indication. IVPs have an advantage over CT and ultrasound in the evaluation of obstruction as excretion is directly evaluated on IVPs, whereas it is only implied on CT and ultrasound due to the presence of dilation of the collecting system (hydronephrosis).

☐ Evaluation of bladder abnormalities. IVPs have slightly improved resolution for the evaluation of bladder masses compared to CT. This is due to the very dense contrast that is excreted on CT; this can obscure a small mass in the bladder lumen.

CONTRAINDICATIONS

☐ Previous IV hydration will dilute the contrast and will make it more difficult to visualize.

LIMITATIONS

☐ Renal masses cannot be characterized and may not be visible if they are small or obscured by overlying bowel gas/stool. A mass is suspected if there is an area of the kidney that does not enhance with contrast or if there is contour deformity of the collecting system or renal cortex. CT and MR are the studies of choice for the evaluation of renal masses.

☐ Ureters are muscular and therefore demonstrate peristalsis. Because of this action, the ureters may not fill with contrast or they may empty the contrast from some segments in between films. This renders these segments of the ureters unevaluable.

☐ Small lesions in the collecting system, ureters, and bladder may be below the resolution of the study. These lesions may be obscured if contrast is too dilute or if there are overlying structures such as bowel.

☐ If there is poor or no renal function, that kidney and its respective collecting system and ureter cannot be evaluated.

CT Urography

▪ CT urography is performed without oral and with IV contrast.

▪ It allows for evaluation of the renal cortex (i.e. for renal masses such as renal cell carcinomas) and also allows for evaluation of the collecting systems and ureters for lesions such as transitional cell carcinoma.

▪ The study is performed with different protocols depending upon the institution. One protocol involves scanning the abdomen and pelvis from the level of the kidneys through the bladder without contrast then administering IV contrast and scanning the kidneys, ureters, and bladder in different phases of contrast enhancement.

■ The study is for the purposes of initial diagnosis only and should not be requested to follow up known lesions.

INDICATIONS

☐ Evaluation of patients with hematuria

☐ Evaluation for metachronous or synchronous sites of disease in patients with known transitional cell carcinoma (due to the increased risk of additional lesions in patients with transitional cell carcinoma)

☐ Presurgical planning for partial nephrectomy (for renal cell carcinoma in order to determine if a partial nephrectomy can be performed or if a total nephrectomy must be performed)

CONTRAINDICATIONS

☐ Young patients with hematuria. The likelihood of a genitourinary malignancy is relatively low in this population, thus benign etiologies of hematuria should be considered. Depending upon the clinical question, a decision should be made to image the patient using the least radiation (e.g. ultrasound for renal stones or obstruction).

☐ No residual renal function in patients with renal failure. If there is poor renal function, the kidneys cannot take up or excrete IV contrast, causing the study to be of no benefit as the renal parenchyma and ureters cannot be evaluated due to the lack of contrast opacification.

☐ Renal transplant recipients. In many institutions, patients who have undergone renal transplantation are not candidates for IV contrast-enhanced examinations. This decision is often at the discretion of the transplant surgeon or nephrologist. IV contrast is not administered in order to protect the transplanted organ from complications of contrast-induced nephropathy.

LIMITATIONS

☐ Due to the technique of the imaging and the density of the contrast, occasionally there is artifact (streak) from the contrast in the kidneys such that evaluation of the intrarenal collecting system or the renal cortex may be limited.

☐ Patients with large body habitus are poor candidates due to the poor quality of the images, thus, small lesions cannot be detected with this technique.

Nephrostogram

■ The study is performed under fluoroscopy through a preexisting nephrostomy tube or nephroureteral stent.

■ Non-ionic contrast is dripped under gravity into a preexisting nephrostomy tube or nephroureteral stent.

INDICATIONS

☐ Evaluate the size and morphology of the renal collecting system.

☐ Evaluate for residual filling defects (e.g. calculi or hemorrhage).

☐ Evaluate the drainage of the renal collecting system.

☐ The study is often performed to determine if drainage from the intrarenal collecting system into the ureter and bladder is adequate to allow a catheter to be capped or removed.

CONTRAINDICATIONS

☐ Active infection. If there is an active pyelonephritis, pyelitis, or urinary tract infection, there is a theoretic risk of infection spread (including sepsis) by putting the system under increased pressure during contrast injection.

LIMITATIONS

☐ Collecting systems under high pressure cannot be easily opacified and thus only minimal contrast may be introduced into the system. This may limit evaluation of the collecting system.

Loopogram

■ This is a fluoroscopic study performed in patients with ileal conduits.

■ Non-ionic contrast is dripped under gravity into the stoma while fluoroscopic imaging is performed.

INDICATIONS

☐ Visualization of the course and caliber of the postoperative ureters

☐ Evaluation of filling defects, strictures, and areas of obstruction in patients with suspected recurrent or residual neoplasm (typically transitional cell carcinoma)

CONTRAINDICATIONS

☐ Recent conduit formation. This is a relative contraindication. Damage to the conduit by catheter placement for the study may occur in a recently formed conduit.

LIMITATIONS

☐ Due to the retrograde nature of the study and the lack of direct cannulation of the ureters, it may be difficult to get contrast into the loop and ureters, thus limiting the study.

Cystogram/Voiding Cystourethrogram

■ The study is performed under fluoroscopy.

■ A Foley catheter is placed into the bladder and the balloon is inflated. Under gravity, contrast is instilled into the bladder. The bladder is fully distended to optimally evaluate bladder abnormalities. If there is a concern for urethral stricture or trauma, a retrograde urethrogram (RUG) (see, Retrograde Urethrogram, later) may be performed prior to Foley catheter placement to ensure that it is safe to place the catheter.

■ A voiding cystourethrogram (VCUG) differs from a cystogram in that VCUGs evaluate not only the bladder but also the urethra. In a cystogram, contrast is instilled into the bladder through the catheter; however, once the bladder is fully distended and evaluated, the study is complete. In a VCUG, after the bladder is evaluated, the catheter is removed and the patient is evaluated under fluoroscopy while voiding. This allows for evaluation of the urethra. It also allows for the evaluation of vesicoureteral reflux, which may only occur when the intravesicular pressure increases during processes such as voiding.

INDICATIONS

☐ Cystogram:

- The most common indication is evaluation of suspected bladder injury.
- Identification of the presence and location of sites of bladder injury
- Determination of intraperitoneal versus extraperitoneal bladder injury, which subsequently dictates management. CT cystography or combination with CT scanning may be of further benefit in the distinction between intraperitoneal and extraperitoneal bladder rupture.
- Evaluation of suspected fistulas (e.g. vesicocutaneous, vesicovaginal, etc.

☐ VCUG:

- The most common indication is evaluation of suspected vesicoureteral reflux.

- Identification of ureteroceles, bladder diverticula, and vesicoureteral reflux
- Evaluation of possible urethral abnormalities, such as strictures and urethral valves

CONTRAINDICATIONS

☐ If there is a known or suspected urethral injury, a RUG may be required prior to Foley catheter placement.

☐ In the setting of active infection, a cystogram or VCUG generally is not performed. The reasoning behind this is that there is a risk (particularly in patients with vesicoureteral reflux) of spreading infection from the bladder to the kidney or collecting system. In most instances, it is generally preferable to wait to perform the study until after resolution of the infection.

LIMITATIONS

☐ If there is a question of bladder injury, urethral injury must first be excluded. Further urethral damage may be caused by the introduction of a Foley catheter. Therefore, if there is suspicion of a urethral injury on clinical grounds (e.g. a high-riding prostate on rectal examination or blood at the urethral meatus), a RUG (see later) should be performed prior to the cystogram.

☐ Vesicoureteral reflux is often intermittent and may not be demonstrable at the time of the examination. However, if reflux is not demonstrated, it DOES NOT mean that it is not present. It simply means that it was not identified during that examination. Patients may be treated symptomatically and, if need arises, may have the study repeated at a later date to determine if reflux is present.

☐ Small fistulas or bladder leaks may be difficult to visualize with these techniques. CT cystograms may provide more information in patients with negative fluoroscopic examinations with continued high clinical concern for fistula or leak.

☐ Small masses or abnormalities in the bladder mucosa or urethra may be below the resolution of this technique.

☐ Patients may be unable to void during a VCUG; this may be on the basis of bladder outlet obstruction (e.g. urethral stricture), social anxiety, neurogenic bladder, and so on. If patients are unable to void, the study may be limited for the evaluation of vesicoureteral reflux (lack of increased bladder pressure with voiding) or evaluation of the urethra.

- [ ] Patients who are not mobile may have study limitations if they cannot be positioned in such a way that areas of bladder abnormality or the urethra can be evaluated.

Retrograde Urethrogram

- RUG is performed under fluoroscopy.
- A Foley catheter is placed into the distal aspect of the urethra. The balloon is NOT inflated. Contrast is instilled by injection into the urethra via the Foley catheter. This often requires the catheter to be held in place by the patient or physician performing the study. However, there are devices available that circumvent the need to hold the catheter in place.

INDICATIONS

- [ ] Evaluation of traumatic urethral injury
- [ ] Evaluation of urethral strictures

CONTRAINDICATIONS

- [ ] Inability to safely cannulate the meatal orifice

LIMITATIONS

- [ ] If the patient is unstable (e.g. in a trauma setting), the study may be performed with conventional radiography (i.e. pelvic x-rays). However, this limits evaluation of the urethra.
- [ ] If the patient cannot be appropriately positioned for the examination, it may be difficult to evaluate the entire urethra.
- [ ] If there is a high grade stenosis or urethral transection, the urethra proximal to this segment and the bladder base/neck cannot be evaluated for additional sites of injury in a retrograde manner. An alternate imaging study or imaging after repair of the site may be required for complete evaluation.

Hysterosalpingography

- The study is performed under fluoroscopy.
- The cervix is cannulated and contrast is injected through the catheter into the uterine cavity.
- The study allows for evaluation of the uterine cavity for possible fibroids, polyps, or synechiae. The main purpose is evaluation of fallopian tube patency.

■ Hysterosalpingography (HSG) has largely been superseded by MR for the evaluation of congenital uterine anomalies (e.g. septate or bicornuate uteri) and for the evaluation of fibroids. Hysterosonography also has become available for evaluation of endometrial abnormalities such as submucosal fibroids, polyps, and neoplasms without the risk of radiation.

INDICATIONS
☐ Evaluation of couples with primary or secondary infertility

CONTRAINDICATIONS
☐ Pregnancy. All patients should undergo a pregnancy test prior to the examination to exclude early pregnancy.
☐ IV contrast allergy. Even though the contrast is injected into the endometrial cavity of the uterus, if the injection pressure is sufficiently high that contrast leaks into the myometrium, it can be returned into the venous system by draining uterine veins. This can lead to a contrast reaction if the patient is at risk.

LIMITATIONS
☐ Patients with known contrast allergies may not be candidates for HSG. Although contrast is not directly instilled into the systemic circulation, with forcible contrast injection, contrast can traverse the uterus and enter the uterine veins and reach the systemic circulation through the iliac veins.
☐ If the cervix cannot be cannulated, the study cannot be performed.
☐ Some women experience extreme cramping from the distension of the uterus related to contrast administration. Some of these patients are unable to tolerate the entire examination.
☐ The contrast material itself can act as an irritant to the peritoneal cavity. In some women, once the contrast spills from the fallopian tubes into the peritoneum, they may experience nausea and vomiting, which may limit the examination due to motion.
☐ Myometrial processes such as intramural/subserosal fibroids may not be readily detectible with this study; MR is more sensitive for this purpose, as is ultrasound.
☐ If the balloon/catheter is advanced too far into the cavity, it may occlude one horn of the uterus, thus giving the appearance of a unicornuate uterus. If there is an apparent

unicornuate uterus, the catheter should be pulled back and injection repeated.

☐ Uterine anomalies are better characterized with MR than HSG.

☐ The ovaries cannot be visualized with this technique; however, they may be evaluated with MR or ultrasound.

5

Gastrointestinal (Barium) Imaging

Conventional Radiographs

- This is often the first imaging evaluation of abdominal pathology.

- A complete abdominal series (also known as "three way of the abdomen" and "acute abdominal series") includes an erect frontal view of the chest and erect and supine views of the abdomen/pelvis.

- The erect CXR is obtained to evaluate for acute cardiopulmonary disease, such as pneumonia, which may mimic abdominal pain. Additionally, it allows for evaluation of subdiaphragmatic pneumoperitoneum.

- Erect and supine views of the abdomen/pelvis are preferred in order to evaluate for bowel loop dilation and air-fluid levels, which may indicate an obstruction or ileus, as well as to evaluate for pneumoperitoneum. However, if erect radiography is not possible due to the patient's clinical status, tangential beam imaging (i.e. right side up decubitus imaging) may be performed. It should be noted that patients must be kept in the decubitus position for several minutes before radiographs are obtained in order to allow adequate time for the relocation of free intraperitoneal air to the perihepatic space, where it can be visualized.

- Cholelithiasis or nephrolithiasis may be visible radiographically; however, radiography is of little or no value in the evaluation of acute cholecystitis or renal obstruction. Radiographs are, however, useful in the uncommon conditions of gangrenous cholecystitis or emphysematous pyelitis.

Gastrointestinal (Barium) Imaging

INDICATIONS

☐ Evaluation of acute abdominal pain

☐ Evaluation for pneumoperitoneum

☐ Evaluation of suspected small bowel obstruction or colonic ileus or obstruction

☐ Evaluation of pneumonia mimicking abdominal pain

☐ Evaluation of the presence of nephrolithiasis (CT or ultrasound may be performed to evaluate for the presence of renal or ureteral obstruction in the presence of nephrolithiasis)

CONTRAINDICATIONS

☐ If a patient is already scheduled to undergo diagnostic abdominopelvic CT, there is no additional value in conventional radiographs. They simply add additional radiation to the patient for no additional diagnostic yield.

LIMITATIONS

☐ Non-bowel–related pathologies such as abscesses or microperforations related to diverticulitis are typically radiographically occult. CT is required for diagnosis of these entities.

☐ If patients are not appropriately positioned for examinations or are not left in the upright or decubitus positions for adequate amounts of time, small to moderate amounts of pneumoperitoneum may not be recognized.

☐ Obese patients are difficult to image as they often exceed the size of the imaging plate, thus portions of the bowel/soft tissues may not be included on the examination.

☐ Many gallstones are radiographically occult.

☐ Acute inflammatory processes (e.g. acute cholecystitis, diverticulitis, etc.) are radiographically occult. The only true indications for abdominal radiographs in patients with suspected cholecystitis or pyelonephritis who have been imaged previously with ultrasound is to evaluate emphysematous cholecystitis or emphysematous pyelonephritis in which air is present in the gallbladder wall (cholecystitis) or kidney (pyelitis). The air may be difficult to identify on ultrasound (see Chapter 10); however, the air is readily visible on CT.

Esophagography

■ This is a barium study performed with fluoroscopy. It may be performed with sodium diatrizoate (Hypaque)/amidotrizoate and meglumine (Gastrografin) (water soluble contrast agent) to evaluate for esophageal perforation or leak.

- The patient receives barium of two consistencies (thick and thin) as well as an effervescent agent to allow for evaluation of the mucosal lining of the esophagus (i.e. a double contrast study).
- The larynx and pharynx are often evaluated for gross abnormalities such as masses.
- The esophagus is evaluated in its entirety, including the gastroesophageal junction. The stomach is NOT evaluated on an esophogram.
- The study is used to evaluate for intrinsic esophageal motility abnormalities, mass lesions (submucosal, intramural, and extrinsic), strictures, and symptomatic esophageal rings. A double contrast study (i.e. barium plus an effervescent agent) is used to better delineate the mucosal lining, particularly for ulcers.
- In clinically suspected esophageal perforations, Hypaque/Gastrografin used as barium may cause mediastinititis in patients with perforation. Conversely, barium is used to evaluate for suspected aspiration as Hypaque/Gastrografin may induce pulmonary edema if aspirated.

INDICATIONS
- ☐ Evaluation of patients with dysphagia
- ☐ Evaluation of patients with odynophagia
- ☐ Evaluation of suspected gastroesophageal reflux (the stomach is not evaluated in an esophogram). However, provocative maneuvers (e.g. rolling the patient, straight leg raise, etc.) are performed in an attempt to elicit gastroesophageal reflux.
- ☐ Evaluation of suspected caustic ingestion (e.g. lye) in acute phase and chronic (for stricture)
- ☐ Evaluation of esophageal perforation (Hypaque/Gastrografin)
- ☐ Evaluation of motility abnormalities, intrinsic or extrinsic masses, rings, or strictures; mucosal abnormalities
- ☐ Evaluation of postoperative patients with esophageal anastamosis or gastric pull-up for leak

CONTRAINDICATIONS
- ☐ Patients who are suspected or known to aspirate are at risk of aspiration-induced pneumonitis. If patients are known to

aspirate or demonstrate aspiration during the examination, the study should be aborted.

☐ If patients are to undergo CT examination following the esophogram (e.g. for staging of an esophageal tumor), the CT should be performed prior to the GI barium study. CT oral contrast material and contrast material used for fluoroscopic GI studies are not the same. Barium used for fluoroscopic studies is denser than that used for CT. Due to its high density, it causes significant streak artifact on the CT examination and may render the CT uninterpretable if a significant amount of contrast was administered. If there is a likelihood that a CT will be performed in a short time period in relation to the barium study, CT should be performed first as it is possible to differentiate between the two contrast agents when performing the fluoro study. The CT contrast is also less dense than barium for fluoroscopy and thus does not pose as much of a problem with artifacts.

LIMITATIONS

☐ Poor esophageal distension may lead to inadequate evaluation of the esophageal lumen. If there is persistently poor distension, it may be difficult to determine if the underdistension is due to technique or to stricture.

☐ Poor coating of the esophagus by the barium may render the study uninterpretable due to the inability to evaluate the mucosa. Poor coating may result from technique but is more frequently related to recent food or fluid ingestion. Patients should be kept NPO for at least 4–6 hours prior to a GI examination in order to optimize contrast coating and to prevent false-positive results. Adherent particulate matter (e.g. food) can cause an apparent filling defect and may result in a misdiagnosis.

☐ The presence of gastroesophageal reflux is not always identified, even in cases of documented reflux; this is due to the intermittent nature of the entity.

☐ In patients with obstructive esophageal lesions or abnormal esophageal peristalsis, it may not be possible for barium to pass into the stomach. In these cases, the esophagus distal to the abnormality cannot be assessed.

☐ Patients who cannot be positioned for the study or who cannot comply with study directions are not candidates for the examination.

Modified Barium Swallow

- This is a fluoroscopic study used solely for the evaluation of aspiration risk.
- It is often performed in conjunction with the speech pathology service.
- Patients are administered barium in varying consistencies while the oropharynx is evaluated fluoroscopically. The swallowing mechanism is evaluated for motor coordination, efficacy of the swallow to clear barium from the pharynx, and possible aspiration.
- The study does NOT evaluate the esophagus in its entirety.

  INDICATIONS
  - ☐ Evaluation of patients with known or suspected aspiration
  - ☐ Follow-up of patients after treatment for underlying abnormalities causing aspiration (e.g. stroke) to determine if aspiration is still present

  CONTRAINDICATIONS
  - ☐ Unstable patients
  - ☐ Uncooperative/minimally responsive patients who cannot follow commands
  - ☐ Patients with significant lung disease and with suspected aspiration in whom oral contrast aspiration may exacerbate the acute/underlying pulmonary abnormality

  LIMITATIONS
  - ☐ The study does not evaluate the entire esophagus; if there is concern for concomitant esophageal abnormality, the study may be followed by a dedicated esophogram.

Upper GI Series

- An upper GI (UGI) series is performed in a manner similar to esophagography.
- The larynx/pharynx and cervical esophagus are typically NOT evaluated at the time of UGI although they may be if specifically requested.
- The study is used to evaluate for abnormalities of the distal esophagus, stomach, and duodenum.
- The study is usually performed as a double contrast examination (i.e. with oral barium of thick and thin consistency and an effervescent agent to allow for evaluation of the mucosa).

■ It may be performed as a single contrast study in patients unable to ingest the effervescent agent in whom the main clinical concerns are penetrating (deep) ulcers or mass.

INDICATIONS

☐ Esophageal: Motility abnormalities, intrinsic or extrinsic masses, rings, or strictures; mucosal abnormalities

☐ Gastric: Evaluation of erosions, ulcers, masses, extrinsic impressions

☐ Duodenum: Evaluation of fold thickening in inflammation, ulcers, masses; less commonly to evaluate for malrotation as this is typically detected in childhood

CONTRAINDICATIONS

☐ Patients with known or suspected aspiration due to the risks of aspiration pneumonitis. If unsuspected aspiration is identified during the examination, the study is terminated.

LIMITATIONS

☐ Poor coating of the GI tract by barium will significantly limit evaluation.

☐ If patients cannot be mobilized (rolled), gastric coating of the stomach by the barium may be suboptimal.

☐ The study may be performed in combination with a small bowel follow-through (SBFT); however, it is preferred that the two studies be performed at separate times as the effervescent agent may cause difficulty in evaluation of small bowel pathology. Conversely, a UGI performed as a single contrast study (i.e. without the effervescent agent) limits evaluation of mucosal abnormalities.

Small Bowel Follow-Through

■ The patient is administered a total of two 8-oz cups of thin liquid barium. No effervescent agent is administered.

■ The patient is administered the first cup of barium under fluoroscopic guidance to evaluate the duodenum (first portion of the small bowel).

■ If necessary, the barium can be administered through a nasogastric (NG) tube.

■ The small bowel is examined in its entirety to the terminal ileum/ileocecal valve.

■ Transit time to the colon is variable, ranging from 30 minutes to hours. It is particularly advised that patients with clinically suspected or radiographically proven small bowel obstruction be imaged as the first case of the day. Typically, these patients have markedly prolonged transit times and it may take more than 12 to 24 hours for the barium to reach the transition point/point of obstruction. Due to obvious limitations in staffing resources, these patients cannot be followed as closely as warranted if the examination is started late in the day.

INDICATIONS

☐ Evaluation of small bowel obstruction for transition point of obstruction. CT is increasingly performed for this indication as causes of obstruction, points of obstruction, and sequelae of obstruction can be demonstrated. This includes ischemic bowel, internal hernias, obstructing masses, and so on.

☐ Identification of diverticula, fistulas, masses

☐ Diagnosis or follow-up of inflammatory bowel disease or infectious/parasitic enteritis

☐ Diagnosis of diseases such as scleroderma or celiac sprue

CONTRAINDICATIONS

☐ Patients who are at risk for or who have documented aspiration should not be administered oral contrast for the examination. Contrast can be administered through an enteric tube (which may be placed at the time of the study, if necessary).

☐ Patients who are scheduled to undergo or who may require a subsequent CT of the abdomen/pelvis should not be administered barium for the small bowel study prior to the CT. This is due to the relatively high density of the barium that is administered for the small bowel study; it results in significant streak artifacts on the CT examination, which may render the CT uninterpretable. Patients can receive CT contrast prior to a small bowel series without complete interference as the contrast for the small bowel series will appear more dense on fluoroscopy than the CT contrast.

LIMITATIONS

☐ Abnormalities within the small bowel lumen may not be visible (e.g. polyps) if they are small or the contrast is dense. Enteroclysis (see later) is a more optimal study to evaluate for the intraluminal contents of the small bowel.

☐ The cause of a small bowel obstruction may not be identified unless it is due to adhesions. CT is a more optimal study for the determination of small bowel obstruction caused by

Gastrointestinal (Barium) Imaging

extrinsic abnormality as it allows for evaluation of structures outside of the bowel.

☐ Patients with small bowel obstruction may not be able to ingest or keep down the oral contrast. If an adequate amount of contrast is not instilled into the small bowel, it is not adequately distended or opacified. In these patients, the small bowel may not be fully assessed for bowel wall thickening, mass, or distension.

☐ In patients with small bowel obstruction, the contrast is often diluted due to the fluid-filled, obstructed small bowel loops. This may make it difficult to see the contrast if it becomes very dilute.

☐ Patients with small bowel obstruction often have delayed transit of contrast through the small bowel. This may cause the study to be prolonged or may not provide adequate information on the transition point as the contrast may not reach the transition point in high grade obstructions.

Enteroclysis

■ This is a fluoroscopic procedure similar in principle to double contrast upper GI series. A long Frederick-Miller catheter is placed into the proximal jejunum via a nasal approach. Barium and methyl cellulose are given through the catheter into the small bowel. The effect is to distend the small bowel while allowing for detailed evaluation of the mucosa, which is difficult to evaluate on conventional small bowel series.

INDICATIONS

☐ Evaluation of suspected small bowel masses (often suspected on the basis of prior imaging studies such as conventional small bowel series or CT)

☐ Evaluation of possible lead points for intussusceptions in adults

☐ Evaluation of the small bowel mucosa for abnormalities such as erosions

☐ Evaluation of the small bowel folds for evaluation of processes affecting the wall such as celiac disease, scleroderma, and so on

CONTRAINDICATIONS

☐ Acute process involving the small bowel (e.g. infection). The bowel distension may cause pain or trauma to friable walls in susceptible patients.

☐ Patients with small bowel obstruction should not be evaluated with this technique as the installation of additional fluid can result in worsening of bowel loop distension.

LIMITATIONS

☐ Patients may not be able to tolerate the procedure, resulting in procedure failure.

☐ If the study is not performed correctly, it is possible to obscure findings. If the rates of contrast and cellulose administration are not appropriate, the study may be limited.

☐ The radiation dose is higher than standard small bowel series in most cases as the contrast and cellulose must be administered under fluoroscopy in order to perform the study accurately with appropriate doses/rates of administration of each agent.

Single Contrast Barium/Hypaque Enemas

▓ Barium is an inert substance; however, in patients with perforations, it may spill into the peritoneal cavity and cause peritonitis. A single contrast barium enema is one in which barium alone is instilled into the colon through a rectal catheter. This so-called single contrast (or single column) enema allows for evaluation of gross lesions such as masses or of obstruction.

▓ Hypaque is a highly osmolar material that is less radiodense than barium, thus, it is more difficult to visualize radiographically. For this reason, Hypaque is used to answer specific questions related to acute abnormalities and NOT to evaluate lesions such as polyps.

▓ Bowel preparations are not required for these studies.

INDICATIONS

☐ Single contrast barium enema:
  • Evaluation of suspected large colonic masses or large polyps
  • Evaluation of suspected colonic fistulas (e.g. coloenteric, colocutaneous fistulas)
  • Evaluation preoperatively for reanastamosis following diverting colostomy

☐ Hypaque:
  • Evaluation of suspected obstructing colonic lesions such as mass or stricture
  • Evaluation for possible colonic perforation
  • Evaluation of sigmoid or cecal volvulus

Gastrointestinal (Barium) Imaging

- If no gross colonic perforation is demonstrated with Hypaque, additional imaging with single contrast barium may be performed to further evaluate for colonic pathology.
- Therapeutic for some patients with processes such as meconium ileus equivalent in whom there is thick, viscous stool. The high osmolality of the Hypaque draws water into the bowel and assists in evacuation of the bowel contents.

CONTRAINDICATIONS

☐ Patients with pneumoperitoneum demonstrated on prior imaging. This suggests that there is bowel perforation; these patients should (in general) undergo surgical management.

☐ Patients who may require CT examinations. As with oral barium, rectal barium is dense and may cause significant streak artifact, rendering the CT uninterpretable. This is still possible, but less likely to occur with Hypaque.

☐ Patients who cannot be mobilized and cannot be rolled on the imaging table are not optimal candidates for the study as it is difficult or impossible to fill the colon with the patient in one position. It may also be difficult to image these patients with the fluoroscopy unit due to limitations in positioning.

☐ Toxic megacolon is an absolute contraindication to the administration of rectal contrast. The colon is very fragile in toxic megacolon; the colonic distension caused by the addition of the liquid contrast can cause the bowel to perforate.

LIMITATIONS

☐ Masses or polyps within the bowel lumen may not be identifiable on single contrast examinations, particularly if they are small. Single contrast examinations are of benefit mainly for the evaluation of obstruction, volvulus, and other anatomic abnormalities.

☐ Patients may not tolerate the examination, particularly if there is an obstruction. The addition of fluid to dilated bowel may cause significant discomfort.

☐ The cause of a colonic obstruction may not be identified on a single contrast study if it is external to the colon. CT is a better imaging study for extrinsic impression on the colon as it allows for the structures outside of the colon to be assessed.

Double Contrast Barium Enema

- The study is performed with rectal barium in addition to insufflated (i.e. hand pumped in) air.
- A preliminary abdominal radiograph (KUB) is obtained to evaluate the adequacy of the colonic preparation. If there is residual formed stool, the study may be rescheduled following a more rigorous bowel preparation. Residual stool can mimic colonic polyps and masses, thus leading to a false-positive study.
- A digital rectal examination is performed to identify large hemorrhoids or masses. These are contraindications to the placement of the rectal tube as they may be traumatized during tube placement or balloon inflation.
- If there are no contraindications to placement of the rectal tube, a soft-tipped rectal tube is placed and the balloon is inflated under fluoroscopic evaluation. This allows the degree of balloon inflation and positioning to be confirmed without risk of overinflation and bowel perforation.
- Barium and air are administered through the tube while the patient rolls in a 360-degree circle on the fluoroscopy table. This allows the entire colon to be coated with an adequate amount of barium; patients must roll to allow gravity to assist in movement of barium through the bowel. Air is then insufflated (i.e. pumped in by hand) into the bowel to distend the colon and allow the mucosal lining of the bowel to be assessed.
- The study is completed when air or contrast are demonstrated to reflux into the terminal ileum.
- It allows for evaluation of the mucosal lining of the colon.
- The endpoint of the examination is reflux of air and/or contrast into the terminal ileum. The small bowel is not evaluated in the study.
- The study requires an adequate bowel preparation as retained fecal material can simulate pathology such as a polyp. The study also requires a compliant patient who is able to rotate 360 degrees while prone on the imaging table.
- Bowel preparation typically involves the following (although different institutions may use alternate preparations): NPO from midnight the night before, clear liquids for 24 hours, oral laxative such as GoLytely.

INDICATIONS
- ☐ Screening study for colonic polyps and occult neoplasms

Gastrointestinal (Barium) Imaging

☐ Follow-up to unsuccessful or incomplete colonoscopy

☐ Evaluation of diverticular disease to assess extent and chronicity (particularly preoperatively for elective partial colonic resections). This is uncommonly done due to the excellent resolution of CT for diverticulosis.

☐ Evaluation of hematochezia, melena, fecal occult blood. Double contrast barium enema will allow for the detection of benign diseases (e.g. diverticulosis) or malignancy, which may be the cause of symptoms.

☐ Evaluation of anemia. Right colon masses are usually the etiology, although diverticulosis may cause anemia.

CONTRAINDICATIONS

☐ Poor colonic preparation. Retained stool can mimic disease.

☐ Recent polypectomy or colonic biopsy. There is a theoretic risk of bowel perforation during the study at the site of biopsy or polypectomy.

☐ Rectal mass. It may be traumatic or impossible to pass a rectal tube beyond an anal or rectal mass.

☐ Inability to roll 360 degrees on the fluoroscopy table

☐ Inability to lie flat for the examination

☐ Toxic megacolon, bowel perforation, acute colonic inflammation/infection

LIMITATIONS

☐ Poor bowel preparation may result in false-positive studies (retained stool mimicking polyps) or false-negative studies (if the colon is too "wet" [i.e. too much mucus or fluid], the barium will not stick to the mucosa and it cannot be evaluated).

☐ Small polyps may be below the resolution of the study.

☐ It may be difficult to differentiate colonic diverticula from polyps.

Fistulograms

■ This is a barium study performed fluoroscopically with injection of barium through a cutaneous fistula.

■ It evaluates the site to which a cutaneous fistula connects.

■ The study may be performed prior to a small bowel study or enema in an attempt to evaluate the fistula. If the fistulous tract cannot be identified from injection of contrast into the fistula, administration of oral contrast into the small bowel or rectal contrast into the colon may be performed in an attempt to delineate the fistulous connection.

INDICATIONS
- ☐ Evaluation of patients with suspected enterocutaneous or colocutaneous fistulas
- ☐ Evaluation of surgically created fistulas for presurgical planning (e.g. colostomy take down), evaluation of fistula stricture

CONTRAINDICATIONS
- ☐ Cutaneous fistula site cannot be identified.
- ☐ Acute inflammation of the cutaneous site. Antegrade studies (e.g. small bowel series) can be performed in these patients in an attempt to identify a fistula.
- ☐ Bowel perforation known or suspected

LIMITATIONS
- ☐ Small fistulas may be below the resolution of the technology.
- ☐ Some cutaneous fistulas cannot be identified and thus cannot be cannulated in order to inject contrast material.
- ☐ Enteroenteric, coloenteric, or enterovesicular fistulas cannot be evaluated with this technique as an adequate amount of contrast material cannot be injected (in most cases) to allow complete evaluation of the bowel.

Ostomy Studies

- ▪ This is a fluoroscopically guided barium study performed through an ostomy aperture.
- ▪ The balloon of a Foley catheter is inflated OUTSIDE of the ostomy. The tip of the Foley is then placed into the stoma and the balloon is positioned such that occlusion of the stoma is achieved. Due to the limitations of the occlusive seal, only a single contrast study can be performed (i.e. air cannot be insufflated to evaluate mucosal detail).

INDICATIONS
- ☐ Anatomic study (performed in conjunction with a single contrast barium enema) to evaluate the residual bowel prior to ostomy takedown
- ☐ Evaluation of residual or recurrent disease (e.g. inflammatory bowel disease)
- ☐ Evaluation of ostomy stricture

☐ Evaluation of suspected ostomy leak (Hypaque is used for this indication; if no leak is demonstrated, the study can be repeated with barium.)

CONTRAINDICATIONS

☐ Acute inflammation/infection. The friable mucosa may be damaged by the placement of the catheter or by contrast installation.

LIMITATIONS

☐ If there is residual contrast material within the bowel (from prior studies), it may be difficult to evaluate the ostomy.

☐ If a poor seal is achieved of the Foley catheter with the ostomy, it may be difficult to achieve adequate distension of the bowel with contrast as a significant amount of contrast may leak from the ostomy site.

6

Computed Tomography

CT of the Brain and Head and Neck:
Please see Chapter 8.

CT of the Thorax:
Please see Chapter 2.

Abdominopelvic Imaging

▣ CT imaging is being employed with increasing frequency in the evaluation of patients with acute abdominal and pelvic pain, as well as in the evaluation and follow-up of oncologic patients.
▣ Imaging of the abdomen, particularly in the setting of acute abdominal pain, requires the evaluation of pelvic viscera as well as intra-abdominal structures. At most institutions, particularly in the era of managed care, abdominal and pelvic CTs must BOTH be requested by the ordering clinician. If an abdominal CT ONLY is requested, potential bowel pathology or pelvic lesions will not be imaged.
▣ CT examinations may be obtained as follows:
  □ Without oral or IV contrast
  □ With oral and without IV contrast
  □ With IV and without oral contrast
  □ With both oral and IV contrast.
▣ The purpose of this chapter is to clarify the use of oral and IV contrast in abdominopelvic imaging.

General Considerations in CT Imaging

▣ There should be a valid indication for CT examination, particularly given the risks of IV contrast and the significant radiation doses attained. Radiation dose is of even greater concern in the era of multidetector (multislice) detector CT imaging. If a diagnosis may be made on clinical grounds only, a CT may be circumvented if unnecessary. Consideration should also be given to potential imaging studies that require lower doses of or no radiation (e.g. can the question be answered with conventional radiographs or ultrasound).

- Weight limits: Patients whose weight exceeds 350–400 lbs CANNOT be imaged on standard CT tables. CT scanners do exist to image patients who exceed standard table weight limits; however, these scanners are typically found at veterinary hospitals and are often not readily available for clinical imaging. As the weight limits vary from vendor to vendor, it is suggested that you consult your local radiology department to determine their weight limit. Patient girth is also a consideration in CT and MR scanning. The CT and MRI units are effectively large circles; therefore, the patient must be able to fit into the "hole." Again, different manufacturers have different apertures, thus it is advisable to discuss the aperture limit with your local radiology department.

- IV contrast:
  - ☐ IV contrast is often required in the evaluation of suspected abdominopelvic pathology. The indications for IV contrast are discussed here.
  - ☐ For all inpatients, it is recommended that peripheral IV access be obtained on the floor prior to the examination. Most PICC lines CANNOT be used for the administration of IV contrast agents, particularly for arterial phase imaging as rapid infusions are not possible through the small lumens. Additionally, there is a risk of PICC line disruption with high rates of contrast injection. There are PICC lines (often called "power PICCs") that are specifically designed to allow rapid contrast administration. These PICC lines can be used for power injectors. Discuss with the PICC service or interventional radiologists who place the lines to determine which type of PICC line they use.
  - ☐ Institutions vary as to the limit of renal function at which IV contrast may be safely administered. The nephrotoxic effects of IV contrast are well recognized (e.g. contrast-induced nephropathy). For this reason, at our institution, IV contrast is typically not administered to patients with creatinine (Cr) levels >1.5 mg/dL.

□ If patients are on dialysis (either hemodialysis or peritoneal dialysis), attention should be paid to the schedule of dialysis. It is advisable that patients undergoing contrast-enhanced CT (CECT) examinations be dialysed within 24 hours of the contrast dose. This is mainly related to volume and osmotic effects of the IV contrast agents.

□ Patients with diabetes who are on oral hypoglycemic agents such as metformin (Glucophage) require that the agent be discontinued for 48 hours following the administration of IV contrast. Additionally, they require that a repeat Cr level be drawn 24–48 hours following the administration of contrast to evaluate for potential nephrotoxicity.

□ Consideration should be given to the necessity of IV contrast in patients with a history of thyroid carcinoma. If possible, IV contrast should be avoided in these patients as it has effects upon thyroid tissue and thus may affect the uptake of nuclear medicine radiotracers. This, in turn, may have an impact on the restaging and treatment of these patients with radioactive iodine.

□ A history of prior contrast reaction should be obtained prior to a request for a CECT study. Contrast reactions can range from minimal reactions such as hives to full anaphylactoid-type reactions requiring cardiopulmonary resuscitation efforts. The severity of a prior contrast reaction is NOT a predictor of the severity of a future contrast reaction. Patients with hives from a past CECT may go on to manifest a much more severe reaction the next time they have CECT. If a risk of contrast reaction exists, or if there is a documented prior reaction, premedication regimens should be implemented prior to the examination.

Premedication for Patients with IV Contrast Allergies

■ A variety of regimens are in clinical use for the premedication of patients with known or suspected contrast reaction.

■ The need for premedication should be communicated to the scheduler at the time of the imaging request so that the examination may be scheduled for a time when the premedication regimen has been completed. For inpatients requiring premedication, it is suggested that the housestaff stay in communication with the technologists/schedulers to ensure completion of the regimen.

Computed Tomography

☐ The following regimens are suggested:

Regimen 1

* Medication: Prednisone
* Route: Oral
* Dose: 50 mg
* Schedule: 13, 7, and 1 hour prior to CECT
* Diphenhydramine (Benadryl) 50 mg oral or IV is also administered 1 hour prior to CECT
* Cimetidine may also be administered for its H_2 antagonist effects.

Regimen 2

* Medication: Methylprednisolone sodium succinate (Solu-Medrol)
* Route: IV
* Dose: 125 mg
* Schedule: 6 and 1 hour prior to CECT
* Benadryl 50 mg oral or IV is also administered 1 hour prior to CECT.
* IV cimetidine may also be administered for its H_2 antagonist effects.

Hepatic CT Imaging

■ Hepatic lesions are commonly identified on routine abdominal imaging. The majority of these lesions is below the resolution of CT and thus cannot be further characterized. Typically, these lesions do not require further follow-up.

■ If hepatic lesions are suspected on the basis of clinical grounds or have been identified on other imaging studies and require further evaluation, a CT may be obtained. Three-phase hepatic imaging is typically performed in order to characterize lesions. Three-phase hepatic imaging consists of the following:

☐ Non-contrast 5-mm thick images through the liver

☐ Thin section (2.5 mm) axial images through the liver in the arterial, portovenous, and delayed phases of IV contrast enhancement

☐ Oral contrast is not required for the examination.

■ Three-phase contrast imaging is not required for all hepatic lesions. For patients in whom hepatic lesions have previously been documented, routine abdominopelvic CT may be performed with single-phase imaging (portovenous phase) after

IV contrast administration. This is particularly of use in the follow-up of known hepatic metastatic disease.

INDICATIONS

☐ Evaluation of suspected subtle hepatic lesions such as in patients with high clinical suspicion of hepatic metastatic disease

☐ Screening for hepatoma in patients with cirrhosis

☐ Characterization of hepatic lesions demonstrated on alternate imaging modalities (often incidental findings at the time of abdominopelvic imaging performed for alternative reasons)

CONTRAINDICATIONS

☐ Patients who cannot receive IV contrast for reasons of poor renal function, lack of IV access, or allergy are not candidates for this examination.

☐ Young patients with hepatitis or cirrhosis who are at increased lifetime risk of developing hepatoma may be better screened with MRI as it does not involve the use of ionizing radiation. Repeated use of CT increases the lifetime risk of radiation-induced malignancy.

LIMITATIONS

☐ Patients who are not able to lie flat are not good candidates for the examination.

☐ Patients are required to hold their breath for the examination. Due to the multiple phases of scanning, they are required to breath-hold in a similar manner in all phases so that direct comparison of specific locations may be performed to allow for accurate evaluation of perceived masses.

☐ Minimal difference in timing of IV contrast material between follow-up examinations may make it difficult to evaluate for interval change in size or presence of some hepatic lesions. This may make it difficult to determine if the lesion is still present, if it represented a vascular shunt, or if it has increased in size (and is therefore suspicious for a hepatocellular carcinoma).

Biliary Imaging

▪ CT may be helpful in the evaluation of suspected biliary tree obstruction, particularly when evaluating for associated obstructing masses such as cholangiocarcinoma or metastatic disease.

■ CT cholangiography may be performed following percutaneous cholangiography. This allows more accurate evaluation of the biliary anatomy than routine CT imaging.

■ Ultrasound is often the investigation of choice to evaluate the biliary tree for several reasons, including the lack of ionizing radiation, increased sensitivity to early biliary dilation (often prior to CT manifestations of ductal dilation), and more reliable characterization of gallbladder pathology.

■ CT is NOT sensitive for the detection of cholelithiasis or early cholecystitis. However, CECT is superior to ultrasound in the evaluation of suspected common bile duct stones.

INDICATIONS

□ Evaluation of choledocholithiasis (approximately 50%–70% sensitivity)

□ Pre-drainage procedure planning (i.e. "roadmap" to allow the interventionalist to plan the best location for the percutaneous biliary duct puncture)

□ Evaluation of known or suspected obstructing biliary mass (e.g. cholangiocarcinoma, pancreatic head mass, gallbladder carcinoma)

□ CT cholangiography may be performed for evaluation of biliary anatomy prior to partial hepatic resection or liver transplantation.

□ CECT may be performed for the evaluation of an obstructing mass leading to intra- and extrahepatic biliary ductal dilation. Pancreatic ductal dilation also may be seen in the setting of an obstructing pancreatic head mass, leading to the "double duct sign" of pancreatic duct and common bile duct dilation. If evaluation of a pancreatic mass or mass in the porta hepatis is required, the study should be performed as a hepatic mass protocol (porta hepatis mass) or pancreatic mass protocol (pancreatic head mass).

CONTRAINDICATIONS

□ Patients who cannot receive IV contrast are not candidates for CECT.

□ CT cholangiography cannot be performed on patients who cannot undergo percutaneous cholangiograms.

LIMITATIONS

☐ CT is not sensitive for the detection of subtle biliary obstruction; CECT is required as it allows differentiation of vascular structures and periportal edema from ductal dilation.

☐ CT has relatively low sensitivity for the detection of choledocholithiasis, although it is more sensitive than ultrasound for this indication.

☐ CT is of limited usefulness in the evaluation of acute cholecystitis. The diagnosis may be suggested based on enhancement of the gallbladder wall, gallbladder wall thickening, and mesenteric fat inflammation centered on the gallbladder.

☐ CT has poor resolution for the identification of cholelithiasis. Although some stones may be dense and therefore able to be seen on CT, not all stones are visible and it is often not possible to differentiate sludge from small stones. Ultrasound is the imaging modality of choice for this indication.

☐ CECT may not detect infiltrating masses such as cholangiocarcinoma, which tends to enhance late (8–10 minutes following IV contrast enhancement). MR is a more sensitive modality for the evaluation of these late-enhancing masses.

☐ Some pancreatic masses cannot be readily identified on CT or MRI. If there is high clinical suspicion for the presence of a pancreatic mass in the setting of a negative CT or MR, endoscopic ultrasound may be performed for further evaluation. Endoscopic ultrasound involves passage of an ultrasound-mounted endoscope into the stomach. The stomach serves as a good window for high resolution evaluation of the adjacent pancreas. Transgastric biopsies also may be performed via this route if a mass is identified.

Splenic Imaging

■ There are few specific indications for dedicated splenic CT imaging. Indications include suspected splenic trauma, infarction, abscess formation, or autosplenectomy in sickle cell patients. CT also may be useful in the identification or confirmation of residual splenic tissue in patients with idiopathic thrombocytopenic purpura (ITP). IV contrast is required for all of these diagnoses with the exception of suspected autosplenectomy and residual splenic tissue.

■ Splenic lesions are often identified incidentally on routine CT studies.

■ CT often cannot fully characterize splenic lesions.

INDICATIONS

☐ Evaluation of suspected splenic trauma

☐ Evaluation of the presence or absence of the spleen in cases of suspected heterotaxy syndrome (congenital asplenia or polysplenia syndromes)

☐ Evaluation of suspected splenic infarction or abscess

☐ Evaluation of autosplenectomy

☐ Identification of residual splenic tissue in patients with hematopoietic abnormalities such as ITP. Nuclear medicine sulfur colloid studies are more sensitive for the identification of small islands of ectopic splenic tissue.

CONTRAINDICATIONS

☐ Patents who cannot receive IV contrast

LIMITATIONS

☐ Splenic imaging is notoriously difficult. No single imaging modality currently exists that can characterize the majority of splenic lesions. CT is no exception. Although splenic masses can be readily identified on CT, there are no accurate imaging characteristics that will allow for lesion identification. Splenic biopsy is not routinely performed given the highly vascular nature of the organ.

☐ Non-contrast examinations are of limited benefit as splenic infarctions or abscesses cannot be readily detected without IV contrast administration.

☐ Infiltrating splenic processes such as lymphoma, sarcoid, and amyloid cannot be readily distinguished from other splenic abnormalities.

☐ Single-phase imaging may lead to false-positive or false-negative results in the identification of splenic lesions. For example, arterial phase (early) imaging causes the spleen to demonstrate a very bizarre, heterogeneous enhancement pattern that is caused by the different enhancement characteristics of the red and white pulp. This may cause a false-positive diagnosis of a splenic lesion. Late imaging after IV contrast enhancement may lead to false-negative results in that vascular lesions may equilibrate with the splenic parenchyma or washout by the time imaging is performed.

Pancreatic Imaging

- CT is frequently requested for the evaluation of suspected pancreatitis. CT is often unnecessary to confirm a biochemically documented episode of acute pancreatitis as the imaging findings may be minimal or absent.
- Ultrasound is the imaging study of choice in the evaluation of cholelithiasis as a potential cause of pancreatitis.
- CT is useful in the follow-up of patients with documented pancreatitis in whom symptoms persist or worsen. Oral contrast is recommended for the study in order to separate the pancreatic parenchyma from surrounding duodenum. Additionally, because pancreatic inflammation can cause secondary colonic inflammation, oral contrast is required for adequate bowel distension. IV contrast is necessary to evaluate for pancreatic necrosis, which is manifest by regions of decreased or absent pancreatic enhancement.
- CT also may be used to evaluate suspected or known pancreatic masses. Typically, the CT is performed with IV contrast in multiple phases of contrast enhancement. Oral contrast may be useful for the study to allow separation of the duodenum from the pancreas as well as to evaluate for possible duodenal involvement by tumor.
- CT angiography (CTA) may be performed in cases of known pancreatic neoplasm to allow for surgical planning, including vessel involvement.

  INDICATIONS
  - ☐ Evaluation of complicated pancreatitis such as pancreatic necrosis, pancreatic abscess, or hemorrhagic pancreatitis (routine CT of the abdomen and pelvis with oral and IV contrast; single phase of contrast enhancement)
  - ☐ Evaluation of complications of pancreatitis including pseudocyst formation (typically >6 weeks following an acute episode of pancreatitis), splenic vein occlusion, or pseudoaneurysm formation (may be performed either as routine CT of the abdomen and pelvis with oral and IV contrast or as pancreatic mass protocol study with IV contrast in multiple phases of contrast enhancement)

Computed Tomography

☐ Evaluation of known or suspected pancreatic masses. This may be performed to identify suspected pancreatic masses or to determine resectability of a pancreatic mass. The study is performed as a pancreatic mass protocol with multiple phases of IV contrast enhancement. Depending upon the institution, the study may be performed such that only limited portions of the remaining abdomen are imaged so that thin sections of the pancreas may be obtained. If this is the case, liver metastases may not be identified. If liver metastases are suspected, discuss the case with the radiologist so that the liver may be included in the study.

CONTRAINDICATIONS

☐ Patients who cannot receive IV contrast are not candidates for the study.

LIMITATIONS

☐ Small pancreatic tumors may not be identifiable on CT or MRI. Endoscopic ultrasound is the imaging study of choice for the evaluation of suspected pancreatic masses that are occult on CT or MRI.

☐ Resectability of pancreatic tumors can be difficult to determine with certainty on imaging studies. Features that determine resectability include degree of involvement of the superior mesenteric artery and vein, local lymph node involvement, and distant disease (e.g. liver metastases). The degree of vessel involvement can be underestimated with current imaging modalities.

Adrenal Imaging

▪ Small adrenal lesions commonly are incidentally identified on CTs obtained for a variety of clinical indications. These lesions are often benign entities such as myelolipomas or adenomas, which then do not require further imaging or follow-up.

▪ If an adrenal lesion is identified on CECT, which does not demonstrate CT characteristics of a benign lesion, further evaluation may be warranted if there are no prior studies to document stability. This is particularly important in patients with known neoplasms in whom an adrenal metastatic deposit would change staging and management.

▪ Indeterminate adrenal lesions may be evaluated by CT or MRI. CT is a more cost-effective method of evaluating these lesions and involves both non-contrast and IV contrast-enhanced imaging. IV contrast is required for the evaluation of adrenal lesions as it is the percentage rate of washout of IV contrast from the adrenal gland which allows characterization of the lesion.

■ CT is also helpful in the diagnosis and follow-up of adrenal hemorrhage. Non-contrast imaging is adequate to evaluate for adrenal hemorrhages.

INDICATIONS

☐ Evaluation of previously (often incidentally) identified adrenal lesions for the purposes of lesion characterization. If an adrenal lesion measures water or fat density on CT, no additional evaluation is required as this signifies benignity. However, even benign lesions such as angiomyelolipomas can enhance. Thus, they are often indeterminate lesions when incidentally identified on CECT at the time of imaging for unrelated pathology. Adrenal wash-out imaging allows a lesion to be characterized as benign if there is 50% wash-out of contrast material from the lesion in 15 minutes.

☐ Evaluation of suspected adrenal hemorrhage. IV contrast is not required for this diagnosis; however, follow-up imaging may be necessary to evaluate for an underlying adrenal mass once the hemorrhage has resolved.

☐ Evaluation of adrenal trauma. This is often incidentally identified at the time of routine CECT of the abdomen in the setting of acute trauma.

CONTRAINDICATIONS

☐ There is debate as to whether or not it is safe to give IV contrast to patients who have known or suspected pheochromocytoma. It has been proposed that these patients should not be given IV contrast material or, if they require IV contrast, they should first receive alpha-blockade. These proposals are due to the reported risk of precipitating a catecholamine storm with IV contrast administration. It is advisable to discuss these cases with your imaging department in order to determine their policies.

LIMITATIONS

☐ It may not be possible to fully characterize an adrenal lesion on CT. Lipid-poor adenomas, for example (i.e. adenomas in which the amount of fat is so small that it cannot be detected on CT), may not be able to be characterized with this method. Non-contrast MRI may be a more sensitive study to characterize these lesions.

☐ Adrenal masses that contain hemorrhage may not be identified on initial imaging due to the presence of hemorrhage. If there is suspicion of hemorrhage into an underlying mass (e.g. lung cancer metastasis), a follow-up study or contrast-enhanced MRI should be considered in order to evaluate for the presence of a pathologic adrenal mass.

Renal Imaging

■ There is a vast array of renal pathology that may be identified with CT imaging. Communication of the clinical question to the radiologist conducting the examination is of key importance as different types of renal abnormalities must be imaged in different ways (i.e. IV contrast studies versus non-contrast imaging versus other imaging modalities e.g. ultrasound).

Non-Contrast Renal CT Imaging

■ This type of CT study is performed without oral or IV contrast. The patient is placed in the prone position (to allow for differentiation of calculi lodged at the ureterovesical junction and thus less likely to pass versus calculi which have passed into the bladder).

■ The main indication for non-contrast renal imaging is for the evaluation of renal/ureteral or bladder calculi and for the identification of associated renal or ureteral obstruction.

■ Patients should be appropriately screened for the examination. Although other disease entities such as appendicitis or diverticulitis may occasionally be identified with non-contrast imaging, the examination is suboptimal for complete evaluation of bowel pathology, abscesses, and other intra-abdominal/pelvic abnormalities.

INDICATIONS

☐ Evaluation of obstructing nephroureterolithiasis

☐ Evaluation/follow-up of renal stone burden

CONTRAINDICATIONS

☐ Serious consideration should be given to the radiation risks of this study, particularly in young patients. Flank pain protocol CT examinations (non-contrast CTs) are high radiation studies (6–10 mSv). If patients have known nephrolithiasis and the clinical question is simply if there is obstruction or not, an ultrasound should be strongly considered as an alternative investigation. This is particularly the case if patients present repeatedly with the same symptoms.

Ultrasound may be an appropriate alternative as the main clinical question is often one of renal obstruction.

☐ Always determine if the patient with a history of nephrolithiasis has had a recent CT examination. If there has been a recent study that did not demonstrate nephrolithiasis, it is highly unlikely that stones will have formed in a short interval. Consideration thus should be given to alternative diagnoses and alternative imaging studies, if necessary.

LIMITATIONS

☐ There are certain types of stones that are CT-lucent, which means that they are not visible on CT. In patients with these types of stones, only the secondary effects of renal/ureteral obstruction may be identifiable. These type of stones tend to be seen in patients on indinovir and other antiretroviral agents.

☐ Obese patients may be difficult to evaluate for small stones due to artifacts related to their body habitus.

☐ If there is clinical suspicion of alternative pathology (e.g. bowel or gynecologic pathology), consideration should be given to the most appropriate investigation for the patient's symptoms. If bowel pathology is suspected, oral and IV contrast are more appropriate; non-contrast imaging may not be diagnostic. If gynecologic pathology is suspected, ultrasound should be performed as a first imaging step as there is no ionizing radiation involved. If ultrasound is negative and urologic pathology remains of clinical concern, CT may then be considered.

Contrast-Enhanced Genitourinary Imaging

▪ It may be performed to diagnose acute renal/ureteral or bladder disease, or it may be performed to evaluate or follow-up suspected or known renal abnormalities.

▪ Renal abnormalities may be incidentally identified on imaging performed for an alternative diagnosis.

▪ Although a diagnosis of pyelonephritis may be suggested on the basis of a CECT, it is NOT an imaging diagnosis (i.e. it is a diagnosis made upon clinical grounds). Imaging features of infection may be present or absent and thus are not reliable for establishing the diagnosis.

INDICATIONS

☐ Routine CECT of the abdomen/pelvis is used for the evaluation of suspected traumatic renal/ureteral/bladder injury.

This indication requires the administration of IV contrast. Delayed CT imaging is obtained (at >5 minutes) to evaluate for injury to the collecting system or ureter. The time delay allows for the normal filtration and excretion of contrast into the collecting system and ureter, at which time leaks may be identified. Suspected bladder injury may require additional imaging for diagnosis and characterization. Imaging of suspected bladder injury may be performed under fluoroscopic or CT imaging. This process (cystogram/CT cystogram) requires direct instillation of contrast through a Foley catheter into the bladder.

☐ Routine CECT is used for the evaluation of suspected vascular injury, including trauma to the vascular pedicle. Renal infarction may also be identified by the presence of wedge-shaped areas of decreased renal perfusion. CT may also be performed in the subacute period to evaluate the sequelae of renal perfusion abnormalities.

☐ CECT may be performed to grossly estimate renal function. The kidneys normally filter and excrete IV contrast agents. In normally functioning kidneys, excretion should be symmetric. In patients with obstruction, excretion may be delayed or absent. However, nuclear medicine renal imaging is a more sensitive and specific study that allows for quantitation of differential renal function.

☐ CECT is useful to identify suspected perinephric or renal (parenchymal) abscesses. It is a useful study to plan percutaneous drainage of these abscesses as well as to follow the collections to resolution.

☐ CECT may also be performed as a dedicated study to evaluate renal masses identified on prior imaging studies or in at-risk or symptomatic patients. This type of study is commonly termed a *renal mass protocol CT* and is discussed later in this chapter.

CONTRAINDICATIONS

☐ Patients who cannot receive IV contrast material are not candidates for evaluation of renal disease with CT, with the exception of patients with nephroureterolithiasis.

☐ For patients with a solitary kidney, IV contrast is a relative contraindication. If there is normal renal function, the study may be performed with a lower or half dose of contrast in an attempt to protect renal function.

☐ Renal transplant patients with suspected native kidney masses may not be candidates for CECT. This is somewhat institution-dependent; some transplant surgeons will not allow renal transplant patients to receive IV contrast as it may cause acute tubular necrosis or renal impairment in the transplant kidney. It is advisable to discuss these patients with the referring clinician in order to determine if IV contrast should be administered. If it cannot be given, patients should be referred for MR (ultrasound is not the study of choice but may be performed if patients cannot undergo MR or CT examinations).

LIMITATIONS

☐ Routine CT is NOT the imaging modality of choice to evaluate the urothelium for lesions such as transitional cell carcinoma. CT may be performed in conjunction with an IV pyelogram (IVP) in order to evaluate both the urothelium (via the IVP) and the renal parenchyma (CT). Please refer to Chapter 4 for a more detailed description of this study. CT urography has largely supplanted the CT-IVP and will be discussed later.

☐ Patients with poor renal function may not be able to concentrate IV contrast adequately; therefore, enhancement patterns that may be crucial for the characterization of the lesion may not be demonstrable.

☐ In patients in whom urolithiasis is suspected, IV contrast opacification of the kidneys, ureters, or bladder may mask the presence of a small calculus. Secondary signs of obstruction may be recognized (e.g. hydro [uretero] nephrosis, delayed or asymmetric nephrogram, perinephric fat stranding). However, as the size of the stone (>5 mm) often dictates management, it is advisable to perform a non-contrast (flank pain protocol) study in order to optimally identify the presence, size, and location of a stone.

Imaging of Suspected Renal Masses (Renal Mass Protocol CT)

■ This is an abdominal CT performed for the express purpose of evaluating the renal parenchyma. For this reason, the pelvis is NOT imaged and only an abdominal CT should be requested by the ordering clinician.

■ The study is composed of non-contrast CT images through the abdomen followed by thin section images through the kidneys in multiple phases of IV contrast enhancement. No oral contrast is required for the study.

GENERAL CONSIDERATIONS

☐ As IV contrast is required for the study, renal function should be assessed shortly prior to the scheduled examination. This is of particular importance in patients with diabetes, with prior nephrectomy or partial nephrectomy, or with known renal insufficiency. In patients with an elevated Cr (>1.5 mg/dL), a CECT cannot be safely performed due to the renal toxic effects of IV contrast. In these patients, known or suspected masses must be evaluated by ultrasound or MRI.

☐ The study is performed to evaluate known or suspected renal masses for neoplastic lesions. A renal mass protocol is NOT required to follow up a previously documented benign lesion or to follow metastatic lesions or known primary renal malignancies. These patients simply require a routine CECT of the abdomen and pelvis to assess for interval change in size or morphology of the previously documented lesion(s).

INDICATIONS

☐ Evaluation of indeterminate renal masses demonstrated on alternative imaging studies (e.g. ultrasound, routine CECT)

☐ Follow-up of suspicious masses that remain indeterminate on imaging (e.g. Bosniak IIIb lesions)

☐ Screening of patients with prior partial or total nephrectomy for renal cell carcinoma or transitional cell carcinoma involving the kidney. MR may be a better modality for the long-term follow-up of these patients due to the lack of ionizing radiation and iodinated IV contrast.

☐ Surgical planning for partial nephrectomy

☐ Screening of patients with inherited syndromes (e.g. von Hippel Lindau) who are at risk of developing renal cell carcinomas. CT or MR may be performed for this indication.

CONTRAINDICATIONS

☐ As listed earlier in the section Contrast-Enhanced Genitourinary Imaging

LIMITATIONS

☐ The urothelium cannot be adequately assessed with this technique; CT urography is the imaging modality of choice.

☐ A mass is deemed suspicious for malignancy if it demonstrates enhancement of >10 HU. There also may be artifactual causes of apparent enhancement or lack of enhancement including streak artifact related to a patient's arms at the sides when the scan is performed and related to obese patients in whom images tend to be visually noisy and in whom, therefore, accurate attenuation values cannot be assessed.

☐ Small masses may be difficult to characterize on CT.

CT Urogram

▪ CT urography is a relatively new technique that has been made possible largely due to the advent of multidetector CT scanners with improved spatial and temporal resolution.

▪ The study has nearly completely replaced IVPs (see Chapter 4 and CT-IVPs for the evaluation of urothelial abnormalities).

▪ The examination is more time-consuming than a routine CT of the abdomen and pelvis, and the patient incurs a significantly higher radiation dose (30–40 mSv) than during routine CECT (5 mSv) and IVP examinations.

▪ The study consists of both non-contrast and contrast-enhanced sequences and may be performed with IV hydration and IV furosemide (Lasix) in order to distend the urinary collecting system and promote contrast excretion.

▪ The bladder is not optimally evaluated with this technique, and cystoscopy or a cystogram may be required for evaluation of the bladder.

▪ CT urography allows for evaluation of urothelial lesions such as transitional cell carcinoma.

▪ The non-contrast portion of the examination allows for the identification of nephroureterolithiasis as a cause of hematuria.

INDICATIONS

☐ Evaluation of patients with hematuria

☐ Screening of patients with history of transitional cell carcinoma or urothelial tumor. There is an increased risk of synchronous or metachronous lesions in patients with transitional cell carcinoma.

☐ Presurgical planning for patients with known urothelial malignancy

☐ CT urography may be helpful in cases of suspected ureteral injury from trauma or surgery; alternatively, routine abdominal-pelvic CECT with a >3-minute delay can be performed for the evaluation of traumatic ureteral injury (the delay is to allow time for excretion of contrast into the collecting system).

☐ The study may be performed in a variety of ways; however, it often includes a non-contrast CT of the abdomen and pelvis (to identify calculi and to assist in characterization of renal masses, if present), followed by at least two phases of IV contrast enhancement (usually corticomedullary and delayed; this assists in detection and characterization of renal masses, if present). A delayed CT of the abdomen and pelvis in the excretory phase (i.e. when the collecting systems and bladder are opacified with contrast) is performed at >3 minutes following IV contrast administration.

CONTRAINDICATIONS

☐ Younger patients (generally <40 years), for whom nephroureterolithiasis is the main clinical concern as the etiology of hematuria, should undergo ultrasound or non-contrast CT (flank pain protocol). CT urography requires multiple imaging phases over the entire abdomen and pelvis, thus has an extremely high radiation dose (approximately 30–40 mSv in average-sized patients).

☐ The study may not be performed if IV contrast or Lasix is contraindicated.

LIMITATIONS

☐ If there is poor renal function or obstruction of the collecting system (particularly if proximal to the kidney or renal pelvis), masses in the ureter may be difficult to identify as they are not outlined by contrast.

☐ If scanning is not performed with the appropriate timing of the contrast bolus, lesions may be missed or may not be able to be characterized based on their contrast enhancement characteristics.

☐ Subtle, small, or urothelial surface lesions may be below the resolution of CT and may not be identified.

☐ Bladder lesions, particularly if confined to the bladder mucosa, may not be detectable with this method.

☐ The high radiation dose may be prohibitive for routine screening examinations in patients with known transitional cell carcinoma. Consideration should be given to the radiation dose for all patients in whom this study is ordered, particularly in younger patients who are at increased cumulative lifetime risk of radiation-induced malignancy.

☐ The study is limited for evaluation of mucosal lesions in obese patients as there is often significant image degradation due to patient size.

CT Cystogram

■ A cystogram is a retrograde study performed by instilling contrast material into the bladder through a Foley catheter. The contrast medium is diluted with saline and is dripped into the bladder under gravity (typically a total of 250 cc).

■ Cystograms may be performed under fluoroscopy (see Chapter 4) or under CT. CT cystography is increasingly being used due to its superior anatomic detail over conventional cystograms. This superior detail allows accurate assessment of injury location and intra- versus extraperitoneal bladder rupture.

■ CT cystography involves several scans of the pelvis (the abdomen is not imaged), which often include a non-contrast examination (to evaluate for hemorrhage) followed by imaging with the bladder distended. This allows the bladder wall integrity to be assessed. If there is a bladder leak/rupture, contrast will extend across the site of injury (which may be directly visible) and around the bladder. The location of the contrast extravasation can be determined. If the contrast is confined to the retropubic region and perivesicular space, it is determined to be extraperitoneal. If it extends to surround loops of bowel and other structures within the peritoneum, it is deemed to be intraperitoneal bladder rupture.

■ Management of bladder rupture is dependent upon the location of bladder rupture. Extraperitoneal bladder rupture often results from trauma (e.g. pelvic fractures), whereas intraperitoneal injury most often results from injury during pelvic surgery.

■ Extraperitoneal bladder rupture is treated conservatively with Foley catheter placement to maintain the bladder in a constant state of decompression, thus allowing the site of injury to heal.

■ Intraperitoneal bladder rupture is treated surgically with direct repair of the site of injury. Uncommonly, it may be treated conservatively, similar to treatment of extraperitoneal bladder injury.

INDICATIONS

☐ Evaluation of patients with pelvic fractures to assess for associated extraperitoneal bladder injury. It should be noted that if patients experience trauma with a distended bladder, it is possible to have intraperitoneal bladder injury or intra- and extraperitoneal bladder injury.

☐ Assessment of uremic patients who have had recent trauma or surgery. In cases of intraperitoneal bladder rupture, urine leaks into the peritoneal cavity where it is absorbed back into the blood. This causes an elevation of serum BUN/Cr and can present as acute renal failure or uremia. This does not occur in isolated extraperitoneal bladder rupture as the urine is not absorbed.

☐ Evaluation of patients with recent abdominal or pelvic surgery in whom there are symptoms or uremia, abdominal pain, hematuria, or new ascites. Intraperitoneal bladder rupture may present in this fashion.

CONTRAINDICATIONS

☐ Questionable urethral injury. In these patients, the study should be performed under fluoroscopic guidance in order to first evaluate the urethra. A retrograde urethrogram (see Chapter 4) is first performed by placing the tip of the Foley catheter into the urethral meatus and hand injecting contrast under fluoroscopy to evaluate for leak (urethral injury). If there is no leak, the Foley can be advanced and a conventional cystogram can be performed at that time.

☐ Unstable patients. If a trauma patient is unstable at the time of the initial imaging, it is advisable that the patient be managed acutely and stabilized prior to CT cystography.

LIMITATIONS

☐ Small perforations in the bladder wall may not be identified at CT imaging.

☐ If the bladder is not fully distended (e.g. due to patient discomfort or blood clot within the Foley or bladder), small or slow bladder leaks may not be identified. However, small amounts of extravasated contrast material may be visible in the intra- or extraperitoneal space, thus allowing diagnosis.

☐ If patients are imaged after they are stabilized with an external fixation device for pelvic fracture, streak artifact from the metallic device may mask contrast extravasation and may complicate diagnosis.

CT Imaging of Gynecologic Disease

▦ CT has a limited role in the evaluation of suspected or known gynecological abnormalities. MR and transvaginal ultrasound are the imaging modalities of choice. Hysterosalpingography or hysterosonography may also be used in the appropriate setting (see Chapters 4 and 10).

▦ CT may on occasion identify adnexal or uterine abnormalities. This is particularly true in the case of adnexal masses; CT may identify and occasionally characterize an adnexal mass. CT is particularly helpful in the identification of fat contained within an adnexal mass, thus suggesting a diagnosis of benign disease.

▦ CT is very useful in the evaluation of suspected omental disease from gynecological primaries.

INDICATIONS
☐ Identification of fat in an ovarian mass in patients with suspected teratoma
☐ Evaluation of omental and peritoneal spread of malignant disease
☐ Evaluation of solid organ and lung metastatic disease
☐ Evaluation of extension of cervical carcinoma (although MR is a more sensitive imaging modality for this indication)

CONTRAINDICATIONS
☐ Primary evaluation of gynecologic abnormality
☐ Pregnancy, because radiation causes risks to the fetus. If there is a question of gynecologic malignancy or spread of malignant disease, MR may be performed (without IV contrast due to fetal risk) for this purpose.

LIMITATIONS
☐ CT cannot adequately assess the ovaries for the presence of mural nodules or intracystic masses, which would suggest malignancy as it does not have adequate soft tissue (contrast) resolution.
☐ CT cannot assess ovarian flow; therefore, ovarian torsion cannot be excluded on the basis of CT. Ultrasound is the imaging modality of choice for the evaluation of suspected ovarian torsion.

Computed Tomography

☐ Uterine anomalies and endometrial malignancy cannot be assessed on CT as the contrast resolution is not adequate. Extension of uterine or cervical malignancy can, however, be assessed.

☐ Processes such as endometriosis are not well evaluated with CT. Ovarian masses (e.g. endometriomas) cannot be characterized on CT.

CT Imaging of Bowel Pathology

■ CT is increasingly employed in the evaluation of bowel pathology, particularly in the setting of acute abdominal pain or known bowel obstruction.

■ As bowel abnormalities may be manifest by subtle findings such as minimal bowel wall thickening, adequate distension of the bowel by oral contrast is imperative for an optimal study. Patients are required to consume a total of 16 oz of barium or Hypaque. Hypaque is used in patients with suspected acute bowel abnormality in whom the possibility of emergent/urgent surgical intervention may be necessary as Hypaque has less risk of peritonitis and is less viscous than barium.

■ IV contrast is also of the utmost importance in the evaluation of acute bowel abnormality, particularly when there is a suspicion of intra-abdominal/pelvic abscess. In the absence of IV contrast, fluid collections may not be identified or may not be recognized as organized, walled-off collections.

■ Rectal contrast also may be administered for the evaluation of suspected bowel pathology. It may be administered as the only contrast agent, with IV contrast, or with oral and IV contrast (the so-called "triple contrast"). Rectal contrast has the added advantage over oral contrast alone in that it allows for improved colonic distension over oral contrast alone and with less time required for the study preparation. If oral contrast only is administered, the patient is usually not scanned for at least 1.5–2 hours following contrast ingestion to allow normal transit of contrast from the esophagus to the colon; the transit time may be slower in some individuals (e.g. patients on narcotics, patients with small bowel obstruction). Rectal contrast also allows for rapid evaluation of bowel injury in patients with penetrating abdominal or pelvic trauma. If rectal contrast is considered, discuss it with the radiologist.

INDICATIONS

Acute Bowel Pathology

☐ CT is quickly becoming the imaging study of choice in the identification of bowel obstruction, the site of transition, and possible masses or extrinsic abnormalities.

☐ Primary diagnosis or evaluation of complications from diverticulitis. IV contrast is of particular importance in this setting in order to evaluate for walled-off or drainable abscess cavities.

☐ Evaluation of appendicitis

☐ Diagnosis of bowel perforation and pneumoperitoneum

☐ Identification of bowel ischemia. IV contrast is required in this setting, particularly to allow for possible identification of arterial or venous thrombus within the mesenteric vasculature.

☐ Identification of acute bowel infection (e.g. *Clostridium difficile* colitis)

☐ Evaluation of flairs of inflammatory bowel disease (i.e. ulcerative colitis and Crohn's disease)

☐ Evaluation of bowel injury in the setting of trauma

Nonacute Bowel Pathology

☐ Virtual colonoscopy has been heralded as a new method to screen for colonic polyps and neoplasms. The examination involves the instillation of air into the colon via a rectal tube. The colon is distended and CT images are obtained. Reformatted images are then reconstructed in various planes.

☐ Routine CECT may occasionally identify large, predominantly exophytic bowel masses (e.g. in lymphoma, adenocarcinoma)

CT Enterography

☐ This is a relatively new imaging method that uses negative oral contrast (i.e. water or an agent that is less dense than the bowel wall). This allows the bowel to be distended without obscuring the mucosa (which is what occurs with positive contrast agents such as Hypaque or barium). The study is performed with this negative oral contrast agent and IV contrast and images are acquired in thin sections. This allows for evaluation of the mucosa for ulcerations as well as for strictures and fistulas. The drawback to this technique is the relatively high radiation dose. MR enterography may provide similar information in these patients without the use of ionizing radiation (see Chapter 7).

☐ Evaluation of hernias. The main indication for these patients is to identify the location of the hernia, identify the muscles involved, and determine if the fascia is intact. There is little need for CT for the identification of the presence of a hernia or an incarcerated hernia as this diagnosis may be made on clinical grounds without the necessity of CT radiation.

CONTRAINDICATIONS

☐ Oral contrast is recommended for all studies in which bowel pathology is suspected. However, barium is not recommended if there is concern for bowel perforation due to the increased risk of peritonitis and contamination of the surgical field. In patients presenting with suspected acute bowel pathology, Hypaque is administered. Hypaque is not administered for routine abdominal imaging due to its very unpalatable taste!

☐ Rectal contrast may be unsafe in patients with toxic megacolon or severe colitis due to the increased bowel distension and pressure related to the contrast volume.

☐ Patients with known or suspected perirectal abscess may not be optimal candidates for rectal contrast for evaluation of the abscess. Although rectal contrast is clearly more rapid than oral contrast (which requires a 2-hour minimum delay for transit to the rectum in these patients), there is a risk of traumatizing the anus or rectum while placing the catheter and instilling the contrast. If rectal contrast is considered or desired in these patients, it is advisable to discuss the case with the radiologist.

LIMITATIONS

☐ CT is not specific or sensitive for the identification of the cause of GI bleeding. Although processes such as diverticulosis/diverticulitis can be detected on CT and may be the cause of the GI bleed, causes of GI bleeding often go undetected on CT. Nuclear medicine studies (e.g. sulfur colloid or tagged red blood cell studies) or catheter angiography may be necessary to identify causes of GI bleeding.

☐ In patients with small bowel obstruction, the precise site and cause of the obstruction may be difficult or impossible to identify on CT. The majority of small bowel obstructions are the result of adhesions related to prior surgery. However, adhesions cannot be directly visualized on CT and may only be suggested by an angulated appearance of bowel loops with a transition point to decompressed bowel at the site of obstruction.

☐ If patients cannot tolerate oral contrast, it may be difficult to evaluate the bowel, particularly if the bowel is not distended. This may cause false-positive or false-negative results. False-positive results can be seen if the bowel is not fully distended, leading the bowel to appear thick-walled and thus simulating disease. Alternatively, false negatives can occur if the bowel is not adequately distended to allow evaluation of the wall for masses and thickening.

☐ If there is not a long enough delay between the ingestion of oral contrast and the study performance, the entire bowel may not be opacified. This is particularly important in cases where there is a concern for appendicitis or diverticulitis.

☐ It may not be possible to differentiate the cause of bowel wall abnormality. For instance, it is often not possible to differentiate between wall thickening caused by infection (e.g. colitis), inflammation (e.g. inflammatory bowel disease), and neoplasm.

☐ Bowel injury in the setting of trauma is often not identified on CT examination. It is very uncommon to identify direct evidence of bowel injury (e.g. free intra-abdominal air, leakage of oral contrast, IV contrast blush). More often, there is indirect evidence that is not specific (e.g. free pelvic fluid in the absence of a solid organ injury).

Vascular CT Imaging

▣ CECT imaging is employed in the evaluation of acute vascular abnormalities, of known or suspected vascular anatomic variants (e.g. aberrant vessels or a duplicated aortic arch), and of neoplasms preoperatively to allow safe and accurate resection margins.

Aortic Imaging

▣ It may be performed with or without IV contrast, depending upon the indication for the study.

Computed Tomography

INDICATIONS

Non-Contrast Aortic Imaging

☐ It may be performed to identify or follow up the size of an aortic aneurysm

☐ It may be performed prior to certain vascular surgeries, including CABG, to evaluate for calcified atherosclerotic plaque, which may interfere with graft placement.

Contrast-Enhanced Aortic Imaging

☐ The most frequent use of CT for aortic imaging is in the setting of suspected or known aortic dissection. Imaging includes both non-contrast and IV contrast-enhanced images. Non-enhanced images are obtained to allow for identification of high attenuation intramural hematoma (hemorrhage within the wall of the aorta separating the intima from the media), which has prognostic importance. Intramural hematoma is masked once IV contrast is administered (when it will often look like benign atheromatous plaque). Contrast administration is required to evaluate for a dissection flap, which indicates the presence of blood dissecting between the aortic intima and media. For patients who are unable to receive non-ionic IV contrast (either on the basis of renal insufficiency or contrast allergy), high-dose gadolinium may be of benefit to identify the dissection flap. This has fallen out of favor due to the increased risk of development of nephrogenic systemic fibrosis (see Chapter 7).

☐ CECT is also performed to evaluate for ruptured aortic aneurysms, although contrast may not be absolutely necessary in these cases if there is hemorrhage surrounding the aorta secondary to rupture.

☐ CECT may be of use to evaluate for the presence of flow within aortic grafts (e.g. aorto-bifemoral bypass grafts) or to evaluate for complications in aortic stent grafts (e.g. endoleaks).

☐ Congenital vascular abnormalities can be characterized with CECT imaging.

☐ Traumatic aortic injury requires the administration of IV contrast for diagnosis.

CONTRAINDICATIONS

☐ In patients with poor renal function, a lower dose of IV contrast may be considered for evaluation of the aorta. However, MR or echocardiography may be more appropriate imaging modalities in these patients.

LIMITATIONS

☐ If the CT is not gated to the heart rate or if there is a high heart rate, an artifact can occur in the aortic root/ascending aorta. This artifact is due to cardiac motion and presents as a line through the vessel in this location. This can mimic a flap of aortic dissection and can render the examination equivocal or cause a false-positive result. If this occurs on an examination, the study may be repeated (although this puts the patient at risk from the additional IV contrast and radiation). An echocardiogram, MRI, or conventional catheter angiogram may be necessary to confirm or refute these findings. In these cases, confer with the radiologist to determine the best course of action.

☐ IV contrast is required in order to identify a dissection flap; if contrast cannot be administered, an alternate imaging modality should be considered as the sensitivity of non-contrast CT is low for a dissection. If there is concern for aortic aneurysm rupture or aortic transsection, non-contrast CT may be adequate to evaluate for periaortic hemorrhage, which would suggest the diagnosis in the appropriate clinical setting.

☐ If there is blood in the anterior mediastinum in patients with trauma, it may be difficult to determine if it arises from the aorta/great vessels or if it is due to a sternal injury. It is essential to determine if the blood arises from a fracture (e.g. sternum if anterior, vertebral body if posterior) or from a vascular injury.

Renal Vascular CT Imaging

▪ Some institutions advocate the use of CECT with computer generated reformatted images in various planes for the evaluation of renal artery stenosis. This examination CANNOT be performed in patients with Cr levels >1.5 mg/dL due to the risk of contrast-induced nephrotoxicity.

▪ CTA may also be performed in the evaluation of potential renal donors. This allows for identification of the number and position of the renal vasculature prior to transplantation.

▪ The renal donor study involves non-contrast images through the kidneys to allow for stone or mass detection followed by arterial phase IV contrast-enhanced images in thin sections to allow vascular assessment. Delayed images are then obtained to characterize any renal lesions identified and to assess the collecting systems. If the study is performed solely for the evaluation of renal vascular abnormalities such as stenosis, a CECT angiogram is performed with only contrast-enhanced images obtained.

INDICATIONS

☐ Evaluation of known or suspected renal artery stenosis in patients with renal impairment or hypertension

☐ Evaluation of the renal arteries or veins in patients with a history of trauma, prior biopsy, and vascular malformation. This allows for evaluation of the presence, size, and location of a vascular lesion such as an arterial aneurysm. The study may also assist in preprocedure (surgery or percutaneous intervention) planning for repair.

☐ CTA may be performed for evaluation of patients with known renal tumors in whom partial resection is planned. This allows for evaluation of the vascular supply to the tumor as well as assessment of the location of large vessels, which may be traumatized during surgery.

☐ Patients who are planning to donate a kidney are evaluated prior to donation. A CT is performed to evaluate for renal abnormality, which would preclude donation (e.g. tumor, hydronephrosis). The angiographic portion of the examination allows for assessment of the number of renal arteries/ veins as well as their location. The collecting system is also evaluated. This allows for determination of the best kidney for donation and the best surgical approach.

CONTRAINDICATIONS

☐ Patients with borderline or elevated renal function should not receive IV contrast.

LIMITATIONS

☐ Patients previously treated for renal artery stenosis with metallic stents may be difficult to evaluate for recurrent stenosis due to streak artifact related to the presence of the stent. This is becoming less problematic with the implementation of 64-slice multidetector row CT scanners.

☐ In patients with slow flow in a vascular malformation (e.g. a venous varix), it may be difficult to characterize the abnormality as a vascular lesion and it may be difficult to determine if there is still flow in the abnormality (if it is slow flow).

☐ If the study is not appropriately timed, a true arterial phase may not be obtained; therefore, the arterial structures may not be optimally evaluated.

Venous CT Imaging

■ CT plays a limited role in the evaluation of venous abnormalities.

■ Venous thrombus within the inferior vena cava or iliac/femoral venous system may be identified with scanning delays set for optimal venous opacification by contrast material.

■ The study is performed following the administration of IV contrast. The abdomen and pelvis are scanned (unless only pelvic clot is suspected, in which case only the pelvis may be scanned). A delay of 90–120 seconds following IV contrast administration is required to allow time for contrast to opacify the vessels and prevent artifacts.

INDICATIONS
☐ Evaluation of thrombus within the inferior vena cava, pelvic veins, gonadal veins

CONTRAINDICATIONS
☐ IV contrast allergy or impaired renal function

LIMITATIONS
☐ Mixing of contrast-opacified blood with non-opacified blood can cause all or part of the vein to appear dark. This can simulate the presence of partially occlusive or occlusive venous thrombosis. It is therefore imperative to perform the scan after a delay following IV contrast administration to decrease the chance of a false positive.

Computed Tomography

7

Body MRI

General Considerations

■ MRI is often used as a problem-solving tool in body imaging (e.g. lesion identification and characterization of liver lesions).

■ MRI is NOT cost- or time-effective as a screening tool for metastatic disease in the chest/abdomen/pelvis. CT is the imaging study of choice for staging/restaging patients with known malignancies; however, MR is emerging as an alternative screening method for recurrent lymphadenopathy in patients with lymphoma and in children with malignancy in whom radiation considerations are of paramount concern. MR is increasingly requested for the evaluation of metastatic disease for a variety of primary malignancies. With improvements in MR equipment, it is becoming feasible to image patients with MR for metastatic disease. MR remains inadequate for the evaluation of parenchymal pulmonary abnormalities such as metastases and lung nodules.

■ MR is useful in screening for hepatocellular carcinomas (HCC) in patients with known cirrhosis; however, only approximately 50%–70% of HCCs are identifiable with MRI.

■ There are a number of significant advantages/disadvantages of MR versus CT:

ADVANTAGES

□ Absence of ionizing radiation in MR

□ Gadolinium (the MR contrast agent) is significantly less nephrotoxic than CT contrast agents (both ionic and non-ionic contrast). However, nephrotoxic effects have been reported with gadolinium at high concentrations (i.e. triple dose) and in patients with markedly elevated creatinine (Cr) (i.e. >5 mg/dL).

□ Better soft tissue resolution than CT

DISADVANTAGES

□ Length of study: MR examinations can require a minimum of 20 minutes to several hours of imaging time, whereas CT often requires <2–5 minutes (particularly in the era of multislice scanners).

□ Due to the configuration of the magnet, patients who are claustrophobic may be unable to complete the MR examination. The majority of radiology departments do not have the staff or medications available to be able to medicate patients prior to an MR examination. Therefore, it is recommended that patients with known claustrophobia be provided sedatives/anxiolytics by their primary caregivers. These medications should be made available to patients prior to the date of their examination. If patients will require conscious sedation for their examination, this should be made known to schedulers at the time of the study request so that this may be arranged.

□ Patients unable to lie completely supine are difficult to image with MR.

□ Patients with respiratory compromise may not be able to tolerate supine positioning. Patients with an inability to breathhold may be unable to comply with key sequences that may result in suboptimal or uninterpretable studies.

□ There are a number of contraindications to MRI, which are detailed in the following section.

Contraindications to MRI

ABSOLUTE CONTRAINDICATIONS

□ Artificial cardiac valves (now only St. Jude valves) cannot be imaged with MR due to the effect of the magnetic field upon the devices.

□ Metallic foreign bodies within the orbits (patients with exposure history should be screened for metal with orbital radiographs prior to the MR examination) cannot be imaged with MR due to the effect of the magnetic field upon the devices.

□ Patients with ferromagnetic surgical clips (e.g. cerebral aneurysm clips) cannot be imaged with MR due to the effect of the magnetic field upon the devices.

☐ Patients with pacers or automatic implantable cardioverter defibrillators (AICDs) cannot be imaged with MR due to the effect of the magnetic field upon the devices.

RELATIVE CONTRAINDICATIONS

☐ Recently placed cardiac stents (within 1–2 days)

☐ Obesity: The majority of MR scanners have a table limit of 350 lbs. Patients exceeding this limit cannot be imaged on conventional MR scanners. Patient girth is also a limitation; if patients exceed a certain circumference, they will not fit into the bore of the magnet.

☐ Claustrophobia: Many patients are unable to tolerate a complete MR examination based on claustrophobia. If there is a preexisting history of claustrophobia, the patient may be booked for the examination with sedation or may require anesthesia if sedation is inadequate to allow completion of the study.

☐ Inability to lie supine: Patients who are unable to lie completely flat are often poor candidates for MRI. Images may be suboptimal due to patient positioning. Additionally, if patients are unable to be appropriately positioned based upon respiratory compromise when in a supine position, they are often unable to tolerate the examination. MRI of solid organs such as the liver and kidneys often requires the patient to breath-hold for 20–30 seconds. If the patient is unable to do so, the images may be degraded to the degree of being uninterpretable.

MR of the Chest

▨ Chest MRI: Performed without IV contrast, often to evaluate for lymphadenopathy in patients with lymphoma

▪ Chest MRI with IV contrast: Performed to characterize mediastinal masses and evaluate extent of disease and invasion

▨ Aorta MR angiogram (MRA): Performed with IV contrast. Only the aorta and the origins of the great vessels are evaluated. It is performed to evaluate for aortic pathology such as aneurysm or dissection.

MR of the Heart

▨ Due to the long imaging times and the specific nature of the examination, the precise question to be answered must be clearly communicated to the radiologist prior to the examination so that the study may be tailored to answer the clinical question.

▪ Right ventricle (RV) dysplasia: Performed solely to evaluate for this entity. Generally, IV contrast is not required, although it may be administered if the diagnosis is in doubt.

▪ MR of the heart with IV contrast: May be performed to evaluate for the presence of and to characterize cardiac masses suspected or identified on other imaging modalities (e.g. echocardiography or CT). It may be useful to evaluate for constrictive pericarditis versus restrictive cardiomyopathy. It may play a role in identifying infiltrative cardiac disease such as amyloid or sarcoid.

▪ MR of the heart/valvular disease: Does not require IV contrast. It is often performed as part of a more comprehensive cardiac examination. Cardiac MR can determine valvular dysfunction and quantify the degree of insufficiency/stenosis.

▪ MR of the heart/perfusion/viability: Performed without and with IV contrast. Pharmacologic stress imaging is performed, often with adenosine, and myocardial perfusion is evaluated. Delayed images are also obtained in order to evaluate for myocardial viability (i.e. to evaluate for areas of scar).

MR of the Abdomen

▪ Due to the relatively long imaging times required for MR examinations, only limited areas of the body may be imaged at any given time. For this reason, the body region of most clinical interest/concern should be determined prior to the performance of the study in order to optimize the examination. The majority of MR abdominal examinations will image all of the solid organs of the upper abdomen (i.e. liver, gallbladder, spleen, pancreas, adrenal glands, and the majority of the kidneys), whereas thin section imaging of the entire abdomen cannot be performed (unlike CT).

▪ Specific imaging protocols differ between institutions. Representative protocols are listed (specific organ-based discussion follows):

  ☐ MR abdomen: Includes liver, gallbladder (without magnetic resonance cholangiopancreatography [MRCP]), spleen, adrenal glands, pancreas, and portions of the kidneys. The study is performed without and with IV contrast.

☐ MRCP: May be performed as a sole imaging test or may be combined with MR of the abdomen (both studies must be requested). MRCP is NOT performed with IV contrast.

☐ MR adrenal glands: Thin section imaging is performed through the adrenal glands only. The remainder of the abdomen is not imaged. It is typically performed without IV contrast; however, contrast may be administered as warranted (as determined by the radiologist monitoring the examination).

☐ MR kidneys: Performed for the purpose of renal lesion evaluation. The remaining abdominal solid organs are not evaluated. The study is performed without and with IV contrast. The CPT (billing) code for this study does not include an MRA to evaluate for renal artery stenosis.

☐ MRA kidneys: Performed to evaluate the renal arteries in patients with suspected renal artery stenosis. The study is performed without and with IV contrast. The kidneys can often be evaluated at the time of the study.

MR of the Pelvis

▪ Pelvis without IV contrast: Performed as a routine study to evaluate for benign diseases of the pelvis such as fibroids (which are not scheduled to undergo embolization; see next), adenomyosis

▪ Pelvis with IV contrast: Performed to evaluate for fibroids scheduled to undergo uterine artery embolization, to evaluate adnexal masses (contrast may not be required; however, this is determined by the monitoring radiologist at the time of the study), and to stage for gynecologic malignancy

▪ MR prostate: Performed in patients with known prostate malignancy to evaluate for extracapsular extension, neurovascular bundle involvement, and local lymph node involvement. An endorectal coil (i.e. MR coil placed within the rectum) may be used, depending upon the protocol and capability of the local scanner.

MR of the Liver

▪ Requires the patient to be able to breath-hold for 20–30 seconds

▪ Performed both without and with IV gadolinium (non-contrast imaging sequences are obtained prior to the administration of IV contrast)

■ MRCP is not performed routinely as part of the examination and must be requested separately.

■ Often performed based on the recommendations of another imaging study. Lesions that cannot be characterized on CT or ultrasound are often referred for MRI to characterize the lesion.

■ May be performed to identify hepatic lesions that cannot be seen with other imaging modalities; this is particularly useful in patients with known cirrhosis to evaluate for occult hepatocellular carcinomas

■ May be performed for surgical planning to evaluate for lesion location, vascular relationships, and vascular involvement

INDICATIONS

☐ Screening: For patients with a high clinical suspicion of hepatocellular carcinoma or metastatic disease, MR may be performed for lesion detection

☐ Lesion characterization: Hepatic lesions are commonly identified on routine abdominal imaging; however, these lesions are often incidental findings. As incidental findings, the lesions are often not fully characterizable on these studies. MR may be performed to define these masses. If cholangiocarcinoma is a clinical concern, it is important to impart this information to the radiologist prior to the examination as delayed post-contrast imaging (10 minutes following IV contrast administration) is often required to make this diagnosis and this is not routinely performed.

☐ Restaging: MR may be performed to follow hepatic masses (e.g. metastases or hepatocellular carcinoma) after treatment (chemotherapy, chemoembolization).

☐ Surgical planning: MR may be performed on patients with hepatic masses (both benign and malignant) preoperatively in order to determine resectability. MR can also determine vascular anatomy, which will assist the surgeon in preoperative planning.

☐ Vascular invasion: Patients with hepatocellular carcinoma are at increased risk of tumor thrombus formation, which characteristically involves the portal vein. MR not only can identify the presence of thrombus but also can determine thrombus enhancement, which suggests tumor as opposed to bland thrombus (i.e. clot).

CONTRAINDICATIONS

☐ Patients with severe liver dysfunction are at increased risk of developing nephrogenic systemic fibrosis (NSF)

following IV contrast administration. These patients should have a Cr level drawn 24 hours prior to the MR and if the estimated glomerular filtration rate (eGFR) is <40, IV contrast should not be administered. Local imaging center policies on gadolinium may differ, thus it is advised that a discussion occur with the local radiology department to determine the policy.

☐ Patients with significant ascites should not be imaged on a 3-tesla scanner due to an artifact produced by the magnetic field in the presence of ascites. The artifact is called the *dielectric effect* and is seen mainly on T2-weighted sequences, rendering them limited for the evaluation of disease. The effect is present but to a much lesser extent on 1.5-tesla scanners, thus these are the preferred scanners for patients with known or suspected ascites.

LIMITATIONS

☐ Patient factors:

• Breath holding: Respiratory motion causes significant movement of the upper abdominal solid organs. This motion leads to blurring of the MR image, which, in turn, degrades image quality. Lesions may be incompletely characterized due to these limitations. Depending upon the degree of motion artifact, lesions may be completely obscured. To avoid respiratory motion artifact, patients are given verbal instructions regarding breath holding and must be able to suspend respiration for a minimum of 20–30 seconds (for contrast-enhanced imaging). Intubated patients are poor candidates for hepatic imaging due to the difficulty they have suspending respiration.

• Body habitus: As noted previously, obese patients are poor candidates for MR examinations as their abdominal circumference may be as large as or greater than that of the imaging bore (maximum abdominal circumference 52 cm, weight 350 lbs). CT scanners have larger imaging bores and can accommodate slightly larger patients (maximum abdominal circumference 70 cm, weight 400 lbs).

• Venous access: Nearly all MR examinations performed for hepatic abnormalities (be it laboratory derangement or focal mass) require the administration of IV gadolinium (for lesion detection and characterization). Due to the rapid imaging required to evaluate the liver in different phases of contrast enhancement, a tight bolus of contrast is required. This requires a large bore IV (≥ 20 gauge).

Magnetic Resonance Cholangiopancreatography

▪ Patients should be fasting for 4–6 hours preceding the study in order to decrease bowel motility, which may lead to imaging artifacts. Patients should NOT be administered agents such as morphine prior to the examination as this may cause contraction of the sphincter of Oddi, which may in turn produce false-positive results of choledocholithiasis.

▪ It does not require the administration of IV gadolinium.

▪ It involves a relatively short imaging time (10–20 minutes).

▪ The study evaluates the intra- and extrahepatic biliary ducts.

▪ It is often performed in conjunction with MRI of the abdomen (see earlier).

INDICATIONS

☐ MRCP may be performed prior to endoscopic retrograde cholangiopancreatography (ERCP) or percutaneous cholangiography as an anatomic roadmap.

☐ Evaluation of suspected common bile duct (CBD) stones

☐ Evaluation of suspected sites of biliary obstruction

☐ Evaluation of suspected or known biliary strictures

☐ It may be useful to evaluate for ductal involvement by sclerosing cholangitis.

CONTRAINDICATIONS

☐ Recent meal, which may contract the gallbladder and stimulate the sphincter of Oddi

☐ Recent pain medication administration as it may affect the sphincter of Oddi

LIMITATIONS

☐ Of limited usefulness in patients with normal caliber ducts as the ducts are often below the resolution of the MRI

☐ Normal structures such as the sphincter of Oddi may mimic disease (i.e. CBD stones).

☐ In patients with prior cholecystectomy, metallic clips within the surgical bed may produce artifact significant enough to distort the MRCP images, thus rendering them uninterpretable.

☐ Pneumobilia (e.g. in patients with prior papillotomy for choledocholithiasis) may mimic a CBD stone.

☐ As with all MRI, motion and respiratory artifact will substantially degrade image quality and may render studies
uninterpretable.
☐ Without IV contrast, masses or neoplastic strictures (i.e.
cholangiocarcinoma) may not be identified.

MR of the Pancreas

■ It requires the administration of IV contrast following non-
contrast imaging. It is often imaged as part of an abdominal
MR study (see earlier).
■ It is often performed to evaluate for occult pancreatic lesions
or to evaluate pancreatic findings identified on other imaging modalities such as endoscopic ultrasound, CT, or ultrasound.
■ As with other imaging modalities, MR often cannot differentiate
between focal pancreatitis and malignancy.
■ It may be performed for preoperative planning to determine if
a mass is resectable.

INDICATIONS

☐ Identification of suspected pancreatic mass. MR is less sensitive than CT and endoscopic ultrasound for the identification of small pancreatic masses. If an MR fails to demonstrate a pancreatic mass in a patient in whom there is a high
clinical suspicion (e.g. in a patient with hormone-producing
tumors such as insulinoma), additional evaluation with a
pancreatic mass CT (see Chapter 6) or endoscopic ultrasound may be performed.
☐ Staging/restaging of known pancreatic malignancy. MR may
be performed for this indication; however, CT also may be
performed and is often the imaging modality of choice. This
is particularly true in patients with newly diagnosed pancreatic neoplasm who require a determination of resectability.
In these patients, adjacent vascular involvement or nodal
disease will determine if they are candidates for resection;
CT tends to be preferred in these patients. CT angiography (CTA) of the pancreas allows for more accurate and
rapid determination of local invasion than does MR. MR
may become the study of choice in a patient with renal
insufficiency in whom contrast-induced nephropathy is of
concern.

☐ Lesion characterization: Pancreatic lesions are often incidental findings on imaging studies performed for other indications. MRI may be useful in characterizing these lesions;
however, MRI may not be able to determine if a lesion is
neoplastic, thus endoscopic ultrasound with biopsy may be
required.

☐ Preoperative planning: In patients with known pancreatic malignancy who are scheduled for surgical resection,
MR may be performed to evaluate anatomy and vascular
involvement preoperatively. CTA of the pancreas, however,
is often the study of choice for this indication.

CONTRAINDICATIONS

☐ Patients with acute pancreatitis (as determined by laboratory values and clinical presentation) may not be optimally
evaluated with MR due to the active inflammation. It may be
difficult to differentiate between acute mass-like inflammation and a focal pancreatic mass. It may be more appropriate
to allow for subsidence of the acute event prior to imaging.

LIMITATIONS

☐ Patients unable to breath-hold or remain motionless during
the study will produce degraded images, thus decreasing
the quality of the study.

☐ As noted earlier, small pancreatic masses may be below
the resolution of MRI. Thus, in a patient with a high clinical suspicion of pancreatic malignancy, additional imaging
with contrast-enhanced CT (CECT) of the pancreas (pancreatic mass protocol CT) or endoscopic ultrasound may be
required.

☐ Due to the long imaging times and inability to image very
thin sections, CTA may be of greater usefulness than MR in
assessing resectability of the tumor.

☐ Pancreatic lesions may be difficult to characterize as malignant or benign based upon MRI findings. For example, intraductal papillary mucinous neoplasms may not be readily
separable from benign processes such as pancreatic pseudocysts based upon their MRI characteristics. ERCP may, thus,
be required in order to make the diagnosis (i.e. blue mucin
arising from the duct on ERCP).

☐ Preoperative planning for resection of pancreatic neoplasms
may be inadequate with MRI due to the spatial resolution;
CTA may be of more benefit for this purpose.

Body MRI

Body MRI

MR of the Adrenal Glands

■ The study may or may not require the administration of IV contrast.

■ It is often used to characterize adrenal masses identified on other imaging studies (typically CECT)

■ It may be used to identify suspected adrenal lesions (e.g. suspected pheochromocytomas).

■ The study is performed to evaluate the region of the adrenal glands only and thus does not evaluate the remaining solid organs of the abdomen. The relatively small area to be imaged allows for thinner imaging sections and thus higher spatial resolution of the area.

INDICATIONS

☐ Evaluation of adrenal masses incidentally identified at the time of imaging performed for an unrelated indication. This is the most common indication for dedicated adrenal imaging (i.e. the so-called adrenal incidentaloma). These are lesions often seen at the time of abdominal CT imaging that do not meet CT criteria for benign processes such as adrenal adenomas or myelolipomas. These patients are then referred for MR opposed-phase imaging in order to determine if the lesion represents an adenoma. The vast majority of these lesions can be characterized as adenomas without the administration of IV contrast. If the mass is not an adenoma, IV contrast may be administered in order to determine if the mass is a metastasis.

☐ Evaluation of suspected adrenal masses. In patients with symptoms suggestive of pheochromocytoma and elevated urinary catecholamines, MR of the adrenal glands may be performed in an attempt to identify a mass. If, however, the study is negative and there remains a high clinical suspicion for a pheochromocytoma, MRI of the abdomen/pelvis may be performed at another time to evaluate for possible masses along the sympathetic chain. Imaging of the neck may also be performed to evaluate for paragangliomas (extra-adrenal pheochromocytomas). Nuclear medicine imaging (MIBG) may be performed prior to imaging of the neck/chest/abdomen and pelvis as whole body imaging can be performed with a single injection of a radiotracer and may direct further MRI (see Chapter 11).

CONTRAINDICATIONS
- There is debate as to whether IV contrast material is contraindicated in patients with known or suspected pheochromocytomas. There is a theoretic risk of precipitating an adrenergic storm. It is advisable to discuss these patients with the local radiology department prior to performance of the study.

LIMITATIONS
- Motion and respiratory artifact will degrade image quality and may render the study uninterpretable.
- Patients who have undergone prior adrenal/upper abdominal surgery (e.g. contralateral adrenal mass resection) will suffer image degradation due to the presence of surgical clips. This may render the MRIs uninterpretable.

MR of the Kidneys

- It requires non-contrast and contrast-enhanced imaging.
- It requires the patient to breath-hold for 20–30 seconds.
- The study is often used to characterize lesions identified on other imaging studies (CT and ultrasound).
- MR has better contrast resolution than CT, thus MRI allows resolution of lesions that are too small to be evaluated on CT imaging.
- Multiplanar imaging capabilities of MR may be useful in evaluation of lesions.

INDICATIONS
- Characterization of lesions identified on alternate imaging modalities (e.g. CT or ultrasound). MR is the study of choice to evaluate cystic renal masses, which may represent cystic renal cell carcinoma.
- Follow-up of renal masses: Cystic renal lesions that are not clearly malignant but do not represent simple cysts (e.g. Bosniak IIF lesions) may be followed with MRI to assess for stability or progression to malignancy.
- Surveillance: In patients with prior partial or complete nephrectomy for renal cell carcinoma, MR may be performed to evaluate for lesion recurrence or synchronous lesions. MR is preferable to CT in these patients as their renal function is often compromised due to prior renal resection, thus MR contrast (gadolinium) is preferred to the more nephrotoxic CT contrast.

□ Staging: Patients with known or suspected renal cell carcinoma may be staged with contrast-enhanced MRI. This
is particularly important for evaluation of tumor extension
into the renal veins and inferior vena cava (IVC) as this
has obvious prognostic and surgical implications. MR has
the ability to evaluate vascular involvement and to determine if vascular thrombus is bland (i.e. clot only) or tumor
thrombus. It is also of paramount importance to evaluate
for involvement of the IVC and right atrium by thrombus
as this not only will change the patient's staging but also
will determine the surgical approach. If there is thrombus
within the IVC at or above the level of the hepatic veins,
a cardiothoracic surgeon must be part of the surgical team
in order to resect the thoracic extent of intravascular tumor
thrombus.

CONTRAINDICATIONS

□ Patients with renal compromise are at increased risk of
developing NSF following IV contrast administration. If a
patient has a low eGFR and cannot receive IV contrast, MR
is of limited use. IV contrast is often required for evaluation
of known or suspected renal masses.

LIMITATIONS

□ Respiratory and motion artifact will often degrade image
quality and render a study uninterpretable.

□ Surgical clips in patients with prior partial nephrectomy or
complete nephrectomy will produce artifacts, which may
degrade the image quality.

□ Small lesions may be below the resolution of MRI for identification and characterization.

□ MR may not be able to assess the urothelium and ureters for
synchronous or metachronous lesions. MR urography may
be helpful; however, it remains less useful than CT/CT-IVP
examinations.

MR Angiogram of the Renal Arteries

■ This is rapidly becoming a primary indication for MRI.
■ The most common indication is refractory hypertension.
■ It is performed without and with IV contrast.
■ It requires the patient to be able to breath-hold for 20–30 sec-
onds.

- MRA of the renal arteries is optimal for proximal and ostial lesions. It is less sensitive for distal arterial stenoses (i.e. in the distal branch vessels of the renal vasculature).

INDICATIONS
- ☐ Evaluation of patients with hypertension or renal insufficiency, which may be secondary to renovascular disease
- ☐ Follow-up of patients treated for renal artery stenosis (although this may be suboptimal if arterial stents have been placed)

CONTRAINDICATIONS
- ☐ Heavily calcified renal arteries: If it is known that the patient has densely calcified renal vessels, MRA may not be the optimal imaging study. Calcification may cause overestimation of stenosis due to the loss of signal caused by the calcium.
- ☐ Renal artery stents may render the study suboptimal or may overestimate the degree of stenosis. An alternate study such as CTA, ultrasound, or conventional catheter angiography may be more appropriate investigations for these patients.

LIMITATIONS
- ☐ Respiratory and motion artifact will often degrade image quality and render a study uninterpretable.
- ☐ Small accessory renal arteries may be out of the imaging plane or may be diminutive in size and thus not be recognized with MRA imaging. These small accessory vessels may be stenosed and thus may be symptomatic.
- ☐ Distal and branch vessels of the renal arteries may not be adequately evaluated with MRA due to the limitations of spatial resolution. Thus, stenosis in these vessels as a cause of symptoms may be overlooked.

MR of Cardiac Abnormalities

- Increasingly used to evaluate cardiac abnormalities, particularly myocardial ischemia and scar
- The study may be performed without IV contrast, although there are certain indications for the administration of IV contrast (including evaluation of cardiac masses, assessment of myocardial viability).
- It requires the patient to be in normal sinus rhythm as the study is performed with cardiac gating (i.e. the scanner is triggered

Body MRI

to start scanning based upon the cardiac tracing). Patients with arrhythmias are poor candidates for cardiac MRI as the scanner is inconsistently triggered to start scanning.

INDICATIONS

☐ Valvular: Echocardiography remains the gold standard for the evaluation of valvular cardiac disease (typically left heart valves). However, cardiac MR has emerged as a new modality to identify and quantify the amount of valvular disease present. There is good correlation of the quantification of disease with both modalities. Evaluation of valvular disease with MR is time-consuming and not routinely performed unless specifically requested. IV contrast is not administered for this indication.

☐ Vascular (pulmonary artery/aorta):
  • MR can evaluate the location of the main pulmonary artery and aorta and arterial-ventricular relationships in patients with suspected congenital cardiac anomalies. This does not require IV contrast administration.
  • Evaluation of the size of the main pulmonary artery and aorta may be performed in patients with suspected aneurysm. This may be performed without IV contrast; however, it is often performed as part of a contrast-enhanced examination.
  • Patients with suspected supra-cardiac congenital anomalies such as partial or total anomalous pulmonary venous return (PAPVR/TAPVR) are excellent candidates for evaluation with MRI. These patients require the administration of IV contrast material.

☐ Evaluation of intra- and extracardiac shunts including surgical shunts/baffles:
  • Patients with suspected congenital intracardiac or extracardiac shunts (e.g. persistent ductus arteriosis) may be non-invasively evaluated with MRI. IV contrast is not required for this study; however, it may be helpful in certain instances, which are often determined at the time of the study by the monitoring radiologist).
  • Patients with surgically placed conduits, baffles, and shunts may be monitored for stenosis and patency with MR. The degree of shunting can be assessed and monitored with MR. The study is often performed without and with IV contrast.

□ Intracardiac (e.g. congenital anomalies): Patients (particularly infants) with suspected congenital cardiac disease may be non-invasively evaluated with MRI. The study is typically performed without IV contrast unless there is a question of an associated supra-cardiac vascular anomaly.

□ Myocardial: This is one of the most important emerging applications for cardiac MRI. There are two main applications for myocardial imaging:

• Perfusion: This type of study is performed as a monitored examination since pharmacologic vasodilation (typically with adenosine) is performed. The study is performed as part of a complete cardiac imaging study. The perfusion portion of the examination allows for evaluation of myocardial blood flow. Areas with abnormal perfusion are interpreted as regions of ischemia.

• Diffusion (delayed myocardial enhancement): This type of study is performed in conjunction with a complete cardiac MR examination (often with perfusion). The study is performed following the administration of IV contrast such that approximately 8–10 minutes following contrast administration, images are obtained. Areas of myocardium that display areas of late (delayed) enhancement are considered abnormal and represent areas of myocardial scar. There is typically a corresponding perfusion abnormality with regions of abnormal myocardial contraction.

□ Epicardial (e.g. invasion): Mediastinal or pulmonary parenchymal disease such as primary bronchogenic carcinoma may extend into the epicardial region. MR may be performed to evaluate the extent of local invasion.

□ Pericardial:

• As noted earlier for epicardial disease, MR may be performed to evaluate for pericardial involvement by adjacent neoplastic or inflammatory disease. Malignant and benign pericardial effusions may also be identified.

• The primary role for MR in the evaluation of pericardial disease is to differentiate constrictive pericarditis from restrictive cardiomyopathy. Unlike restrictive cardiomyopathy, constrictive pericarditis is a treatable cause of heart failure. Constrictive pericarditis is well evaluated by MR such that even small focal areas of pericardial thickening can be identified and the diagnosis made. The study is performed as part of a complete cardiac examination as other causes of heart failure may be identified. Additionally, secondary signs of constrictive pericarditis such as interventricular septal wall motion abnormalities may be identified and further confirm the diagnosis.

CONTRAINDICATIONS

☐ Patients not in sinus rhythm are not good candidates for cardiac MR as ECG gating cannot be adequately performed, thus the scanner cannot be triggered to scan.

☐ Patients with ECG changes or recent acute MI are not candidates for stress perfusion imaging due to the risks of pharmacologic stress.

☐ Patients with pacemakers and AICDs are not candidates for MR examinations.

☐ There is debate as to whether implanted epicardial pacer leads are contraindicated for cardiac MR examinations due to the risk of heating during the study. This should be discussed with the radiologist prior to the examination.

LIMITATIONS

☐ Patient factors:

• Patients with large body habitus may not be evaluable with MRI.

• Patients who cannot comply with multiple, repeated breath holding imaging sequences are poor candidates for cardiac MRI. Due to the exquisite sensitivity to motion and respiratory artifact, patients must remain motionless and suspend respiration in order for adequate images to be obtained. However, some scanners are able to image patients who are not able to breath-hold for the examination. These cases should be discussed with the radiologist prior to the study.

• Patients with arrhythmias are poor candidates for cardiac MRI as the scanner is triggered to scan based upon the R-R interval. Newer MR scanners may allow for limited studies in patients who are not in sinus rhythm.

☐ Technical factors:

• Due to the mechanics of the MR scanner, the T wave may be enlarged and may mimic an R wave, thus inappropriately triggering the scan and producing significant artifacts.

MR of Vascular Structures

- It is performed without and with IV contrast.
- Patients must be clinically stable enough to undergo the examination (this is particularly important in patients with suspected aortic dissections).
- MR of the aorta is particularly useful in patients with suspected dissection who are unable to receive non-ionic IV contrast for CT imaging (based on poor renal function or documented contrast allergy).
- Peripheral vascular imaging:
  - It is often used to evaluate peripheral vessels of the lower extremities in patients unable to undergo conventional angiography.
  - It is performed without and with IV contrast.
  - It requires the patient to lie supine and immobile for extended periods of time (the examination can require up to an hour of imaging time per extremity).
  - Surgical clips can degrade the study. The artifact can be minimized by using different imaging techniques; however, it is helpful to be aware of the presence of clips prior to commencement of imaging.

INDICATIONS
- ☐ Arterial:
  - Evaluation of the presence and extent of aortic dissection in patients unable to undergo CECT imaging
  - Evaluation of suspected arteritis (e.g. Takayasu arteritis, which affects the large vessels, particularly the aorta and origins of the great vessels)
  - Evaluation of suspected arterial stenosis (e.g. subclavian steal phenomenon, mesenteric ischemia, renal artery stenosis)
  - Evaluation of peripheral vascular disease (e.g. lower extremity claudication)
- ☐ Venous:
  - Evaluation of suspected DVT or thrombosis of the IVC and pelvic vessels in patients with negative or suboptimal lower extremity DVT ultrasound studies
  - Evaluation of suspected upper extremity or SVC thrombosis
  - Evaluation of the presence and extent of tumor thrombus (e.g. into the renal veins/IVC in patients with renal cell

Body MRI

carcinoma, portal vein thrombus in patients with hepatocellular carcinoma)

CONTRAINDICATIONS

☐ Patients who cannot receive IV contrast are not candidates for MRA.

☐ Patients who cannot remain immobile are not candidates for the examination as it is essential that the patient be in exactly the same position for multiple image acquisitions in order to obtain diagnostic information.

☐ Patients who are unstable should not be placed in the magnet.

LIMITATIONS

☐ Patient factors:

- Patients unable to remain motionless are poor candidates for the examination as motion artifact significantly degrades the images and can simulate or obscure areas of stenosis.

- Patients unable to breath-hold are poor candidates for studies such as evaluation of mesenteric or renal artery stenosis as respiratory motion may mask areas of stenosis.

- Patients in whom a large bore IV cannot be placed are not eligible for contrast administration by power injector. These patients are administered the contrast by hand injection, thus a tight bolus of contrast cannot be obtained and suboptimal imaging often occurs.

- Patients with IVC filters, renal artery stents, arterial stents, or metallic surgical clips are suboptimal candidates for MRA as these devices cause significant artifact and areas of disease may be obscured.

■ Technical factors: Older MR scanners may not be able to adequately image the entire vascular system (e.g. for evaluation of the aortopopliteal system as the images cannot be acquired rapidly enough to prevent venous contamination). This renders areas of arterial disease difficult to identify.

MR of the Pelvis (for Gynecology/Obstetrics)

■ It may be performed with or without IV contrast dependent upon the study indication.

■ Patients may not eat 4–6 hours prior to the examination, and caffeine must be avoided for 24 hours (to decrease bowel peristalsis and thus decrease artifacts).

INDICATIONS

- ☐ Fibroids: MR is exquisitely sensitive for the identification and characterization of uterine fibroids. It is particularly useful when ultrasound is equivocal or cannot differentiate between a pedunculated fibroid and a pelvic mass.
  - If identification of fibroids is the clinical question, IV contrast is not required.
  - If the patient is a candidate for or has previously undergone percutaneous uterine fibroid embolization, IV contrast is administered as enhancement is an indicator that the procedure will likely be successful.
  - MR is the study of choice for the identification of adenomyosis.
- ☐ Uterine anomalies: In the evaluation of infertility or recurrent pregnancy loss, MR may be definitive for the identification and characterization of congenital uterine anomalies. Limited renal imaging should be performed at the same time due to the associations of renal and genitourinary anomalies.
- ☐ Endometrium: MR is NOT useful to evaluate endometrial abnormalities (e.g. polyps); however, it is sensitive for the local staging of known endometrial or cervical carcinoma. IV contrast is required for this study.
- ☐ Ovarian: MR is very useful to evaluate known or suspected ovarian pathology.
  - This is particularly true for known or suspected endometriosis. IV contrast is NOT required for the imaging of endometriosis.
  - MR is a valuable study for ovarian masses that do not demonstrate characteristics of endometriosis. A diagnosis may be suggested or confirmed with MR. IV contrast may be required, depending upon the imaging appearance of the ovarian mass; however, this is often not predictable until the study is performed. Therefore, it is suggested that the study be requested WITH IV contrast. If it is not required, it will not be administered.
  - Placenta: MR is useful for the evaluation of suspected placental abnormalities (i.e. placenta accreta, percreta, and increta). IV contrast is not required for the study.
- ☐ Appendicitis in pregnancy: MR may be performed for the identification of suspected appendicitis in pregnancy if ultrasound is unsuccessful.

☐ Fetal MR: This is an emerging indication for MRI. Currently, the main indication is for the evaluation of CNS abnormalities identified or suspected on ultrasound. If there is concern for other fetal abnormalities, discuss the case with the radiologist to determine if MR may be useful to answer the clinical question.

CONTRAINDICATIONS

☐ IV contrast should not be administered in pregnancy as the risk to the fetus is unknown.

LIMITATIONS

☐ Endometrial disease is not well evaluated with MRI, with the exception of evaluation of the extent of disease in patients with endometrial carcinoma.

☐ Placental disease (i.e. acreta, percreta, increta) may be difficult to identify and characterize.

☐ Appendicitis: The appendix is not always readily identifiable, thus, a diagnosis of appendicitis may not always be possible.

☐ Small peritoneal implants of endometriosis are often below the resolution of MR and may not be identified.

MR of the Breast

■ This is an emerging use of MRI.

■ Depending upon the type of scanner, it may be possible to evaluate only one breast during a session, although this is becoming less common as technology evolves.

■ It is NOT routinely performed as a screening study for breast carcinoma unless the patient is high risk and/or has contralateral breast carcinoma.

INDICATIONS

☐ Implant rupture: MR is only performed for silicone or silicone/saline hybrids. (Saline-only implants deflate! Thus, rupture can be determined clinically.) No IV contrast is required.

☐ Tumor staging/extent: For patients with known breast carcinoma, MR is exquisitely sensitive for evaluation of the extent of tumor. MR is particularly valuable to interrogate potential chest wall involvement. IV contrast is required.

☐ Problem-solving: In patients with indeterminate mammographic findings, MR may be a useful adjuvant for lesion characterization or evaluation. The study must be interpreted in conjunction with the mammogram. IV contrast is required for the study.

☐ Screening: MR screening for breast carcinoma is controversial. As noted earlier, it may be considered in patients at high risk or with contralateral breast carcinoma. Patients with dense breasts in whom the sensitivity of lesion detection with mammography is lower may also be candidates for MR screening.

CONTRAINDICATIONS

☐ Patients who are recently postoperative may experience discomfort from the prone positioning and coils needed for the study. These patients may be poor candidates for the study in the perioperative period.

LIMITATIONS

☐ Motion artifact can significantly degrade images and may mask small lesions.

☐ MR is a sensitive modality to identify lesions. However, MR is not specific to characterize lesions. This may lead to unnecessary biopsies and follow-up examinations.

MR of the Prostate

▪ MR is increasingly being used for the evaluation of patients with elevated prostate-specific antigen levels and biopsies positive for prostate cancer.

▪ Patients are often diagnosed based on ultrasound-guided sextan biopsies; however, no good imaging modality exists to localize the primary tumor and to evaluate the extent of local disease.

▪ Prognosis and therapy are dependent upon local staging of the tumor, mainly if there is extracapsular extension of tumor. MR is increasingly being used for this purpose.

▪ MRI of the prostate may be performed with externally positioned surface coils or with endorectal coil placement. For an endorectal coil, a digital rectal examination is first performed to determine if there are contraindications to coil placement. If there are no contraindications, the coil is placed into the rectum and a balloon inflated to maintain its positioning.

▪ IV contrast is required for the examination.

INDICATIONS

☐ Identification of the primary malignancy

☐ Determination of spread of tumor, particularly extracapsular spread of tumor

CONTRAINDICATIONS

☐ It is recommended that a patient who has undergone biopsy not be imaged within 3–4 weeks in order to allow adequate time for the blood produced by the biopsy to resorb.

☐ Patients who have a contraindication to endorectal coil placement should not be imaged with the coil; surface coil imaging should be performed in these patients.

LIMITATIONS

☐ MR is not sensitive for the detection of the primary tumor and its extension. This leads to false-negative results.

☐ Residual blood from a biopsy may complicate interpretation.

☐ Poor coil contact may limit imaging.

Neuroradiology

Conventional Radiographs

- Conventional radiographs have little role in current modern-day neuroimaging.
- Skull radiographs are often obtained with chest and abdominal radiographs as part of a shunt series to evaluate for possible shunt disruption as an etiology for shunt dysfunction.
- Orbital films are obtained in all patients with a history of prior metal exposure (e.g. welding) prior to MRI. Orbital metal may move during MRI, causing ocular damage.
- In the past, conventional radiographic series (i.e. multiple films of the same region in different orientations) were acquired for imaging of the paranasal sinuses, orbits, facial bones, nasal bone, and mandible. There are a few considerations to be made prior to ordering these films:
  - There are few, if any, indications for nasal bone films. Treatment will not be altered based upon radiographic evidence of a fracture. The only alteration that will occur to treatment is if there is a submucosal hematoma, which can cause necrosis of the nasal septum. However, this is a *clinical* diagnosis, not a radiologic diagnosis.
  - Many films are required to evaluate the bones of the head and face, with relatively low sensitivity. CT has a comparable radiation dose with a significantly higher sensitivity. If these regions require evaluation, CT is the superior method for evaluation.

Non-Contrast CT of the Brain

■ This is the initial imaging study for evaluation of acute neurological abnormality. It is a readily available modality with rapid image acquisition (on the order of 15–30 seconds of scan time). It is the study of choice for identification of subarachnoid, subdural/epidural, and parenchymal hemorrhage. Early ischemic events (stroke) may not be detected with CT.

■ Routine imaging for acute events or trauma does not require the administration of IV contrast.

■ The lens is the most radiation-sensitive cranial structure; cataract formation is a well-recognized complication of cranial CT. Efforts should be made to minimize the necessity for repeat CT examinations. Extrinsic shields also are available for orbital protection from the radiation; efforts should be made to use these shields if they are available.

INDICATIONS

□ Evaluation of acute stroke

□ Evaluation of acute change in mental status

□ Evaluation for intraparenchymal hemorrhage, subarachnoid hemorrhage (SAH), and epidural or subdural hemorrhage

□ Evaluation of traumatic injury

□ It is commonly used in the evaluation of new or increased frequency of seizures; however, non-contrast CT is of low yield and MRI is the study of choice

□ Identification of hydrocephalus or cerebral edema, both of which would preclude spinal tap (lumbar puncture)

CONTRAINDICATIONS

□ Patients who are actively seizing should be stabilized prior to the examination, if possible.

□ There is an increased risk of cataract formation from the radiation used for the CT examination. The necessity and benefits of the CT should be carefully weighed against the risks of the radiation exposure before the scan is performed. Patients with a history of seizure or headache with multiple prior studies may not require a CT examination, thus decreasing the risk of radiation exposure.

LIMITATIONS

□ Patient motion may produce significant artifacts, thus decreasing sensitivity for abnormalities.

Neuroradiology

☐ Dense vessels may mimic areas of pathology (i.e. intracranial hemorrhage). This is particularly true in children and patients with hyperviscosity syndromes such as polycythemia vera as the increased iron content of the blood renders intravascular blood more dense on CT.

☐ Patients with prior surgical or endovascular treatments for processes such as aneurysm repair may have suboptimal examinations due to the significant streak artifact related to the clips.

☐ Early ischemia (infarcts) may not be visible on CT. Areas of infarction are often not visible on CT for 12–24 hours after the onset of symptoms. The major role that CT plays in patients with clinical symptoms of acute stroke is to exclude intracranial hemorrhage, which would contraindicate antithrombolytic therapy.

☐ Patient motion may limit the examination as small lesions may not be well visualized through the artifact.

☐ Artifacts related to patient apparel (e.g. earrings, hairpins) may cause significant artifact, thus limiting evaluation of adjacent areas of the brain.

☐ For patients with seizures, MR is the imaging modality of choice as subtle lesions (e.g. heterotopic gray matter) are not detectable on CT.

☐ Masses within the brain may not be identifiable on noncontrast CT imaging unless there is associated edema or mass effect. If there is concern for the presence of a mass, contrast-enhanced CT or MR is recommended.

Contrast-Enhanced CT of the Brain

▪ The study is performed following the administration of IV contrast.

▪ IV contrast is not administered for routine cases; the majority of brain CT examinations are performed as non-contrast examinations. In general, contrast-enhanced CT of the brain is performed following a non-contrast examination.

▪ Lesions such as intracranial metastases, primary neoplasms, and infections often are not detected on non-contrast imaging. These lesions are often recognized due to their enhancement properties with or without surrounding parenchymal edema.

■ Meningitis is NOT routinely detected with contrast-enhanced imaging. Although meningeal enhancement may be seen, it is not sensitive or specific for the identification of meningeal disease. In cases of suspected meningeal irritation (i.e. meningitis), CT typically is performed as a non-contrast examination to exclude contraindications to lumbar puncture (e.g. brain herniation).

INDICATIONS

☐ Evaluation of intracranial masses and suspected or known metastatic lesions

☐ Evaluation of suspected intracranial infection

☐ Contrast administration may be useful to confirm the presence of isodense subdural hematomas as they displace vessels away from the calvarium. However, MR is a more sensitive modality for the identification of these subdural hematomas.

☐ Contrast-enhanced CT may demonstrate meningeal enhancement in patients with meningitis, particularly tuberculous or fungal.

CONTRAINDICATIONS

☐ IV contrast allergy

☐ Elevated creatinine (Cr)

☐ Acute trauma. IV contrast may mask or mimic SAH. If SAH is suspected, IV contrast should not be administered before a head CT is performed. This includes contrast-enhanced CT of the neck, chest, abdomen, or pelvis. If IV contrast is administered, it will take at least 6 hours to clear the contrast from the subarachnoid space.

LIMITATIONS

☐ Patient motion may limit the examination as small lesions may not be well visualized through the artifact.

☐ Artifacts related to patient apparel (e.g. earrings, hairpins) may cause significant artifact, thus limiting evaluation of adjacent areas of the brain.

☐ Hemorrhagic masses that have acutely bled may not be readily identifiable as solid/cystic masses due to the presence of blood products. Subacute imaging following evolution of the hemorrhage or MRI may prove more diagnostic.

☐ Meningeal processes (e.g. infection) may not be detected with contrast-enhanced CT imaging. In cases of fungal or tuberculous meningitis, thick meningeal enhancement may be identified.

☐ Contrast should not be administered to patients in whom SAH is suspected as contrast within vessels may mimic or mask the hemorrhage. Similarly, as contrast may circulate within the intracranial vasculature for several hours after administration, patients with SAH should not be imaged for several hours after contrast administration for any imaging study.

CT Angiography of the Neck and Circle of Willis

▨ The study is performed with a timed bolus of IV contrast.

▨ The area of interest (i.e. carotid arteries or circle of Willis) must be defined prior to commencement of the examination as the images are acquired differently for the two examinations. Although it is possible to evaluate both the carotid arteries and circle of Willis with the same contrast bolus, dedicated imaging of each area is recommended to optimize image quality. This is particularly true if an older CT scanner is used (i.e. single-slice scanner).

▨ A large bore IV is required (≥20 gauge as a rapid contrast infusion is required for the examination).

▨ A non-contrast CT of the brain may or may not be performed prior to the CT angiography (CTA) depending upon the institutional protocol. In the acute setting, a preceding CT may have been performed. demonstrating the acute abnormality (i.e. SAH). In this case, if the non-contrast CT was obtained within a few hours of the CTA, a repeat non-contrast CT may not be required, thus limiting the radiation dose to the patient.

INDICATIONS

☐ Carotid CTA (CTA neck):
  • Evaluation of carotid injury following trauma (e.g. penetrating injury, seatbelt injury, vertebral artery injury in the presence of a cervical vertebral fracture)
  • Evaluation of carotid stenosis
  • Follow-up of carotid dissection or stenosis

☐ CTA of the circle of Willis:
  • Evaluation of patients with suspected aneurysm (e.g. acute SAH in the absence of trauma). CTA is becoming

the study of choice in these patients due to its high sensitivity and non-invasive nature.

- Follow-up of known aneurysm. In some patients who are poor treatment risks, CTA may be performed to evaluate for interval growth of a previously demonstrated aneurysm.
- Evaluation of known or suspected vascular malformation (e.g. arteriovenous malformation)
- Preoperative planning. In patients with known vascular abnormalities (e.g. aneurysm or arteriovenous malformations), CTA may be performed prior to surgery or endovascular therapy (e.g. coiling, glue).
- Postoperative evaluation. In patients treated for intracranial vascular abnormality, a postprocedural CTA may be performed to evaluate for the efficacy of treatment. Surveillance over the longer term may also be performed with CTA in order to avoid more invasive procedures (i.e. angiography).

CONTRAINDICATIONS

☐ IV contrast allergy

☐ Elevated Cr

LIMITATIONS

☐ CTA of the neck:
  - Motion may produce artifacts, which can obscure disease or mimic areas of stenosis.
  - Metallic objects within the neck (e.g. bullet fragments, surgical clips) may render portions of the vessel uninterpretable due to streak artifact.
  - Heavily calcified plaque may lead to overestimation of carotid stenosis due to "blooming" of the calcification. This artifact may be less problematic with 64-slice CT scanners.
  - Poor timing of the contrast bolus may lead to a poor study in which areas of disease may not be identified; this is more problematic on CT scanners with less detectors (e.g. 4-slice or 8-slice scanners).

☐ CTA of the Circle of Willis:
  - Motion may produce artifacts, which can obscure disease or mimic areas of stenosis.
  - Metallic objects within the cranium (e.g. clips or coils from prior vascular abnormality treatment) may render portions of the vessel uninterpretable due to artifact.

- Poor timing of the contrast bolus may lead to a poor study in which areas of disease may not be identified; this is more problematic on CT scanners with less detectors (e.g. 4-slice or 8-slice scanners).
- Difference in imaging slices or patient positioning may make direct comparison of aneurysm size and shape difficult or suboptimal.

CT of the Sinus

▨ The study is performed to evaluate acute and chronic sinus disease.

▨ The examination is typically performed without IV contrast unless there is a suspicion of fungal sinusitis or intracranial spread of infection.

▨ Routine sinus imaging includes ONLY imaging of the sinuses and does NOT image the entire cranium unless specifically requested.

▨ There is a significant radiation dose involved with CT of the sinuses, particularly to the lens. Therefore, if sinusitis can be diagnosed on clinical grounds, which it generally can, CT should be avoided unless there is concern about complications of sinusitis. In cases of complications of sinusitis, IV contrast is typically necessary in order to evaluate for ascending infection causing an intracranial epidural abscess.

INDICATIONS
- ☐ Evaluation of acute or chronic sinus disease
- ☐ Preoperative planning for sinus surgery
- ☐ Evaluation of the postsurgical sinus
- ☐ Contrast-enhanced CT of the sinuses is performed if there is suspicion of invasive sinusitis (e.g. mucormycosis or aspergillus in immunosuppressed patients).
- ☐ Contrast-enhanced CT of the sinuses and brain are performed if there is concern that the sinus infection has extended into the epidural space of the brain.

CONTRAINDICATIONS
- ☐ Radiation exposure should be avoided if possible.

LIMITATIONS
- ☐ Patients who have undergone multiple surgeries may have distorted anatomy, which may render interpretation of acute abnormalities difficult, particularly if prior images and studies are not available for comparison.

□ Patients who cannot be appropriately positioned (e.g. with the head hanging over the gantry) may be difficult to image adequately as direct coronal imaging cannot be performed, thus, evaluation of the ostiomeatal units may not be possible.

□ In the postoperative patient, it may be difficult to differentiate surgical changes from recurrent sinusitis. Comparison studies are highly useful in the interpretation of the postoperative sinus as it allows for more accurate depiction of residual/recurrent disease as opposed to postoperative change.

CT of the Facial Bones

■ The study is performed as a non-contrast examination for routine imaging.

■ The examination evaluates the osseous structures of the face including the mandible and orbits. With multidetector CT, images are acquired in the axial plane and the data is reformatted into sagittal and coronal planes.

INDICATIONS

□ Non-contrast images are most commonly obtained for the evaluation of acute facial trauma.

□ Contrast-enhanced images may be obtained to evaluate for possible sites of infection and drainable abscess collections.

CONTRAINDICATIONS

□ IV contrast allergy

□ Elevated Cr

LIMITATIONS

□ Motion artifact will significantly degrade image quality and may obscure or mimic sites of disease.

□ Metallic artifacts (e.g. metallic teeth fillings, tongue piercings, prior fracture fixation hardware) will cause significant artifact and may obscure disease.

CT of the Orbits

■ The study may be obtained without or with IV contrast, depending upon the indication.

■ The study provides dedicated imaging of the orbits only; it does NOT evaluate the entire face.

▪ Images are obtained in the axial plane. With multirow detector CT, the data are reformatted into sagittal and coronal images.

INDICATIONS

☐ Non-contrast CT of the orbits:
  • This study is routinely performed for the evaluation of direct orbital trauma. Coronal reformatted images are of particular value in the assessment of orbital floor injury and possible muscle entrapment. The study does not evaluate the remainder of the facial bones; if there is concern for a second site of injury, a non-contrast CT of the facial bones should be obtained.

☐ Contrast-enhanced CT of the orbits:
  • Evaluation of ocular muscular abnormalities such as orbital pseudotumor and thyroid ophthalmopathy
  • Evaluation of orbital or facial cellulitis to look for the presence and extension of abscess
  • Evaluation of known or suspected orbital or ocular masses (e.g. retinoblastoma, melanoma metastases)

CONTRAINDICATIONS

☐ IV contrast allergy
☐ Elevated Cr

LIMITATIONS

☐ Motion artifact will significantly degrade the images; this is of particular importance in the identification of orbital trauma (fractures) as a fracture may be obscured by motion or false-positive results may be obtained.

☐ Patient positioning. If patients are obliquely positioned within the CT gantry, sites of disease may be obscured.

☐ Metallic foreign bodies (e.g. bullet fragments) may produce artifact, which can render the study uninterpretable.

☐ It may be difficult to differentiate between a phlegmon and a mature walled off orbital abscess.

CT of the Petrous/Temporal Bone

▪ The study may be performed without or with IV contrast, depending upon the indication for the examination.

▪ There are highly specific indications to evaluate pathology of the temporal bone, vestibular system, middle and inner ear.

■ Imaging is performed in thin section axial and coronal projections of the petrous apex only. This specific study does NOT image the entire brain.

■ If the clinical indication is infection or cholesteotoma, particularly mastoiditis, the study requires the administration of IV contrast. For all other indications (e.g. evaluation of the ossicles, inner ear anatomy, fractures), IV contrast is not required.

INDICATIONS

☐ Non-contrast:
  • Evaluation of petrous bone fracture
  • Evaluation of hearing loss (i.e. evaluation for otosclerosis)
  • Preprocedure planning for cochlear implants

☐ Contrast enhanced:
  • Evaluation of cholesteotoma
  • Evaluation of masses
  • Evaluation of infection

CONTRAINDICATIONS

☐ IV contrast allergy
☐ Elevated Cr

LIMITATIONS

☐ Due to the small size of the structures of the petrous bone (e.g. ossicles), volume averaging with adjacent structures may limit evaluation.
☐ Motion artifact can limit the examination.
☐ Fractures may be in the plane of the scan, thus may not be easily evaluated; this is typically not a significant limitation as the images are reconstructed into different planes, thus the fracture line often becomes evident.

CT of the Neck

■ The study may be performed with or without IV contrast. Contrast-enhanced CT is preferable because it increases conspicuity of lymph nodes and areas of pathology.

■ The study differs from CTA in several ways. CTA requires a timed bolus of IV contrast to be administered followed by scanning at a specific timed delay. Routine contrast-enhanced CT of the neck does not require contrast bolus timing; a scan is usually performed a few minutes after the contrast is administered. CTA is also performed as thin section axial images, which are then reformatted into different planes; CT of the neck is performed in 3–5 mm sections and usually is not reformatted into different imaging planes.

INDICATIONS

☐ Evaluation of possible infectious processes such as retropharyngeal abscess

☐ Evaluation of palpable abnormalities (e.g. extent of multinodular goiters, branchial cleft cysts, thyroglossal duct cysts). Ultrasound may be useful for the evaluation of palpable abnormalities; however, CT allows for better characterization of the anatomic relationship of the abnormality to adjacent structures, which may allow for a definitive diagnosis. Retrosternal masses cannot be adequately evaluated with ultrasound as the sternum reflects the ultrasound beam; thus, they cannot be evaluated. CT is the study of choice for these lesions.

☐ Evaluation of suspected masses such as paragangliomas. Primary head and neck neoplasms are often occult on imaging; however, associated lymphadenopathy may be identified.

☐ Evaluation of lymphadenopathy (e.g. melanoma, lymphoma)

CONTRAINDICATIONS

☐ IV contrast allergy

☐ Elevated Cr

LIMITATIONS

☐ Metallic artifact related to dental repair (e.g. fillings, bridges) or piercings will cause significant artifact, thus limiting evaluation.

☐ Motion artifact may obscure or mimic disease.

☐ Patients who lack fat may be difficult to evaluate for lymphadenopathy due to lack of soft tissue contrast.

☐ Head and neck cancers may be radiologically occult. Patients who have undergone prior resection with reconstruction (e.g. free fibular flaps) may have radiologically occult recurrence; direct comparison with prior studies is essential to evaluate for recurrence as it allows for detection of change in the appearance of the surgical site.

CT of the Cervical Spine

▪ The study is performed as a routine without IV contrast. It may be combined with CTA of the neck/carotid arteries in the setting

Neuroradiology

of acute trauma. The study is performed with IV contrast as a CTA of the carotid arteries, and the data are reformatted into thicker axial images in a bone window for evaluation of the cervical spine.

■ It is typically performed in the setting of acute trauma or to evaluate for cervical disc disease.

■ The study is performed as direct axial images with reformatted images provided in the sagittal and coronal planes.

■ It requires patient cooperation as motion artifact can render a study non-diagnostic, particularly in the setting of subtle fractures.

■ Cervical spine CT may be performed with IV contrast in a very specific setting, that is, the evaluation of infection. CT with IV contrast is helpful in the evaluation of epidural abscess formation or soft tissue collections, particularly in postoperative patients. MR, however, is more sensitive for the evaluation of small epidural collections and is the study of choice for the evaluation of osteomyelitis/discitis.

INDICATIONS
☐ Non-contrast cervical spine CT:
  • Evaluation of traumatic injury: The study may be performed in the acute setting to evaluate for acute fracture, disc herniation, or epidural hematoma. The study does NOT evaluate for ligamentous injury.
  • Follow-up of known cervical spine fracture: This allows for assessment of the degree of healing and allows assessment of changes in alignment of fracture fragments, which may require further surgical intervention or external fixation.
  • Evaluation of cervical disc disease or osteoarthritic change as a source of neck pain
  • Evaluation of known or suspected congenital bony anomalies of the cervical spine
  • Evaluation of known or suspected bone lesions (e.g. aneurysmal bone cyst, lymphoma)
☐ Contrast-enhanced CT of the cervical spine:
  • Evaluation of discitis/osteomyelitis
  • Evaluation of epidural abscess

CONTRAINDICATIONS
☐ IV contrast allergy
☐ Elevated Cr

LIMITATIONS

☐ Non-contrast CT of the cervical spine:
   - Motion artifact can significantly degrade images and may obscure subtle fractures or produce artifacts that mimic fracture.
   - Streak artifact related to patient jewelry or cervical spine collars may degrade images.
   - In patients with prior surgical fixation, artifact related to the metal hardware may render images uninterpretable.
   - Patients poorly positioned within the CT gantry may be difficult to evaluate as the vertebrae may not appear aligned; this is particularly difficult in older patients with a significant kyphosis who cannot be laid flat for the study.
   - Ligaments and muscles are not well delineated on CT, thus ligamentous injury cannot be assessed. MR is the study of choice to evaluate ligamentous injury.
   - CT is insensitive for evaluation of the spinal cord; MR is the study of choice for the evaluation of spinal cord injury.

☐ Contrast-enhanced CT of the cervical spine:
   - In patients with surgical hardware, artifact related to the hardware may render the study uninterpretable.
   - Early changes of discitis/osteomyelitis may be occult on CT; MR is a more sensitive study for the early detection of these entities.

CT of the Thoracic/Lumbar Spine

▥ It is performed as a routine without IV contrast.

▥ It may be performed in the setting of acute trauma or to evaluate for disc disease.

▥ It is performed as direct axial images with reformatted images provided in the sagittal and coronal planes.

▥ It requires patient cooperation as motion artifact can render a study non-diagnostic, particularly in the setting of subtle fractures.

▥ Reconstructed images of the thoracic and lumbar spine (sagittal and coronal images) may be obtained in the trauma setting from data obtained of the chest, abdomen, and pelvis. The data are reconstructed into thinner slices, and the reformats are performed.

■ There is a high radiation dose involved in scanning the entire spine; effort should be made to localize the level of concern so that only that limited area may be scanned.

■ Thoracic/lumbar spine CT may be performed with IV contrast in a very specific setting, that is, the evaluation of infection. CT with IV contrast is helpful in the evaluation of epidural abscess formation or soft tissue collections, particularly in postoperative patients. MR, however, is more sensitive for the evaluation of small epidural collections and is the study of choice for the evaluation of osteomyelitis/discitis.

INDICATIONS

☐ Non-contrast:
  • Evaluation of acute traumatic injury
  • Evaluation of disc disease in the setting of radiculopathy
  • Evaluation of suspected or known bony masses (e.g. enchondroma, giant cell tumor, chondroblastoma). CT allows for evaluation of the extent of the tumor as well as characterization of the location and matrix, which may allow for the diagnosis to be made.

☐ Contrast enhanced:
  • Evaluation of infection (osteomyelitis)
  • Evaluation of suspected tumors involving the paraspinal soft tissues, nerve roots, or spinal cord

CONTRAINDICATIONS

☐ IV contrast allergy
☐ Elevated Cr

LIMITATIONS

☐ Motion artifact can significantly degrade the images.
☐ Metallic hardware such as spinal fusion rods and surgical clips can produce streak artifact and limit evaluation of adjacent structures.
☐ Unlike MRI, CT cannot evaluate for the presence of edema in the muscles, nerve roots, or spinal cord, which may occur due to compression of the nerves in trauma or disc disease. MR is the imaging study of choice for these patients.
☐ CT has poor contrast resolution compared to MR; therefore, CT is not adequate to evaluate for the presence of ligamentous or muscle injury in the setting of infection.
☐ CT cannot evaluate for edema in or replacement of the bone marrow in processes such as osteomyelitis or metastatic

disease; therefore, changes of osteomyelitis or tumor may not become apparent until late in the disease. MR is the study of choice for these indications.

MRI of the Central Nervous System

General Considerations

■ There are a number of significant advantages/disadvantages of MR versus CT.

  □ Advantages:
  • Absence of ionizing radiation
  • Gadolinium (the MR contrast agent) is significantly less nephrotoxic than CT contrast agents (both ionic and non-ionic contrast). Nevertheless, nephrotoxic effects have been reported with gadolinium.
  • Better soft tissue resolution than CT

  □ Disadvantages:
  • Length of study: MR examinations can require a minimum of 20 minutes to several hours of imaging time, whereas CT often requires less than 2–5 minutes (particularly in the era of multislice scanners).
  • Due to the configuration of the magnet, patients with claustrophobia may be unable to complete the examination. The majority of radiology departments do not have the staff or medications available to be able to medicate patients prior to an MR examination. Therefore, it is recommended that patients with known claustrophobia be provided sedatives/anxiolytics by their primary caregivers. These should be made available to patients prior to the date of their examination. If patients will require conscious sedation for their examination, this should be made known to schedulers at the time of the study request so that this may be arranged.
  • Patients unable to lie completely supine are difficult to image.
  • Patients with respiratory compromise may not be able to tolerate supine positioning. Patients with an inability to breath-hold may be unable to comply with key sequences, which may result in suboptimal or uninterpretable studies.
  • There are a number of contraindications to MRI, which will be detailed in the following section.

Contraindications to MRI

ABSOLUTE CONTRAINDICATIONS

- ☐ Cardiac valves (typically St. Jude valves)
- ☐ Metallic foreign bodies within the orbits (patients with exposure history should be screened for metal with orbital radiographs prior to the MR examination)
- ☐ Patients with ferromagnetic surgical clips (e.g. cerebral aneurysm clips)
- ☐ Patients with pacemakers or automatic implantable cardioverter defibrillators cannot be imaged with MR due to the effect of the magnetic field upon the devices.

Relative Contraindications to MRI

- ▪ Recently placed cardiac stents (within 1–2 days)
- ▪ Obesity: The majority of MR scanners have a table limit of 350 lbs. Patients exceeding this limit cannot be imaged on conventional MR scanners.
- ▪ Claustrophobia: Many patients are unable to tolerate a complete MR examination based on claustrophobia. If there is a preexisting history of claustrophobia, the patient may be booked for the examination with sedation or may require anesthesia if sedation is inadequate to allow completion of the study.
- ▪ Inability to lie supine: Patients who are unable to lie completely flat are often poor candidates for MRI. Images may be suboptimal due to patient positioning. Additionally, if patients are unable to be appropriately positioned based upon respiratory compromise when in a supine position, they often are unable to tolerate the examination. MRI of solid organs such as the liver and kidneys often requires patients to breath-hold for 20–30 seconds. If patients are unable to do so, the images may be degraded to the degree of being uninterpretable.

MRI of the Brain

- ▪ It may be performed as a contrast-enhanced or non-contrast study, depending upon the indication for the examination. Due to increasingly stringent insurance precertification requirements, it is essential to be aware of the type of study being requested prior to scheduling so that examination cancellation due to billing errors does not occur. If a question arises as to whether or not IV contrast may be required, it is

Neuroradiology

advisable to contact the imaging center prior to scheduling so that the appropriate examination may be scheduled and conducted.

Non-Contrast MRI of the Brain

▨ It is performed as a routine without IV contrast unless an abnormality requiring contrast administration is identified while the examination is in progress.

▨ All non-contrast examinations may be ordered in the same manner, regardless of the indication (including evaluation of seizures).

▨ The protocol prescribed by the radiologist will depend upon the indication for the examination. For the most part, routine sequences are performed for all of the indications listed earlier, with the exception of patients with seizures. In these patients, high-resolution images are obtained with a surface coil.

INDICATIONS

☐ Evaluation of headaches (in children and adults)

☐ Evaluation of patients with a history of trauma. MR is NOT indicated in the evaluation of patients with suspected SAH, as it is often not detectable with MRI unless it is recurrent, chronic, or long-standing. MRI may be helpful in dating the age of subdural/epidural hemorrhage, although this is less clear-cut than dating parenchymal hemorrhage. The main advantage of MRI in sub/epidural collections is determination of acute or chronic hemorrhage, which may be of value in suspected non-accidental trauma in children.

☐ Follow-up of ventricular size in patients with known hydrocephalus

☐ Evaluation of patients with seizures

☐ Evaluation of patients with known or suspected cerebrovascular accident

CONTRAINDICATIONS

☐ Patients who are actively seizing should not be placed in the magnet due to the inability to fully monitor the patient's clinical status.

☐ General contraindications for MRI

LIMITATIONS

☐ Areas of abnormal diffusion will normalize over time, thus yielding false negatives for areas of subacute ischemia.

□ Small or subtle masses or areas of infection may not be identifiable on non-contrast imaging unless there is surrounding
parenchymal edema; IV contrast should be administered if
there is concern for intracranial infection or mass.

□ Small areas such as the internal auditory canal or pituitary
are not adequately imaged with routine brain protocols; if
there is concern for pathology in these regions, dedicated
imaging should be performed.

□ If patients are unable to hold still, imaging may be uninterpretable. Unlike CT imaging where only a portion of the
study is affected if a patient moves, in MRI, patient motion
for even a portion of the image acquisition will affect the
whole sequence. This is due to the manner in which data
are acquired and processed in MRI.

□ Small lesions may be below the resolution of MRI.

□ It may be difficult to differentiate between infection and
tumor.

Contrast-Enhanced MR of the Brain

■ It is performed as routine non-contrast images followed by
contrast-enhanced images.

■ Although non-contrast images are obtained in addition to
contrast-enhanced images, the study is ordered as a contrast-
enhanced MR of the brain (not as a without/with contrast
study).

■ The study requires a durable IV.

INDICATIONS

□ Evaluation of patients with altered mental status to evaluate
for underlying structural or mass lesion

□ Evaluation of patients with known or suspected metastatic
disease. MR has a higher sensitivity for detection of parenchymal and leptomeningeal metastatic disease. However,
CT is superior to MR for identification of osseous metastatic
disease.

□ Characterization of masses identified with CT

□ Follow-up of known primary central nervous system neoplasms

□ Evaluation of intracranial infection. It is most useful for parenchymal lesions (i.e. abscess) or epidural collections. Meningeal enhancement may be seen in cases of meningitis (particularly tuberculous, fungal, or aseptic); however, meningeal

enhancement may be seen following lumbar puncture, thus leading to false-positive results. It is advisable to defer lumbar puncture if MRI is planned for the evaluation of suspected meningitis or leptomeningeal spread of tumor.

☐ Evaluation of demyelinating disease (e.g. multiple sclerosis). Although the majority of these studies may be performed without IV contrast to confirm a suspected diagnosis of demyelinating disease, IV contrast is helpful in the identification of active foci of demyelination as these tend to demonstrate peripheral enhancement.

CONTRAINDICATIONS

☐ Patients who are actively seizing should not be placed in the magnet due to the inability to fully monitor the patient's clinical status.

☐ General contraindications for MRI

LIMITATIONS

☐ It may not be possible to differentiate between infection and tumor.

☐ It may not be possible to differentiate among postsurgical changes, radiation-induced change, and recurrent tumor. MR spectroscopy and diffusion imaging may be useful additional imaging sequences in these cases.

☐ Areas of subacute ischemia can be masslike and will demonstrate enhancement in this phase; this may make it difficult to differentiate from tumor or infection.

☐ Small areas such as the internal auditory canal or pituitary are not adequately imaged with routine brain protocols; if there is concern regarding pathology in these regions, dedicated imaging should be performed.

☐ If patients are unable to hold still, imaging may be uninterpretable. Unlike CT imaging where only a portion of the study is affected if a patient moves, in MRI, patient motion for even a portion of the image acquisition will affect the whole sequence. This is due to the manner in which data are acquired and processed in MRI.

☐ Small lesions may be below the resolution of MRI.

MR of the Nasopharynx

▓ It is performed as a routine with IV contrast.

▓ It does not image the brain parenchyma; dedicated images of the nasopharynx are obtained. Imaging does include sequences to evaluate for the presence of lymphadenopathy within the neck.

INDICATIONS

☐ Identification of suspected nasopharyngeal mass
☐ Restaging of known nasopharyngeal malignancy
☐ Evaluation of aggressive sinus infection in the setting of immunocompromise

CONTRAINDICATIONS

☐ Patients with known or suspected gas-forming organisms are better imaged with CT. This is due to the poor imaging capabilities of MR in the presence of air.
☐ General contraindications for MRI

LIMITATIONS

☐ Air within the sinuses creates artifact that makes it difficult to image the region.
☐ A primary head and neck malignancy may be occult on imaging; only metastatic disease may be identifiable.
☐ Subtle areas of vascular involvement may be below the resolution of MRI; CT may be useful for this purpose.
☐ Artifacts from surgical clips may make image acquisition and interpretation difficult.

MR of the Orbits

▪ It is routinely performed with IV contrast.
▪ It may include imaging of the brain parenchyma as it is often performed for evaluation of demyelinating disease.

INDICATIONS

☐ Evaluation of involvement of the orbits in demyelinating disease
☐ Evaluation of suspected ophthalmopathy (particularly Graves)
☐ Evaluation of nerve entrapment or involvement by masses
☐ Evaluation of metastatic disease (particularly melanoma and breast)
☐ Evaluation of primary intraocular tumors (e.g. retinoblastoma, ocular melanoma) and inflammatory lesions (e.g. orbital pseudotumor)

CONTRAINDICATIONS

☐ Surgical clips or metal within the eye may move in the magnetic field. The type of clip should be cleared with a physicist for safety prior to imaging.

☐ General contraindications to MRI
LIMITATIONS
☐ Ocular movement or patient movement may render images uninterpretable.
☐ It may be difficult to differentiate tumor from infection or demyelination.
☐ If masses are large, it may be difficult to determine if they arise from the intraconal or extraconal space. This affects determination of what is the likeliest tumor or infection to cause the abnormality.
☐ Artifacts from surgical clips may make image acquisition and interpretation difficult.

MR of the Pituitary

▪ It is performed as a routine with IV contrast.
▪ It includes evaluation of the brain parenchyma as well as high resolution images of the sella turcica/pituitary with dynamic contrast enhancement.
▪ The indication for the study and the patient's symptoms are critical pieces of information to have prior to performing the examination as the study is performed in a different manner dependent upon the indication (e.g. pituitary microadenoma versus macroadenoma).

INDICATIONS
☐ Evaluation of patients with suspected pituitary macroadenoma (mass effect/visual changes)
☐ Evaluation of suspected microadenoma (hormonal stimulation)
☐ Evaluation of suspected mass in the sella turcica
☐ Evaluation of absent or ectopic pituitary
☐ Evaluation of suspected pituitary infundibular lesion (e.g. diabetes insipidus, sarcoid, eosinophilic granuloma)
☐ Evaluation of pituitary hemorrhage (e.g. postpartum/Sheehan syndrome)
☐ Evaluation of hypothalamic dysfunction
☐ Evaluation of hypothalamic masses (e.g. hypothalamic hamartomas, gelastic seizures, optic gliomas
CONTRAINDICATIONS
☐ General contraindications to MRI
LIMITATIONS
☐ Small masses may be below the resolution of MR.

- [ ] Subtle areas of enhancement may be difficult to recognize, which may make diagnosis of an abnormality difficult.
- [ ] It may be difficult to differentiate tumor from demyelination and granulomatous disease.
- [ ] Artifacts from the adjacent paranasal sinuses and surgical clips may render image acquisition and interpretation difficult.
- [ ] Areas of hemorrhage may complicate interpretation as it may be difficult to differentiate hemorrhage from a mass unless blood products and enhancement characteristics are considered.

MR of the Neck

- It may be performed without or with IV contrast depending upon the indication for the study.
- If the study is performed for evaluation of lymphadenopathy or for localization of parathyroid adenomas, no IV contrast is required.
- If the study is performed as an MR angiogram (MRA) for the purposes of evaluation of carotid or basivertebral disease, IV contrast is required.
- Non-contrast MR of the neck:
  INDICATIONS
  - [ ] Evaluation of suspected lymphadenopathy in patients with a history of head and neck malignancy. This is of particular importance in patients with a history of thyroid malignancy, as CT of the neck requires the administration of IV contrast to identify lymphadenopathy. This is disadvantageous in patients with thyroid neoplasms as the iodine containing contrast may interfere with other imaging modalities or even with planned therapy.
  - [ ] Evaluation of orthotopic or ectopic parathyroid adenomas.
- Contrast-enhanced MR of the neck (MRA):
  INDICATIONS
  - [ ] Evaluation of suspected extracranial carotid/basivertebral disease including stenosis and dissection
  - [ ] Preoperative evaluation of vessel involvement by tumor

CONTRAINDICATIONS
- [ ] General contraindications to MRI

LIMITATIONS
- [ ] Small masses may be below the resolution of MRI.
- [ ] Ectopic thyroid or parathyroid glands may be located within the mediastinum. This region is generally not imaged at the time of imaging of the neck.
- [ ] Lymphadenopathy is deemed pathologic on the basis of size criteria only (short axis >1.5 cm). However, microscopic disease that does not enlarge the lymph node is not recognized on routine MR of the neck.
- [ ] Motion artifact will limit image interpretation.
- [ ] Heavy vascular calcification can cause overestimation of stenosis or may render some segments of the vessel uninterpretable.
- [ ] Subtle areas of vascular involvement by tumor may be below the resolution of MRI.

MR Angiography/MR Venography

- ▣ It may be performed without or with IV contrast.
- ▣ It is typically performed in conjunction with complete imaging of the brain parenchyma to assess for areas of ischemia or infarction.
- ▣ It must be ordered as a separate study from MRI imaging (for billing/insurance purposes).

INDICATIONS
- [ ] Evaluation of known or suspected cerebrovascular accident to evaluate vessel occlusion or stenosis
- [ ] Evaluation of known or suspected aneurysms of the Circle of Willis
- [ ] Evaluation of suspected or known vascular malformations
- [ ] Evaluation of suspected venous occlusion (MR venography [MRV]. It must be specifically requested as it is not performed routinely with MRA imaging. The indication for MRV should be clearly stated at the time of the request for the examination. It is often requested in patients with mastoiditis and in patients who are pregnant or hypercoagulable.

CONTRAINDICATIONS
- [ ] General contraindications to MRI

LIMITATIONS

- ☐ Calcified vessels can lead to under- or overestimation of the degree of stenosis. If the calcification is very severe, it can mimic vessel occlusion.
- ☐ Very slowly flowing blood can mimic thrombus and vessel occlusion.
- ☐ Slow flow in vascular malformations may make it difficult to determine what type of malformation the lesion represents.
- ☐ Motion artifact can limit the examination.

MR Spectroscopy

- ■ It is performed as a routine without IV contrast.
- ■ It is typically performed in conjunction with complete MRI of the brain.
- ■ It must be requested as a separate study in conjunction with a routine MR examination.
- ■ It is not performed routinely due to the length of the imaging sequence as well as the fact that it remains a research tool to some extent with limited application in clinical settings.

INDICATIONS

- ☐ Evaluation of mass lesions in the brain to help differentiate neoplasm from non-neoplastic conditions
- ☐ Evaluation of suspected toxic/metabolic conditions (e.g. Leigh disease)

CONTRAINDICATIONS

- ☐ General contraindications to MRI

LIMITATIONS

- ☐ The lesion must be large enough for an adequate amount of the lesion to be sampled with spectroscopy.
- ☐ MR spectroscopy is not sensitive; it may remain difficult to differentiate between tumor and other processes such as radiation change.
- ☐ It is a relatively time-consuming sequence during which patients must lie still. Due to the length of the image acquisition, it is not routinely used.

MR of the Spine

- ■ It may be performed as a non-contrast or a contrast-enhanced study dependent on the indication for the study.

- As with MRI of the brain, it is essential to request the appropriate study at the time of scheduling so that insurance precertification may be obtained appropriately.

Non-Contrast MR of the Spine

- It is routinely performed without IV contrast unless an abnormality requiring contrast administration is identified while the examination is in progress.
- It requires prolonged immobility and supine positioning. For patients with significant pain in these settings, some degree of sedation or pain relief may be required.

INDICATIONS
- ☐ Evaluation of disc disease
- ☐ Evaluation of acute spine trauma (particularly the cervical spine). MR is the imaging study of choice for the evaluation of ligamentous injury and cord contusion.
- ☐ Evaluation of demyelinating disease (although contrast may be required to evaluate the extent of active disease; see the earlier section, MRI of the Brain)
- ☐ Evaluation of cord pathology due to disc disease, trauma, XRT, congenital malformations (e.g. tethered cord, Chiari malformation, meningomyelocele), cord compression from disc disease

CONTRAINDICATIONS
- ☐ General contraindications to MRI

LIMITATIONS
- ☐ Surgical hardware may cause artifact, which will render image acquisition and interpretation difficult.
- ☐ Motion artifact can significantly limit interpretation.
- ☐ It may be difficult to differentiate cord pathology due to ischemia, infection, and infarction.

Contrast-Enhanced MR of the Spine

- It is performed as a routine with IV contrast.
- It requires prolonged immobility and supine positioning. For patients with significant pain in these settings, some degree of sedation or pain relief may be required.

INDICATIONS
- ☐ Evaluation of suspected osteomyelitis/discitis
- ☐ Evaluation of suspected arachnoiditis

☐ Evaluation of suspected epidural abscess (surgical emergency)
☐ Evaluation of neoplasm, including vertebral body metastases, drop metastases, leptomeningeal spread of tumor
☐ Evaluation of cord compression from neoplasm/osseous metastatic disease
☐ Evaluation of primary tumors of the spinal cord
☐ Evaluation of the postoperative back for recurrent pain

CONTRAINDICATIONS
☐ General contraindications to MRI

LIMITATIONS
☐ Patient motion may limit the examination.
☐ It may not be possible to differentiate among infection, inflammation, and tumor.
☐ It may not be possible to differentiate between recurrent disc disease and scar tissue in the postoperative patient.

9

Cardiac Imaging

General Considerations

■ Cardiac imaging is a rapidly evolving field with much promise for future developments.

■ There is currently much rapid advancement in the field of cardiac imaging. This text is written about the most current cardiac imaging studies available at the time of publication.

■ As with any field in which there are numerous modalities available to image a single organ, no single imaging modality is the optimal study for every patient. The clinical question being posed and the information being sought should be carefully considered for each patient, and the most appropriate imaging modality should be employed. This may require sometimes lengthy conversations with the imager in order to ensure that the correct study is performed.

■ All cardiac evaluations begin with the clinical history, physical examination, family history, and assessment of cardiac risk factors. ECGs are often a part of the workup of suspected cardiac disease.

■ One of the initial imaging studies performed in the evaluation of suspected cardiac disease is conventional radiography, which is discussed later.

■ Currently available imaging studies for the evaluation of suspected cardiovascular disease include the following:
  □ Chest radiography
  □ Echocardiography
  □ Stress testing (with or without nuclear imaging)

- [ ] Nuclear stress/rest perfusion imaging (201-thallium, technetium 99m [^{99m}Tc] sestamibi/tetrofosmin/teburoxime)
- [ ] Nuclear viability imaging (fluorodeoxyglucose [FDG] PET)
- [ ] Nuclear medicine PET CT stress/rest imaging
- [ ] Coronary artery calcium (CAC) scoring
- [ ] Cardiac CT (coronary CT angiography [CCTA])
- [ ] MRI
- [ ] Conventional catheter angiography

■ With the exception of echocardiography and MR, all other imaging modalities involve ionizing radiation. Radiation doses for CT and nuclear studies can reach high levels for purely diagnostic studies and should be carefully considered prior to performance.

■ There are some contraindications for some imaging studies, which are considered individually next, based on modality.

Chest Radiography

■ Chest radiographs are the first step in the imaging of cardiopulmonary disease.

■ A wealth of information can be obtained about a patient's underlying cardiac disease based on the chest radiograph; this includes cardiac chamber enlargement, pulmonary blood flow (increased, normal, or decreased), pericardial abnormalities, and support apparatus. Information obtained about any or all of these findings may lead to the diagnosis without the need for additional imaging.

■ Chest radiographs should always be interpreted in conjunction with the clinical history to ensure that the appropriate interpretation is rendered.

■ Comparing current with prior radiographs is of great value, particularly in patients with known heart disease. The comparison allows for assessment of changes in vascularity and cardiac size in a short time, which suggests the presence of a pericardial effusion.

INDICATIONS

- [ ] Evaluation of acute heart failure
- [ ] Evaluation of chest pain, which can be due to myocardial infarction (MI), aortic dissection, pulmonary embolism, or non-cardiopulmonary abnormalities

☐ Evaluation of cardiac chamber size (echocardiography, CT, and MR are more sensitive and specific for this indication)

☐ Evaluation of pericardial disease (e.g. pericardial effusion, pericardial calcification, pneumopericardium)

☐ Evaluation of cardiac morphology and pulmonary blood flow patterns (normal, increased, or decreased) in children with suspected congenital heart disease (CHD) or adults with surgically corrected CHD

☐ Evaluation of rib abnormalities (e.g. rib notching in coarctation of the aorta)

☐ Evaluation of positioning of cardiac devices (e.g. pacer leads, automatic implantable cardioverter defibrillator [AICD], sternotomy wires)

CONTRAINDICATIONS

☐ Relative: Early pregnancy. Verbal consent should be obtained from the patient after explanation of the risks of the radiation dose. The patient should be shielded for the study, and only a frontal view of the chest obtained.

LIMITATIONS

☐ Radiography is subject to a number of limitations, including magnification of structures with AP films (this is most notable when determining cardiac enlargement).

☐ Radiography offers limited evaluation of pericardial effusion, particularly when only a frontal view of the chest is obtained and there are no recent prior films for comparison. If the size of the cardiac silhouette increases markedly from a recent prior study, it is highly suggestive that a pericardial effusion is present. Echocardiography is the study of choice in these patients.

☐ Interpretation of pulmonary blood flow and edema is highly interpreter-dependent; one reader may call the vascularity normal, whereas another might interpret the film as pulmonary edema.

☐ Specific chamber enlargement may be difficult to evaluate on radiographs, particularly if only a frontal view is provided. Echocardiography, CT, and MR are more sensitive and specific.

☐ Associated findings such as rib notching may not be easily identified, particularly if film quality is suboptimal or the patient is obese.

☐ Cardiac function cannot be assessed on radiographs.

Echocardiography

■ Echocardiography involves the use of ultrasound with specialized probes ("cameras") for evaluation of the heart and pericardium.

■ As with all ultrasound, no radiation is involved with echocardiography.

■ Air is the enemy of ultrasound! It causes the beam to be reflected, thus, no structures can be seen. Ultrasound gel is used on the patient's skin to provide a good interface for the ultrasound beam so that the beam penetrates into the patient's body.

■ There are two main approaches to the evaluation of the heart with echocardiography: transthoracic echocardiography (TTE) and transesophageal echocardiography (TEE). There are two main differences between these two techniques, the most significant being the manner in which the studies are performed.

  □ For TTE, the probe is placed on the chest wall and imaging is performed in multiple projections. This has inherent limitations including poor imaging windows in patients with chronic obstructive pulmonary disease (COPD) (as the lung will reflect the ultrasound beam), kyphosis, obesity, and large breasts. The right heart (i.e. right atrium and right ventricle) is not well visualized with this approach.

  □ For TEE, the patient must be sedated. A specialized ultrasound probe is passed through the mouth into the esophagus in order to evaluate the heart. This technique is technically superior to TTE due to the closer proximity of the ultrasound beam to the heart without the need to scan through the chest wall. The esophagus is anatomically directly posterior to the left atrium, thus allowing excellent visualization of the cardiac structures. There are clear drawbacks to this technique, the most significant of which is the invasiveness and risk of aspiration from sedation and esophageal manipulation.

■ Echocardiography has many benefits for the evaluation of known or suspected cardiac disease:

  □ Relatively low expense
  □ Portability of the machine. Ultrasound machines, although cumbersome, are easily portable. Portability allows echocardiograms to be performed at the bedside if patients are unable to travel to the imaging suite for an examination.

This is particularly important in the acutely ill patient who has hemodynamic compromise that is thought to have a cardiac or pericardial etiology. It is also useful in the trauma setting when patients have pulseless electrical activity in order to determine if spontaneous cardiac activity is present or if resuscitation efforts should be halted.

☐ There is a lack of radiation with ultrasound.
☐ Echocardiograms are reliable, although interobserver variability does occur.

INDICATIONS

☐ Evaluation of cardiac valvular disease (i.e. stenosis or regurgitation). Echocardiography is the gold standard for the evaluation of cardiac valvular abnormalities; MR has comparable sensitivity but takes longer.
☐ Evaluation of cardiac chamber size. Echocardiography allows the evaluation of chamber sizes, although evaluation of the right heart (right atrium and right ventricle) is often limited due to imaging windows and techniques. MR and CT have the advantage over echocardiography for evaluation of the right heart.
☐ Evaluation of known or suspected atrial or ventricular clot
☐ Evaluation of valvular vegitations in infective endocarditis (this is the gold standard)
☐ Evaluation of known or suspected intracardiac masses (although CT and MR are often superior to echocardiography for this indication and allows evaluation of the mass in relation to adjacent structures)
☐ Assessment of CHD for diagnosis of the cardiac abnormality in the pediatric population or as follow-up of patients with treated CHD for acute decompensation or routine surveillance
☐ Evaluation of left ventricular hypertrophy and subvalvular aortic stenosis in patients with hypertrophic obstructive cardiomyopathy
☐ Evaluation of left ventricular muscle mass in patients with hypertension
☐ Evaluation of global and regional wall motion abnormalities in patients with known or suspected coronary artery disease (CAD) or MI
☐ Evaluation of cardiac contractility and calculation of ejection fraction (EF). Echocardiography is the gold standard for

the evaluation of the EF. The EF may be calculated based on ventricular measurements and other parameters; however, EF is often estimated based on observer experience.

☐ Evaluation of pericardial effusion. Echocardiography is the gold standard for the identification and quantification of pericardial effusion. Although cardiac tamponade is a clinical emergency and is often diagnosed on clinical grounds, echocardiography can be used to confirm the diagnosis if readily available.

☐ Echo "bubble" studies (i.e. studies with IV echocardiographic contrast [usually agitated saline]) may be used to evaluate for intracardiac or supracardiac shunts if these are known or suspected (e.g. atrial septal defect, patent ductus arteriosus).

CONTRAINDICATIONS

☐ Patients who are unstable or at significant risk of aspiration are poor candidates for TEE.

☐ Patients with sternal wound infections or open chest walls are not good candidates for the study; if an echocardiogram must be performed, sterile ultrasound gel should be used.

☐ In patients with known large intracardiac or supracardiac shunts, "bubble" studies should be assessed prior to contrast administration to decrease the risk of embolization of the material through a left to right shunt to the pulmonary vascular bed (less likely given that the contrast is administered IV) or through a right to left shunt to the systemic circulation.

LIMITATIONS

☐ As with all ultrasound, echocardiography is dependent upon the operator. A high degree of skill is required to acquire and interpret the images.

☐ There is a significant degree of operator variability with respect to image acquisition and interpretation. This is particularly true with respect to estimation of regional wall motion abnormalities and EF.

☐ Due to the approximation of the EF by visual inspection as opposed to true measurement/calculation, there is significant interobserver variability in EF determination. The EFs obtained with echocardiography, although considered the gold standard, are not always accurate or reproducible. MUGA is a more reproducible manner in which to determine EF.

□ Echocardiography is dependent upon patient factors, including COPD and obesity. Some patients are not good candidates for echocardiography simply based upon their body habitus.

□ Some patients are not candidates for stress echocardiography (either they cannot exercise or cannot receive pharmacologic stress).

Exercise Stress Testing

- This type of study is performed to evaluate for ischemia, left ventricular dysfunction, and left ventricular ectopy.
- For an exercise stress test, a patient walks on a treadmill or exercises on a stationary bike while ECG monitoring, blood pressure response, and/or oxygen consumption are monitored.
- The test is finished when symptoms occur, the patient cannot continue due to physical limitations (e.g. fatigue or leg or chest pain), the exercise protocol is completed, ECG changes occur, or the target heart rate is reached.
- Patients are typically exercised for 6–15 minutes; the entire study requires approximately 30–40 minutes.
- The level of activity is determined based on metabolic equivalents (METs). Exercise work load is typically considered poor, fair, good, or excellent.
- The advantages of exercise stress testing are as follows:
  □ It is non-invasive.
  □ It is reliable and reproducible.
  □ It is safe and does not involve radiation or contrast administration.
  □ An IV is not required unless pharmacologic stress testing is performed.
  □ It is readily available, particularly in chest pain centers of ERs.
- Study preparation is as follows:
  □ Light breakfast or lunch 2 hours prior to the test
  □ Rubber soled heels are worn for safe exercise
  □ Loose, comfortable clothing is worn
  □ Body lotion is not permitted as it prevents the monitoring electrodes from sticking to the skin surface.
  □ Men may require a shaved chest in order for the electrodes to stick.

INDICATIONS
- ☐ Evaluation of chest pain
- ☐ Risk stratification for CAD
- ☐ Evaluation of the severity of CAD (e.g. ischemia)

CONTRAINDICATIONS
- ☐ Patients who are hemodynamically compromised should not undergo stress testing.
- ☐ Patients with clinical, biochemical, and ECG findings of acute MI should not undergo stress testing and should be treated for an acute coronary event (medical or angioplasty).

LIMITATIONS
- ☐ It is relatively expensive.
- ☐ If not combined with perfusion imaging (i.e. SPECT), the extent of ischemia with or without scar may not be determined. The vascular territory also may not be easily identified without perfusion imaging.
- ☐ Because exercise stress testing is based on ischemic ECG changes, patients with baseline abnormal ECGs are not candidates for exercise stress testing.
- ☐ There is a relatively high false-positive rate (15%–40%), particularly in young women.
- ☐ There is a relatively high false-negative rate (15%–30%), particularly in men.

Preparation for Nuclear Stress Tests

SPECT Study

- ▪ The patient must be able to raise both arms above the head and maintain this position throughout the study. Significant artifacts occur when patients are unable to keep their arms above their heads; this can lead to false-positive results of perfusion defects.
- ▪ The patient must be able to remain completely immobile on the imaging table for at least 20 minutes during image acquisition. Movement during imaging results in motion artifacts, which can render the study uninterpretable.
- ▪ Patients receiving dipyridamole studies MUST refrain from all caffeine intake on the day of the study, including coffee, hot or cold tea, soda, hot chocolate, chocolate pudding, and decaffeinated beverages. The caffeine will interfere with the heart rate and uptake, leading to misinterpretation.

- Persantine is contraindicated in asthmatic patients; these patients should be scheduled with dobutamine if pharmacologic stress testing is required.
- There are weight restrictions for nuclear stress imaging:
  - □ Patients who are >400 lbs cannot undergo SPECT imaging. Planar imaging (i.e. the whole heart is imaged in several projections as one unit and not as slices) is available for morbidly obese patients; however, it is significantly less sensitive than SPECT imaging (i.e. slices of the heart are imaged, allowing for evaluation of regional and subtle perfusion abnormalities).
  - □ Male patients >275 lbs require 2-day studies.
  - □ Female patients >175 lbs require 2-day studies.

Nuclear Stress/Rest Perfusion Imaging (201-Thallium, ^{99m}Tc Sestamibi/Tetrofosmin/Teburoxime)

- There are two main types of radiotracer used for SPECT imaging: 201-thallium and ^{99m}technetium-labeled agents (e.g. ^{99m}Tc sestamibi, ^{99m}Tc tetrofosmin).
- The mechanisms of uptake and distribution of the two agents differ, which affects the manner in which studies are performed.
- Both agents may be used with exercise or pharmacologic stress.
- Thallium is a potassium analog, thus it acts on the Na^+-K^+ ATPase pump. This leads to initial distribution of the tracer to be related to regional blood flow. Areas with relatively decreased blood flow (e.g. in vascular territories where coronary stenosis exists) demonstrate decreased uptake (e.g. a perfusion defect) on initial imaging. After a delay (at least 4 hours), if there is stenosis in the vessel that produces exercise-induced ischemia, with redistribution of blood flow, the perfusion defect will resolve. This is so-called rest-redistribution imaging in which initial perfusion imaging is performed followed by delayed imaging (from 4–24 hours following injection; repeat injection of thallium may be required depending upon patient weight). If there is a perfusion defect on initial imaging that resolves on redistribution imaging, a reversible defect is said to be present, indicating an area of reversible ischemia.
- For technetium-labeled agents, the study is performed as a 1- or 2-day study (depending upon patient weight, see earlier) with

stress and rest imaging. Stress images can be obtained with exercise or with pharmacologic stress.

■ Exercise stress testing is performed by having the patient walk on a treadmill or ride a stationary bike according to standard cardiac exercise protocols (the Bruce protocol is the most common); exercise workload is calculated in METs.

■ Pharmacologic stress may be performed with dipyridamole, adenosine, or dobutamine. Protocols exist for dose, endpoint for infusion of the agent, and time after peak stress response; the radiotracer (thallium or technetium) protocol varies by agent.

INDICATIONS FOR PHARMACOLOGIC STRESS

☐ Patients unfit for exercise stress testing
☐ Patients unwilling to exercise
☐ Patients with physical impairment precluding prolonged exercise
☐ Recent MI where excess exercise is contraindicated

CONTRAINDICATIONS FOR PHARMACOLOGIC AGENTS

☐ Dipyridamole: Unstable angina, acute MI, critical aortic stenosis, hypertrophic cardiomyopathy, hypotension, asthma
☐ Adenosine: Unstable angina, acute MI, critical aortic stenosis, hypertrophic cardiomyopathy, hypotension, asthma
☐ Dobutamine: Underlying cardiac arrhythmias due to risk of ventricular tachycardia and atrial fibrillation

LIMITATIONS (OFTEN RELATED TO SIDE EFFECTS)

☐ Dipyridamole: Side effects include dizziness, headache, hypotension, flushing, myocardial ischemia
☐ Adenosine: Similar to dipyridamole, heart block
☐ Dobutamine: Premature ventricular contraction, ventricular tachycardia

INDICATIONS FOR MYOCARDIAL PERFUSION IMAGING

☐ Risk stratification for CAD
☐ Preoperative risk stratification for noncardiac surgery
☐ Identification of CAD
☐ Prediction of outcomes from recent MI
☐ Evaluation of acute chest pain (atypical chest pain)
☐ Evaluation of stable angina

CONTRAINDICATIONS

☐ As listed earlier for recent caffeine intake, contraindication to exercise or pharmacologic stress, pregnancy/breastfeeding

☐ Obesity

LIMITATIONS

☐ Submaximal stress response. If the target heart rate is not met, inducible ischemia may not be identifiable as there is relatively maintained perfusion to the ischemic area and a perfusion defect is not appreciated.

☐ Patient factors

- Obese patients are difficult to image due to artifacts related to attenuation of the photons (x-rays) by breast, pannus, and adipose tissue.
- The hemidiaphragms can cause significant artifacts, which can render a study false positive.
- Motion artifact can produce significant artifact.
- If the patient does not have a regular rhythm, cardiac gating of the study cannot be performed, thus global and regional wall motion abnormalities and EF cannot be assessed.
- Gastrointestinal activity. Some of the tracers are normally taken up by bowel. This bowel activity can be very pronounced and can cause a relative scaling of the activity in the myocardium such that it produces an apparent perfusion defect in the adjacent myocardium. This can lead to equivocal studies or false-positive results. In these patients, cardiac PET CT (see later) may be of use.

Nuclear Viability Imaging (FDG PET)

■ Nuclear viability imaging is typically performed in conjunction with nuclear perfusion imaging (cardiac PET CT; see later).

■ There are two main indications for cardiac FDG PET imaging: evaluation of cardiac sarcoid and cardiac viability imaging.

■ FDG is taken up in the myocardium, which is actively involved with sarcoidosis. There are inherent limitations of the technique for this indication, and contrast MR is the study of choice for evaluation of cardiac sarcoidosis. If sites of active disease are identified, it may help to direct myocardial biopsy, thus allowing confirmation of the diagnosis. It may also be helpful to follow patients with known cardiac sarcoidosis to determine response to therapy.

■ Cardiac viability imaging is performed in order to determine if areas of myocardial ischemia demonstrated on perfusion imaging are viable and thus would be amenable to revascularization. This is of significant clinical importance as ischemic, nonviable myocardium will not respond to revascularization. Indeed, revascularization may be of increased risk in these patients with poor myocardial reserve. Conversely, if the ischemic myocardium is viable, the patient would likely benefit from revascularization (angioplasty with or without stenting; CABG).

■ Patients often fast for the study and then are given a predetermined glucose load in order to enter into a specific serum glucose range, which is required for myocardial uptake of the tracer to occur.

INDICATIONS
☐ Evaluation of cardiac sarcoidosis
☐ Evaluation of myocardial viability in ischemic myocardium

CONTRAINDICATIONS
☐ Patients with uncontrolled diabetes
☐ Pregnancy

LIMITATIONS
☐ If there is poor myocardial uptake due to poor patient preparation, the study may yield a false-negative result.
☐ Areas of sarcoidosis that are not active may not demonstrate radiotracer uptake, even if wall motion abnormalities are present (on gated images).

Nuclear Medicine PET CT Stress/Rest Imaging

■ Cardiac PET CT examinations are performed with rubidium 82, which is a short-lived PET radiotracer that rapidly decays. Therefore, a study must be performed quickly to avoid decay of the tracer.

■ The studies are performed as pharmacologic rest/stress examinations. Exercise stress testing is not possible with this technique due to the short life of the radiotracer.

■ The CT component of the examination is performed for the purposes of attenuation correction, that is, to correct for the PET images so that artifacts do not occur. The CT is performed as a diagnostic examination from which a significant amount of information such as coronary calcium presence and location and pulmonary disease can be obtained.

■ Images are obtained as slices through the heart and are displayed in the same manner as rest/stress SPECT images. Gated images are obtained if the patient is in sinus rhythm, allowing for determination of global and regional wall motion abnormalities and estimation of EF.

■ Perfusion abnormalities are assessed to evaluate for the presence of CAD and ischemia/scar.

■ Images from the PET are manipulated with the CT data to obtain a fused image of the CT and PET images. This allows for the data to be corrected for artifacts produced by the photons from the PET.

■ If misregistration of the CT and PET images occur, significant artifacts may result, which can render the study equivocal. Alternatively, false-positive or false-negative results may occur.

■ The technique is better for the evaluation of CAD in obese patients due to the higher energy photons of the rubidium tracer, leading to more penetration of the body with photons to reach the detectors and produce an image.

INDICATIONS
☐ Evaluation of patients with chest pain
☐ Evaluation of CAD in obese patients
☐ Evaluation of CAD in patients with equivocal SPECT imaging due to artifacts such as breast attenuation, GI activity, and diaphragmatic attenuation
☐ Risk stratification for CAD in patients who are poor candidates for standard SPECT imaging or who have had equivocal SPECT studies

CONTRAINDICATIONS
☐ Patients weighing >500 lbs or whose girth exceeds the width of the CT scanner aperture (approximately 52 inches)
☐ Patients with metabolic derangement in whom insulin levels cannot be controlled (thus preventing appropriate uptake of radiotracer)
☐ Pregnancy
☐ Young patients (relative) due to the high radiation dose of the combination of rest/stress PET with radioactivity and rest/stress CT images (even though low dose)
☐ Recent caffeine consumption
☐ Patients unable to mount a heart rate response to pharmacologic stress

LIMITATIONS

☐ Artifacts can occur with cardiac PET CT imaging, particularly if there is misregistration of PET and CT images. Even if the CT is repeated in an attempt to improve registration, misregistration may remain. This misregistration can lead to false-positive results in that the area that is misregistered may show a relative decrease of tracer activity, leading to the appearance of a perfusion defect.

☐ Patient motion may result in uninterpretable examinations or may lead to false-positive or false-negative results.

☐ Studies on morbidly obese patients may be complicated by attenuation of the photons by their adipose tissue, leading to false-positive results or equivocal studies.

☐ Due to the short half-life of the radiotracer, imaging must be performed quickly following the IV administration of the tracer. The tracer must be "milked" from a generator shortly before administration.

☐ If there is balanced disease (e.g. three-vessel CAD), it may be difficult to identify unless there is subendocardial ischemia, leading to transient ischemic dilation with stress. This results in an apparent increase in the size of the left ventricular cavity with stress due to lack of tracer uptake by the ischemic subendocardium.

☐ The resolution of PET CT is greater than SPECT imaging; however, the resolution of PET CT remains less than that of MR and CT coronary angiography. This can result in false-negative results if areas of ischemia are small or are subendocardial. Small, non-transmural areas of ischemia may also be masked due to this limitation.

Coronary Artery Calcium Scoring

■ Coronary artery calcification is a well-established risk factor for the presence of CAD.

■ CAC has been in use since the 1980s, when it was first performed on electron beam CT.

■ It is now also performed on MDCT with the use of ECG gating techniques.

■ It requires a 4-slice or higher scanner.

■ Patients must be in sinus rhythm for the ECG gating to be performed.

- It is a rapid, low radiation dose study (1–3 mSv) that can be used to diagnose, quantify, and follow the amount of calcium present in each of the coronary arteries.
- It is a reliable and reproducible study, although significant variation in actual CAC values occurs depending upon the scanner type.
- It is a non-contrast examination and can be performed as an independent study or at the time of CT coronary angiography (see later) or cardiac PET CT (see earlier).
- There is no patient preparation for the study with the exception of abstinence from caffeine the day of the examination to maintain the heart rate <90 beats per minute.
- The patient is placed on the CT scanner, ECG leads are positioned, and the scan is performed. Scan time is ≤30 seconds; the whole study can be completed in as little as 10–15 minutes.
- Post-processing is performed by the radiologist on a workstation to determine the CAC score.

INDICATIONS
- ☐ Risk stratification for CAD
- ☐ Evaluation of chest pain in low-risk patients
- ☐ Follow-up of CAC score in patients with known coronary calcification to assess stability or progression, particularly if they are on lipid-lowering agents
- ☐ Some institutions perform CAC scoring prior to CCTA in order to determine the calcium load. If the CAC (Agatston) score is >1000, many institutions will not precede with the CTA as the calcification will cause artifacts that will render many segments of the coronary arteries uninterpretable (see later).

CONTRAINDICATIONS
- ☐ Pregnancy (due to the radiation exposure)
- ☐ Very elevated heart rates
- ☐ Morbid obesity (if patients are too large for the CT scanner)

LIMITATIONS
- ☐ Interscan variability can be as much as 30%, leading to the possibility of inaccurate results for follow-up studies.
- ☐ Obese patients may have streak artifact related to their body habitus, which can mask or mimic calcification, thus leading to inaccurate results.
- ☐ Very small amounts of calcification may be below the resolution of the imaging or may not be of sufficient CT density

to be counted in the CAC score. This is of doubtful clinical significance.

☐ Only calcified plaque is identified with this technique. Calcified plaque is (generally) stable plaque that leads to stable angina. It is atheromatous or fibrofatty plaque, which is more likely to rupture and lead to an acute myocardial event; this type of plaque is not identified with CAC. CCTA and conventional catheter angiography are the studies of choice for the evaluation of non-calcified plaque.

CT Coronary Angiography

■ CCTA/cardiac CT is an exciting new area that has developed since the late 1990s.

■ This technique allows the coronary arteries to be evaluated, along with the remainder of the heart.

■ It is a CT examination that is performed with IV contrast and ECG gating. The technique allows the lumen and the walls of the coronary arteries to be evaluated for the presence and extent of atheromatous or calcified plaque, the presence and degree of coronary stenosis, native coronary artery, or coronary bypass graft occlusion and allows for an estimation of cardiac contractility and function (EF and regional wall motion abnormalities).

■ The study involves a high radiation dose (7–20 mSv), hence it should not be requested without careful consideration of the risks and benefits of the study to the patient.

■ Patients must have normal sinus rhythm in order for the study to be performed (the CT scanner is triggered to scan at 70% or 75% of the R-R interval; therefore, patients must have a normal rhythm for the scanner to be triggered). The heart rate must also be steady and slow (<65–70 beats per minute); patients with frequent atrial or ventricular ectopy are poor candidates for the study.

■ The examination may be performed with or without CAC scoring (see earlier); this should be made clear to the imager at the time of the study request.

■ The study involves the following:
☐ The patient is administered oral with or without IV beta blockade to achieve a heart rate <65–70 beats per minute.
☐ Sublingual nitroglycerin is administered while the patient is on the CT table in order to dilate the coronary arteries for optimal visualization.

☐ ECG leads are placed on the patient and the rhythm is determined; additional beta blockade may be administered at this point to control the heart rate.

☐ A large bore (18 gauge) IV is placed for IV contrast administration through a "power injector."

☐ A non-contrast CT of the heart is performed (as a routine CT or as a CAC scoring study) to localize the coronary artery for timing of the contrast bolus.

☐ The contrast enhanced portion of the examination is performed.

☐ The study is reconstructed on the CT scanner and the images are sent to a separate 3-D workstation for processing to be performed by the radiologist.

INDICATIONS

☐ Evaluation of low- to intermediate-risk patients for the identification of CAD

☐ Evaluation of suspected anomalous coronary arteries

☐ Evaluation of coronary artery anatomy in relation to aortic aneurysm or dissection for the purposes of surgical planning

CONTRAINDICATIONS

☐ Patients who are not in sinus rhythm are not candidates for the study as the CT scanner will not be triggered to scan if a normal rhythm is not present. Patients with sustained or chronic atrial fibrillation, bundle branch block, or frequent atrial or ventricular ectopy are not candidates for the examination.

☐ Patients who cannot receive beta blockade (e.g. asthmatics) are not candidates for the examination unless their baseline heart rate is slow and regular. If patients cannot receive beta blockade, alternative medications exist for heart rate control, including calcium channel blockers.

☐ Patients who do not have IV access are not candidates for the study.

☐ Patients with impaired renal function (Cr >1.5–1.8 mg/dL) or who have contrast allergies (unless premedication can be administered) are not candidates for the study.

☐ Patients with pacers are not candidates for the examination as the right ventricular lead will produce significant artifacts that will preclude evaluation of the right coronary artery.

☐ Patients with previously known high CAC scores (>1,000) are poor candidates as the calcium will render significant segments of the coronary arteries uninterpretable due to the streak artifact related to the calcification.

☐ Morbidly obese patients (particularly women with large or pendulous breasts) are poor candidates for the examination due to limited penetration of the x-ray beam through the adipose tissue, leading to suboptimal visualization of the coronary arteries.

☐ Pregnant patients should not undergo the examination due to the risk of contrast and radiation to the fetus.

☐ Patients with an acute coronary event documented by clinical history, physical examination, biochemical markers, and ECG changes should NOT undergo CT; they should proceed directly to cardiac catheterization for rapid diagnosis and treatment.

LIMITATIONS

☐ Patients with rapid or abnormal rates or rhythms are not candidates for the study.

☐ Motion artifact can render the study uninterpretable.

☐ Sudden, unexpected changes in heart rate (beat to beat variability) can significantly limit the examination.

☐ False-positive and false-negative results can occur.

☐ The study has an excellent negative predictive value (97%–100%), meaning that if no coronary disease is identified on the CT, it is unlikely to be present. However, the positive predictive value is not as high (approximately 95%), thus it is less likely to identify significant coronary disease when it is present. This limits its usefulness somewhat.

Cardiac MRI

■ It increasingly is used to evaluate cardiac abnormalities, particularly myocardial ischemia and scar.

■ The study may be performed without IV contrast, although there are certain indications for the administration of IV contrast (including evaluation of cardiac masses and assessment of myocardial viability).

■ It requires the patient to be in normal sinus rhythm as the study is performed with cardiac gating (i.e. the scanner is triggered to start scanning based upon the cardiac tracing). Patients with arrhythmias are poor candidates for cardiac MRI (CMRI) as the scanner is inconsistently triggered to start scanning.

INDICATIONS

☐ Valvular: Echocardiography remains the gold standard for the evaluation of valvular cardiac disease (typically left heart valves). However, CMRI has emerged as a new modality to identify and quantify the amount of valvular disease present. There is good correlation of the quantification of disease with both modalities. Evaluation of valvular disease with MR is time-consuming and not routinely performed unless specifically requested. IV contrast is not administered for this indication.

☐ Vascular (pulmonary artery/aorta):
  • MR can evaluate the location of the main pulmonary artery and aorta and arterial-ventricular relationships in patients with suspected congenital cardiac anomalies. This does not require IV contrast administration.
  • Evaluation of the size of the main pulmonary artery and aorta may be performed in patients with suspected aneurysm. This may be performed without IV contrast; however, it is often performed as part of a contrast-enhanced examination.
  • Patients with suspected supracardiac congenital anomalies such as partial or total anomalous pulmonary venous return are excellent candidates for evaluation with MRI. These patients require the administration of IV contrast material.

☐ Evaluation of intra- and extracardiac shunts including surgical shunts/baffles:
  • Patients with suspected congenital intracardiac or extracardiac shunts (e.g. persistent ductus arteriosus) may be non-invasively evaluated with MRI. IV contrast, although not required for this study, may be helpful in certain instances. (The decision to use IV contrast is often made at the time of the study by the monitoring radiologist.)
  • Patients with surgically placed conduits, baffles, and shunts may be monitored for stenosis and patency with MR. The degree of shunting can be assessed and monitored with MR. The study is often performed without and with IV contrast.

☐ Intracardiac (e.g. congenital anomalies): Patients (particularly infants) with suspected congenital cardiac disease may be non-invasively evaluated with MRI. The study is

Cardiac Imaging

typically performed without IV contrast unless there is a question of an associated supracardiac vascular anomaly.

☐ Myocardial: This is one of the most important emerging applications for CMRI. There are two main applications for myocardial imaging:

- Perfusion: This type of study is performed as a monitored examination as pharmacologic vasodilation (typically with adenosine) is performed. The study is performed as part of a complete cardiac imaging study. The perfusion portion of the examination allows for evaluation of myocardial blood flow. Areas with abnormal perfusion are interpreted as regions of ischemia.

- Diffusion (delayed myocardial enhancement): This type of study is performed in conjunction with a complete cardiac MR examination (often with perfusion). The study is performed following the administration of IV contrast such that approximately 8–10 minutes following contrast administration, images are obtained. Areas of myocardium that display late (delayed) enhancement are considered abnormal and represent areas of myocardial scar. There is typically a corresponding perfusion abnormality with regions of abnormal myocardial contraction.

☐ Epicardial (e.g. invasion): Mediastinal or pulmonary parenchymal disease such as primary bronchogenic carcinoma may extend into the epicardial region. MR may be performed to evaluate the extent of local invasion.

☐ Pericardial:

- As for epicardial disease, MR may be performed to evaluate for pericardial involvement by adjacent neoplastic or inflammatory disease. Malignant and benign pericardial effusions may also be identified.

- The primary role for MR in the evaluation of pericardial disease is to help differentiate constrictive pericarditis from restrictive cardiomyopathy. Unlike restrictive cardiomyopathy, constrictive pericarditis is a treatable cause of heart failure. Constrictive pericarditis is well-evaluated by MR such that even small focal areas of pericardial thickening can be identified and the diagnosis made. The study is performed as part of a complete cardiac examination as other causes of heart failure may be identified. Additionally, secondary signs of constrictive pericarditis such as interventricular septal wall motion abnormalities may be identified and further confirm the diagnosis.

CONTRAINDICATIONS

☐ Patients not in sinus rhythm are not good candidates for cardiac MR as ECG gating cannot be adequately performed, thus the scanner cannot be triggered to scan.

☐ Patients with ECG changes or recent acute MI are not candidates for stress perfusion imaging due to the risks of pharmacologic stress.

☐ Patients with pacemakers and AICDs are not candidates for MR examinations.

☐ There is debate as to whether implanted epicardial pacer leads are contraindicated for cardiac MR examinations due to the risk of heating during the study. This should be discussed with the radiologist prior to the examination.

LIMITATIONS

☐ Patient factors:
  - Patients with large body habitus may not be evaluable with MRI.
  - Patients who cannot comply with multiple, repeated breath holding imaging sequences are poor candidates for CMRI. Due to the exquisite sensitivity to motion and respiratory artifact, patients must remain motionless and suspend respiration in order for adequate images to be obtained. However, some scanners are able to image patients who are not able to breath-hold for the examination. These cases should be discussed with the radiologist prior to the study.
  - Patients with arrythmias are poor candidates for CMRI as the scanner is triggered to scan based upon the R-R interval. Newer MR scanners may allow for limited studies in patients who are not in sinus rhythm.

☐ Technical factors:
  - Due to the mechanics of the MR scanner, the T wave may be enlarged and may mimic an R wave, thus inappropriately triggering the scan and producing significant artifacts.

Conventional Catheter Angiography

■ This is an invasive procedure that involves puncturing an artery within the groin, passing a wire and catheter through the aorta into the left ventricle (if ventriculography is requested) and aortic root to inject contrast into the coronary arteries.

■ The procedure is performed under fluoroscopy and may be lengthy, resulting in a relatively high radiation dose.

■ During the procedure, IVUS (intravascular ultrasound) may be performed. This involves passing a small ultrasound probe into the artery mounted on a catheter in order to evaluate the wall of the coronary artery. The procedure is expensive and time consuming, thus, only one or two arteries can be evaluated at the time of catheterization. The benefit of IVUS is that the amount and type of coronary artery plaque and the degree of luminal stenosis can be readily determined.

■ Coronary angiography is the gold standard for the evaluation of CAD; however, it too is a flawed study. Another term that could be used for angiography is *luminography* because only the lumen of the vessel can be assessed with this technique. This has inherent drawbacks because so-called subclinical disease or atheromatous disease, which causes changes in the wall of the coronary artery without causing significant narrowing of the coronary artery lumen, may not be detected. Although this degree of disease will likely not change management at the time of catheterization (because angioplasty and stenting are typically performed when a 60%–70% stenosis is present), it is important to identify this disease. These plaques are the early manifestations of coronary disease and, as such, are the so-called vulnerable plaques that have not yet calcified. These plaques are more prone to rupture and lead to acute vessel occlusion. CCTA and IVUS are more useful studies for the detection of coronary disease, which does not affect the lumen of the vessel and cause angiographically visible stenosis.

INDICATIONS

☐ Diagnosis and treatment of patients presenting with acute MI

☐ Patients presenting with stable angina

☐ Patients presenting with unstable angina

☐ Patients with atypical chest pain in whom nuclear stress testing, CT, or MR are non-diagnostic or equivocal

CONTRAINDICATIONS

☐ Uncorrected coagulopathy

☐ Patients on heparin (Coumadin). These agents should be discontinued and reversal of anticoagulation performed prior to the procedure unless emergent.

☐ Pregnancy
☐ Chronic renal insufficiency (unless the study is necessary)
☐ Contrast allergy (unless the patient can be safely premedicated prior to the study)

LIMITATIONS

☐ Lesions that do not cause significant narrowing of the lumen of the vessel may not be identified with this technique.
☐ Patients with heavily calcified vessels or occluded arteries in the groin may not be able to undergo femoral arterial puncture. In these patients, brachial artery (i.e. upper extremity) access may be required.
☐ Catheter-induced arrhythmias can occur and may, rarely, cause significant morbidity or mortality.
☐ Complications from the procedure include the following:
  • Femoral artery pseudoaneurysm
  • Arteriovenous fistula (from groin puncture)
  • Local hemorrhage
  • Retroperitoneal hemorrhage
  • Contrast-induced nephropathy
  • Coronary artery dissection
  • Coronary artery pseudoaneurysm
  • Coronary artery occlusion
  • Coronary artery rupture
  • Death

10

Ultrasound

General Considerations

■ Ultrasound is an inexpensive, readily available imaging tool with a vast array of applications.

■ Unfortunately, ultrasound is highly dependent upon a number of factors, which can render examinations non-diagnostic:

    ☐ Operator skill: Ultrasound is highly dependent upon high quality technologists/sonologists to provide adequate images for interpretation. Subtle lesions are easily overlooked in the absence of high quality scans.

    ☐ Equipment: Due to the physics of the ultrasound beam and the various factors that may impede imaging, high-quality ultrasound equipment is essential for optimal studies.

    ☐ Patient factors: The physical principles of ultrasound imaging are dependent upon the generation and receipt of a pulse wave of sound. This physical principle has clear implications for patients of larger body habitus whom the sound wave may not penetrate. Some patients of average body habitus may not be well imaged due to poor acoustic windows related to their anatomy. Patients with contractures or in extremis may not be readily positioned for imaging, thus a study may be compromised.

■ There are a number of advantages and disadvantages to ultrasound examinations:

    ADVANTAGES

    ☐ Lack of ionizing radiation: This is of obvious benefit, particularly in patients requiring multiple follow-up examinations.

- [ ] Availability: Due to the decreasing cost of equipment and examination costs, ultrasound has clear benefits from an economic perspective.
- [ ] Access: Due to the relative portability of the equipment, ultrasound is of great value in unstable patients who cannot be safely transported for other imaging modalities (e.g. CT).
- [ ] Vascular imaging: Due to its physical principles, ultrasound is of great value in the evaluation of vascular abnormalities, such as carotid stenosis, vascular graft patency, and DVT.

DISADVANTAGES

- [ ] Operator-dependent: As already noted, ultrasound is highly dependent upon the skill of the sonologist.
- [ ] Patient factors: Ultrasound examinations can be rendered uninterpretable based upon a multitude of patient factors, including patients of larger body habitus, patients in extremis, and patients with contractures. Venous studies for thrombosis can be suboptimal in the presence of central venous catheters and overlying bandages.
- [ ] Technical limitations: Due to the small sector width of the transducers, large areas cannot be imaged as a single unit. Additionally, structures deep within the peritoneal cavity often cannot be visualized. Air is a strong reflector of the ultrasound beam; therefore, air within bowel markedly limits evaluation of adjacent and deep structures.

Vascular Ultrasound

- As previously noted, ultrasound plays a large role in the evaluation of vascular structures, although this role may diminish with the advent of newer imaging techniques in CT and MR.
- It allows for non-invasive imaging of suspected or known vascular abnormalities, both venous and arterial.
- Evaluation may be limited by poor visualization of the vessel in question, based on the previously noted limitations of ultrasound.
- It allows for quantification of degrees of stenosis in various arterial systems, as well as evaluation of direction of vascular flow and vascular patency.
- It often requires high degrees of patient compliance, particularly in studies such as renal artery stenosis ultrasound, which require patients to cooperate with instructions on suspension of respiration.

Carotid Ultrasound

- It is the non-invasive imaging study of choice for evaluation of carotid plaque, vessel patency, and degree of stenosis of the extracranial carotid system. Intracranial carotid disease can be suggested on the basis of the examination; however, it is not adequately evaluated with this study and required dedicated imaging with CT angiography (CTA) or MR angiography (MRA) (less commonly with conventional angiography).
- The direction of blood flow in the vertebral arteries is routinely evaluated on carotid ultrasound. If there is reversal of flow in the vertebral artery, a subclavian steal phenomenon may be suggested and, if feasible, the origin of the subclavian artery can be evaluated. However, due to patient factors, this may not be possible, and dedicated imaging of the subclavian artery with CTA or MRA may be required.
- It requires patients to comply with positioning of the head and neck, which is generally well tolerated.
- The study is performed with routine gray scale images as well as pulsed Doppler examination and should be requested as a Doppler examination for billing purposes.

INDICATIONS
- ☐ Evaluation of patients with syncope for carotid disease as the source of syncope
- ☐ Evaluation of ischemic stroke
- ☐ Evaluation of thromboembolic stroke
- ☐ Screening for carotid disease in patients with known coronary artery disease
- ☐ Evaluation of carotid dissection: CTA and MRA are the imaging modalities of choice for the identification of carotid dissection.

CONTRAINDICATIONS
- ☐ Patients who are recently postoperative may have bandages or sutures that preclude ultrasound probe positioning.
- ☐ Active infection requires sterile probe covers.
- ☐ In patients with known heavy calcification of the carotid system, ultrasound may be of no use as the beam is reflected by the calcium and the vessel cannot be evaluated. CT and MR are more optimal imaging techniques for these patients.

LIMITATIONS
- ☐ Patient body habitus: Patients with short or large necks can be difficult to image.

☐ Vessel anatomy: Vessels that are tortuous or dive deep within the neck can be difficult to visualize and may lead to erroneous velocity measurements.

☐ Flow dynamics: Vessels with extremely sluggish flow may be difficult to distinguish from occluded vessels. This obviously is of great importance in any vascular system, particularly in the carotid. In the carotid, the differentiation of extremely slow flow from vessel occlusion is important as it may alter management and render a patient inoperable for carotid disease (if the vessel is occluded). In these settings, further imaging with MRA or conventional angiography may be necessary.

☐ Carotid dissections can be very difficult to identify if the dissection flap is not readily visible; CTA and MRA are the imaging modalities of choice.

☐ Patients with heavily calcified vessels are not well evaluated as the ultrasound beam cannot penetrate the calcium. This may lead to false positives for occlusion (as no flow can be detected through the calcium) or false negatives for stenosis (as accurate flow velocities cannot be obtained).

Abdominal Aorta Ultrasound

■ It is typically performed without pulsed Doppler imaging.

INDICATIONS

☐ Identification and surveillance of abdominal aortic aneurysms

☐ Identification of aortic dissection: Ultrasound plays a limited role in the evaluation of aortic dissection; CT is the imaging modality of choice.

☐ Identification of aortic aneurysm rupture: Ultrasound plays a limited role in the evaluation of aneurysm rupture as active hemorrhage is characteristically of the same appearance (isoechoic) as surrounding structures and thus is not readily identifiable; CT is the imaging modality of choice.

CONTRAINDICATIONS

☐ Recent abdominal surgery; residual postoperative air and skin staples typically obscure evaluation of the aorta and retroperitoneum

LIMITATIONS

☐ Patient body habitus and clinical condition: Patients with large body habitus or extensive bowel gas (particularly an ileus in the setting of aneurysm rupture) may demonstrate limited evaluation of the aorta. Patients with peritoneal symptoms may not tolerate the examination.

☐ As just noted, evaluation of aneurysm rupture or dissection is suboptimal with ultrasound.

☐ The thoracic aorta is not readily evaluable with transthoracic ultrasound imaging.

Splanchnic Vasculature (Celiac Axis/Superior and Inferior Mesenteric Arteries) Ultrasound

■ It may be performed with or without pulsed Doppler interrogation, depending upon the indication.

■ It requires a high degree of patient cooperation in that compliance with breathing instructions is often necessary for the examination.

INDICATIONS

☐ Acute vessel occlusion: Ultrasound for mesenteric artery occlusion may be performed in a limited patient population (i.e. patients with a strong clinical suspicion of acute mesenteric vessel occlusion who are unable to receive IV contrast for CT or who are unable to undergo MRA or conventional angiography). Typically, only the ostia and proximal main arteries (celiac, superior mesenteric artery [SMA], inferior mesenteric artery [IMA]) can be evaluated. Distal embolic occlusion cannot be evaluated with ultrasound

☐ Chronic intestinal angina (stenosis): In patients with symptoms of chronic intestinal ischemia, ultrasound may be performed to identify and quantify a vessel stenosis. Pulsed Doppler interrogation is required. Again, only the proximal vessels can be interrogated; however, this is the characteristic location for a stenosis due to atherosclerotic disease.

CONTRAINDICATIONS

☐ Arterial velocities in the mesenteric vessels will increase in the setting of a recent meal as the blood flow to the bowel increases during digestion. This may mimic pathology such as arterial stenosis.

LIMITATIONS

☐ Patient body habitus

☐ Patient compliance with breath holding instructions

☐ The study is limited to proximal vessels only.

Renal Artery Stenosis Ultrasound

- It is performed with pulsed Doppler interrogation and must be ordered as such.
- It is often performed as a screening study for the presence of renal artery stenosis. Due to limitations of the study, results are often inconclusive or merely suggestive of the presence of renal artery stenosis. Definitive imaging with CTA, MRA, or conventional angiography is often required.
- It requires a high degree of patient cooperation in that compliance with breathing instructions is necessary for the examination. Ventilated patients are NOT candidates for the examination as appropriate imaging cannot be performed without patient compliance.

INDICATIONS
- ☐ Screening for renovascular hypertension
- ☐ Surveillance of known renal artery stenosis prior to or following revascularization (i.e. stenting)
- ☐ Screening for acute or chronic renal failure; if renal failure is acute, renal vein thrombosis should be considered. Ultrasound is sensitive and specific for renal vein thrombosis.

CONTRAINDICATIONS
- ☐ Ventilated patients as they cannot comply with breath holding instructions
- ☐ Uncooperative or poorly compliant patients as they do not comply with breath holding instructions

LIMITATIONS
- ☐ Large patient body habitus
- ☐ Patient compliance with breath holding instructions
- ☐ Limited sensitivity and specificity for renal artery stenosis. It is sensitive and specific for renal vein thrombosis.
- ☐ It is highly operator-dependent.

Ultrasound Doppler Evaluation of the Hepatic Vasculature/Evaluation of TIPS

- It is performed with pulsed Doppler interrogation.
- It requires a high degree of patient cooperation in that compliance with breathing instructions is necessary for the examination.
- The indication for initial placement of the transjugular intrahepatic portosystemic shunts (TIPS) should be made known to

the sonologist at the time of the examination as the study should include evaluation for this abnormality (i.e. varices, ascites, pleural effusion).

INDICATIONS

☐ Evaluation of vessel flow dynamics to identify the presence of portal hypertension (typically in the setting of known cirrhosis)
☐ Evaluation of vessel patency
  • Pre-TIPS
  • In suspected Budd-Chiari syndrome
☐ Evaluation of TIPS
  • Evaluation of TIPS patency
  • Evaluation of TIPS failure
  • Evaluation of TIPS stenosis

CONTRAINDICATIONS

☐ Acute clinical decompensation: These patients should go directly to angiography if they are unstable and there is high clinical concern for acute TIPS occlusion.

LIMITATIONS

☐ Patient factors:
  • Large body habitus
  • Ascites (it limits evaluation of the vessels due to increased distance from the transducer)
  • Patient compliance with breath holding instructions
  • Severely cirrhotic livers may have diminished caliber vessels, limiting evaluation.
☐ It is highly operator-dependent.
☐ Ventilated patients are NOT candidates for the examination as appropriate imaging cannot be performed without patient compliance.

Vascular Graft Ultrasound

■ It is performed with pulsed Doppler interrogation and must be ordered as such.
■ The type of graft must be made known to the sonologist at the time of the study. Information required includes the following:
  ☐ Type of graft material (i.e. vein or Gore-Tex)
  ☐ Site and type of anastamosis (e.g. femoral to popliteal end to side)
  ☐ Prior angioplasty/surgical revision; presence of known persistent stenosis

■ Ultrasound is NOT the imaging modality of choice for disease of the native vessels of the lower extremities as these cannot be well visualized or evaluated. These studies are highly operator-dependent and should be performed in limited settings with careful physician supervision of experienced technologists.

INDICATIONS
☐ Routine surveillance of graft patency
☐ Surveillance or identification of graft stenosis
☐ Evaluation of graft patency
☐ Evaluation of an acutely cold foot in patients with vascular bypass grafts to evaluate for graft occlusion

CONTRAINDICATIONS
☐ Evaluation of native vessel arterial disease; CTA, MRA, or conventional catheter angiography are the studies of choice for this indication

LIMITATIONS
☐ It is operator-dependent.
☐ Flow dynamics: Vessels with extremely sluggish flow may be difficult to distinguish from occluded vessels. Further evaluation with CTA/MRA or conventional angiography may be required in this setting.
☐ If the anatomy of the graft is not known, it may be difficult to locate the graft and evaluate the anastamoses.

Arteriovenous Graft/Fistula Ultrasound

■ It may be performed with or without pulsed Doppler interrogation depending upon the indication.
☐ If the clinical question is one of graft infection and evaluation is requested to identify a perigraft collection, pulsed Doppler interrogation is not required and the graft will only be evaluated with color Doppler interrogation to assess patency.
☐ If the clinical question is one of arteriovenous graft (AVG)/ arteriovenous fistula (AVF) patency, pulsed Doppler interrogation is required and blood flow and velocities throughout the graft will be obtained.
☐ If the clinical question is one of vascular steal phenomenon (e.g. parasthesias in the hand in a patient with an upper extremity AVF/AVG), this should be clearly communicated to the sonologist at the time of the request as a more detailed

examination is required, including pulsed Doppler evaluation of the graft and the native arteries.

■ The type of graft must be made known to the sonologist at the time of the study. Information required includes the following:
  □ Type of graft or fistula (e.g. Gore-Tex graft or native vein fistula)
  □ Site and type of anastamosis (e.g. brachial artery to brachial vein graft; cephalic vein to radial artery AVF)
  □ Prior angioplasty/surgical revision and if there is a known persistent stenosis

INDICATIONS
  □ Routine surveillance of AVG/AVF patency
  □ Surveillance or identification of AVG/AVF stenosis
  □ Evaluation of AVG/AVF patency
  □ Evaluation of vascular steal phenomenon
  □ Evaluation of perigraft collections (infected graft; performed without pulsed Doppler, as noted earlier)

CONTRAINDICATIONS: None

LIMITATIONS
  □ It is operator-dependent.
  □ Flow dynamics: Vessels with extremely sluggish flow may be difficult to distinguish from occluded vessels. Further evaluation with CTA/MRA or conventional angiography may be required in this setting.

Ultrasound Evaluation of Pseudoaneurysm or Arteriovenous Fistula Following Arterial Puncture

■ It is performed with pulsed Doppler interrogation.
■ It is performed in patients following arterial puncture for angiographic procedures to evaluate for the presence of pseudoaneurysm (PSA) or AVF.

INDICATIONS
  □ Post-catheterization decrease in hematocrit
  □ Post-catheterization increase in pain and bruising at the puncture site
  □ Post-catheterization bruit auscultated at the puncture site
  □ Follow-up of PSA or AVF to evaluate for thrombosis or resolution. Note that graded ultrasound-guided compression is no longer the standard of care for treatment of PSA. Currently, PSA is treated by thrombin injection

under ultrasound guidance (performed by the interventional radiology service in most institutions). AVFs often require surgical correction.

CONTRAINDICATIONS

☐ Active bleeding may make it unsafe or difficult to evaluate the groin.

☐ If the patient has a "fem-stop" compression device on the groin to maintain hemostasis, it may not be safe to remove it to perform imaging until hemostasis is achieved.

☐ Extreme patient discomfort may preclude examination.

LIMITATIONS

☐ It is operator-dependent.

☐ Due to variations in measurement between sonographers, precise comparison between studies may be difficult.

☐ Small AVFs may be difficult to fully interrogate, and it may be difficult to determine the site of origin and entry of the fistula.

☐ It may not be possible to differentiate PSAs with thrombus or very slow flow from an avascular hematoma, even with pulsed Doppler interrogation.

☐ Significant groin hematomas/swelling/bruising may make it difficult to evaluate the groin.

☐ Obese patients with significant pannus may be difficult to evaluate.

☐ High arterial punctures resulting in PSA or AVF formation deep in the pelvis may be difficult to evaluate with ultrasound, particularly in obese patients.

DVT (Upper or Lower Extremity) Ultrasound

■ It is performed with pulsed Doppler interrogation.

INDICATIONS

☐ Unilateral extremity swelling

☐ Surveillance in patients with prolonged bed rest

☐ Screening in patients with documented or highly suspected pulmonary embolism

☐ Documentation of thrombus resolution following therapy

CONTRAINDICATIONS: None

LIMITATIONS

☐ Patient body habitus: In patients with deeply positioned vessels or extensive adipose tissue, a lower frequency transducer may be required to visualize the vessels. Due to the physics of lower frequency transducers, non-occlusive thrombus cannot be excluded.

☐ Patient compliance: If patients are unable to tolerate compression of the vessels, non-occlusive thrombus cannot be excluded.

☐ Access: For patients with surgical dressings, orthopedic hardware, and central venous catheters the vessels may not be accessible to imaging.

☐ Vessels evaluated: In most institutions, only the deep veins of the thigh are evaluated for DVT. Thus, thrombus within the calf is not excluded. If there is persistent concern for calf thrombus, follow-up imaging of the thigh vessels may be performed within 7 days to evaluate for thrombus propagation.

☐ Non-occlusive thrombus may be difficult to differentiate from thick-walled veins due to remote DVT.

Neck Ultrasound (Nonvascular)

Thyroid Ultrasound

■ It is a non-invasive imaging method for patients with palpable abnormalities or abnormal thyroid function studies.

■ The study is complementary to physical examination and nuclear medicine imaging (thyroid uptake and imaging).

■ Minimally invasive, ultrasound-guided percutaneous biopsy of nodules may be performed. This is often performed after correlation with nuclear medicine studies if multiple nodules are present. If there is a solitary nodule, correlation with nuclear medicine imaging may not be necessary prior to decision for biopsy.

INDICATIONS

☐ Evaluation of palpable thyroid nodules
☐ Surveillance of known multinodular goiter
☐ Evaluation of patients with abnormal thyroid function studies (e.g. suspected Hashimoto's thyrotoxicosis, multinodular goiter, Graves' disease)
☐ Pre-biopsy images

CONTRAINDICATIONS: None

LIMITATIONS

☐ Patient factors: Patients with short or large necks can be difficult to image.

☐ Imaging features: Unfortunately, there are no reliable distinguishing features between benign and neoplastic thyroid nodules (this is true for all imaging modalities). It is for this reason that percutaneous tissue sampling is required. As noted already, this is often performed in conjunction with the results of nuclear medicine imaging.

☐ Technical factors: Due to differences in scanning technique and measurement between technologists, direct comparison of measurements may be difficult.

Parathyroid Gland Ultrasound

▪ This is a non-invasive imaging method to evaluate for the presence of parathyroid adenoma.

▪ It is complementary to laboratory investigations and nuclear medicine imaging. It is often employed in parallel with nuclear imaging studies.

▪ It may obviate the need for exploratory neck dissection and direct surgical intervention.

▪ Minimally invasive, ultrasound-guided percutaneous biopsy of adenomas may be performed in limited settings.

INDICATIONS

☐ Primary imaging performed for the identification of parathyroid adenomas in patients with a high clinical suspicion

☐ Performed in conjunction with nuclear medicine imaging to interrogate regions of abnormal radiotracer uptake and localize the adenoma

CONTRAINDICATIONS: None

LIMITATIONS

☐ Patient factors: Patients with short or large necks can be difficult to image.

☐ Technical factors: Due to the often diminutive size of the adenomas, they may be difficult to identify. Additionally, as the parathyroid glands can be ectopic and may be found in locations such as the mediastinum, they may not be amenable to imaging with ultrasound.

Soft Tissues of the Neck Ultrasound

▪ The study may be performed with or without pulsed Doppler interrogation dependent upon the indication for the examination.

▪ It is often performed for palpable abnormalities within the soft tissues of the neck.

- It may be performed prior to planned biopsy or drainage of the palpable abnormality.

INDICATIONS

- ☐ Evaluation of suspected lymphadenopathy to confirm the diagnosis and to evaluate for possible necrotic lymphadenopathy or drainable abscess. Unfortunately, benign and neoplastic lymph nodes cannot be reliably distinguished with ultrasound imaging.
- ☐ Evaluation of a palpable abnormality, including cutaneous lesions believed to represent vascular abnormalities, lymphangiomas, hemangiomas, and so on. Ultrasound (which often requires pulsed Doppler interrogation in this setting) may be performed to confirm the diagnosis and to evaluate extent of the lesions and possible involvement of surrounding structures such as muscle.
- ☐ Evaluation and biopsy guidance for drainable collections.

CONTRAINDICATIONS: None

LIMITATIONS

- ☐ Patient factors: Patients with short or large necks can be difficult to image.
- ☐ It may not be possible to make a definitive diagnosis of a soft tissue lesion (e.g. a hematoma cannot reliably be differentiated from an infected hematoma or abscess).
- ☐ Air within a collection may reflect the ultrasound beam, rendering the examination uninterpretable.

Breast Ultrasound

- It is often performed with pulsed Doppler interrogation; however, this may not be required.
- It is characteristically performed in conjunction with mammography, although it may be requested for evaluation of a palpable abnormality in young patients.
- Ultrasound plays a controversial role in screening for breast carcinoma. Currently, it is NOT advocated for primary screening for malignancy.

INDICATIONS

- ☐ Adjunct to mammography to distinguish cysts (simple and complex) from solid masses
- ☐ Therapeutic planning: In patients with mammographically suspicious lesions that require biopsy, ultrasound may be

requested to evaluate if the lesion is amenable to biopsy with ultrasound guidance (as opposed to mammographic x-ray guidance). Ultrasound is a less expensive, easily performed biopsy procedure.

☐ In young, premenopausal women (<40 years old), ultrasound is the imaging method of choice for the evaluation of palpable abnormalities. These patients have dense breasts, which are not easily evaluable with mammography, thus masses can often be difficult to identify.

☐ Evaluation for abscess formation in patients with mastitis. Ultrasound-guided drainage of breast abscesses may also be performed.

CONTRAINDICATIONS: None

LIMITATIONS

☐ Patient factors:
  • Patients with pendulous breasts are often difficult to evaluate and lesions may be of a depth or position where they cannot be identified or readily evaluated.
  • Patients with predominantly fatty replaced breasts are difficult to evaluate with ultrasound as lesions may be obscured in the fatty parenchyma.

☐ Technical factors:
  • Ultrasound is a valuable tool in the evaluation of masses; however, it is NOT able to evaluate or reliably identify calcifications. Calcifications must be evaluated with mammography.
  • Breast ultrasound is highly operator-dependent.

Chest Ultrasound

■ It has limited applications.

■ Echocardiography is the purview of cardiologists in most institutions and will not be considered further in this section.

■ For the majority of indications (excluding cardiac), studies are performed without pulsed Doppler interrogation.

INDICATIONS

☐ Identification of pleural fluid and marking or guidance for thoracentesis.

☐ There are recent reports of identification of pneumothoraces with ultrasound (highly operator-dependent).

☐ Evaluation of soft tissue abnormalities of the chest wall

CONTRAINDICATIONS: None

LIMITATIONS

☐ It is operator-dependent.

☐ Positioning may make it difficult to image the patient. This is particularly true in pleural effusions. In patients who are able to sit erect or mobilize, pleural effusions will be located dependently in the pleural space (i.e. costophrenic angles). However, in recumbent patients, the fluid will follow gravity and be distributed along the posterior pleural surface and will not be located in the costophrenic angles. Thus, it may be difficult to identify and sample if the patient cannot be repositioned.

Abdomen Ultrasound

Right Upper Quadrant Ultrasound

■ It is performed without pulsed Doppler interrogation. If a pulsed Doppler study of the hepatic vasculature is desired (see indications listed previously), right upper quadrant ultrasound must be requested separately.

■ It involves evaluation of the hepatobiliary tree (i.e. liver, intra-hepatic biliary ductal dilation, common bile duct, and gallblad-der), pancreas, and right kidney.

■ It is the imaging study of choice for acute cholecystitis.

INDICATIONS

☐ Evaluation of right upper quadrant pain, particularly attri-buted to the hepatobiliary tree. It is the imaging study of choice for acute cholecystitis (although there are limita-tions).

☐ Evaluation for intra/extrahepatic biliary ductal dilation for pre-endoscopic retrograde cholangiopancreatography (ERCP)/percutaneous biliary drainage planning

☐ Evaluation of masses (hepatic/pancreatic/renal) identified with other imaging modalities (typically CT)

☐ It may identify right hydronephrosis, calculi, or masses, although this should be further evaluated with a dedicated renal (retroperitoneal) ultrasound.

CONTRAINDICATIONS

☐ Recent meal (within 4–6 hours) as this will contract the gallbladder, limiting evaluation for gallstones. It may lead to false-positive findings of wall thickening as the gallbladder will be contracted.

☐ Recent administration of analgesics (e.g. morphine); this will cause the gallbladder and sphincter of Oddi to contract. It will also mask the presence of a sonographic Murphy's sign, which may render diagnosis of acute cholecystitis difficult, particularly in equivocal cases.

LIMITATIONS

☐ Patient factors:

- Obese patients may be suboptimally evaluated due to limitations of ultrasound beam penetration.
- In patients with fatty infiltration of the liver, masses may be obscured and thus may go undetected.
- In patients with co-morbidities such as ascites, hepatitis, and HIV, cholangiopathy may manifest ultrasound features, mimicking acute cholecystitis although the disease is not present. In these patients, nuclear medicine imaging (HIDA) may be required to confirm or refute the diagnosis of cholecystitis.
- Patients with significant bowel gas have limited evaluation of the pancreas.

☐ Operator factors: Image quality is dependent upon the sonologist.

☐ Technical factors: Due to the presence of bowel gas as well as patient factors, the common bile duct often cannot be visualized in its entirety. This clearly limits evaluation for choledocholithiasis. Additionally, ultrasound has a low sensitivity for the presence of choledocholithiasis (ERCP and MR cholangiopancreatography [MRCP] are the imaging modalities of choice although CT may be performed in an attempt to identify the presence of a stone).

☐ Ascending cholangitis may be suggested based on the appearance of the liver and the portal triads; however, it remains a clinical diagnosis.

Abdominal Ultrasound

▪ It is performed without pulsed Doppler interrogation. If a pulsed Doppler study of the hepatic vasculature is desired (see indications listed previously), abdominal ultrasound must be requested separately.

■ It involves evaluation of the hepatobiliary tree (i.e. liver, intra-hepatic biliary ductal dilation, common bile duct, and gallbladder), pancreas, both kidneys, and the spleen. Depending upon the institution, limited evaluation of the aorta and inferior vena cava at the level of the liver may be performed as part of the routine study.

■ It is a more comprehensive examination than a right upper quadrant ultrasound.

INDICATIONS

☐ Surveillance of patients with hepatitis B and C. The study is performed to screen for focal hepatic masses that may represent early hepatocellular carcinomas. The abdominal ultrasound also allows for evaluation of splenic size in patients with known or suspected portal hypertension in the setting of cirrhosis or hepatitis infections.

☐ In patients unable or unwilling to undergo CT or MR examinations for surveillance of metastatic disease, ultrasound may be performed, although sensitivity for metastatic disease (particularly to bowel) is significantly lower than that of CT or MR.

☐ Evaluation of pregnant patients with trauma or history of malignancy. These patients are unable to undergo CT examinations due to the radiation and contrast risks to the fetus. MR has as yet unknown risks to a fetus.

☐ Evaluation of clinically suspected organomegaly or surveillance of known organomegaly (particularly in patients with known deposition disorders such as Gaucher's).

CONTRAINDICATIONS

☐ Recent meal (within 4–6 hours) will contract the gallbladder, limiting evaluation for gallstones. It may lead to false-positive findings of wall thickening as the gallbladder will be contracted.

☐ Recent administration of analgesics (morphine) will cause the gallbladder and sphincter of Oddi to contract. It will also mask the presence of a sonographic Murphy's sign, which may render diagnosis of acute cholecystitis difficult, particularly in equivocal cases.

LIMITATIONS

☐ Patient factors:
  • Obese patients may be suboptimally evaluated due to limitations of ultrasound beam penetration.

- In patients with fatty infiltration of the liver, masses may be obscured and thus may go undetected.
- Patients with co-morbidities such as ascites, hepatitis, and HIV cholangiopathy may manifest ultrasound features mimicking acute cholecystitis, although the disease is not present. In these patients, nuclear medicine imaging (HIDA) may be required to confirm or refute the diagnosis of cholecystitis.
- Patients with significant bowel gas have limited evaluation of the pancreas.

☐ Operator factors: Image quality is dependent upon the sonologist.
☐ Technical factors: Due to the limitations of sector width of the transducers, it may be difficult to obtain a precise measurement of enlarged organs such as the spleen.

Limited Abdominal Ultrasound

▪ It may be performed without or with pulsed Doppler interrogation, depending upon the indication for the examination.
▪ It does NOT evaluate the entire abdomen nor does it evaluate the visceral structures.

INDICATIONS
☐ Evaluation for free fluid in trauma
☐ Identification and marking for paracentesis
☐ Evaluation of palpable soft tissue masses in the abdomen (may require pulsed Doppler interrogation)
☐ Evaluation of muscle tears (highly operator-dependent; not routinely performed at all institutions)
☐ Evaluation of suspected appendicitis or intussusceptions (pediatric population)

CONTRAINDICATIONS: None

LIMITATIONS
☐ It is operator-dependent.
☐ Excessive bowel gas may make it difficult to evaluate the appendix.
☐ Acute hemorrhage is echogenic and cannot be reliably identified among the normally echogenic bowel gas.
☐ Thin patients are good candidates for evaluation of appendicitis with ultrasound; larger patients are difficult to image for appendicitis. In these patients, CT is the study of choice.

Retroperitoneal (Renal) Ultrasound

■ It is performed without pulsed Doppler interrogation. If a pulsed Doppler study of the renal vasculature is desired (see indications listed previously), retroperitoneal ultrasound must be requested separately.

■ It involves evaluation of the kidneys and bladder.

INDICATIONS

☐ Evaluation of obstruction (hydronephrosis) in patients with acute renal failure

☐ Evaluation of patients with chronic renal insufficiency

☐ Evaluation of renal masses demonstrated on other imaging modalities (e.g. CT)

☐ Evaluation for renal infection (e.g. fungal disease). Pyelonephritis is NOT an imaging diagnosis although ultrasound can (occasionally) suggest the diagnosis.

CONTRAINDICATIONS: None

LIMITATIONS

☐ Patient factors:
   • Obese patients may be suboptimally evaluated due to limitations of ultrasound beam penetration.
   • Patients unable to comply with breath holding instructions may not be optimally imaged. (Due to the retroperitoneal location of the kidneys, inspiration is required to reposition the kidneys where they may be imaged.)

☐ Operator factors: Image quality is dependent upon the sonologist.

☐ Technical factors: Small masses may be below the resolution of ultrasound; therefore, it is often not possible to differentiate between a cyst and a solid lesion in masses <1 cm in diameter. This is also true for larger lesions in obese patients.

Renal Transplant Ultrasound

■ It is performed with pulsed Doppler interrogation.

■ It involves evaluation of the renal transplant and bladder only. The native kidneys are NOT evaluated.

INDICATIONS

☐ Immediate postoperative baseline study

☐ Immediate postoperative study in operatively complicated cases to evaluate vascular patency (e.g. evaluate for renal vein thrombosis, renal artery dissection, or thrombosis)

☐ Surveillance of transplants

☐ Evaluation of transplant complications (e.g. rejection, vascular compromise, cyclosporine toxicity) in transplant patients with worsening renal function

☐ Evaluation of peritransplant collections

CONTRAINDICATIONS: None

LIMITATIONS

☐ Patient factors: Immediately postoperatively, patients may not tolerate imaging due to local pain at the incision site. Additionally, dressings and extensive edema may limit visualization of the transplant.

☐ Operator factors: Image quality is dependent upon the sonologist.

☐ Technical factors: Due to the limitations of sector width of the transducers, it may be difficult to obtain a precise measurement of the size of a peritransplant collection.

Pancreatic Transplant Ultrasound

▪ It is performed with pulsed Doppler interrogation.

▪ It evaluates the pancreatic transplant only.

▪ Pancreatic transplant ultrasound has a less well-defined role for pancreatic transplants than renal transplant ultrasound. Ultrasound plays a limited role in the evaluation of rejection. Unlike a renal transplant, there is no role for resistive indices or blood flow patterns to suggest the presence of rejection. The main role for ultrasound is the evaluation of pancreatitis.

INDICATIONS

☐ Immediate postoperative baseline study

☐ Immediate postoperative study in operatively complicated cases to evaluate vasculature

☐ Surveillance of transplants

☐ Evaluation of transplant pancreatitis

☐ Less well-defined role in the evaluation of rejection than renal transplant ultrasound. MR is an emerging tool for the evaluation of pancreatic transplants.

CONTRAINDICATIONS: None

LIMITATIONS

☐ Patient factors: Immediately postoperatively, patients may not tolerate imaging due to local pain at the incision site. Additionally, dressings and extensive edema may limit visualization of the transplant.

☐ Operator factors: Image quality is dependent upon the sonologist.

☐ Technical factors: Due to the limitations of sector width of the transducers, it may be difficult to obtain a precise measurement of the size of a peritransplant collection.

☐ Limited use in the evaluation of transplant failure

Pelvic Ultrasound (Females)

▪ It may be performed without or with pulsed Doppler interrogation, depending upon the indication for the examination.

▪ It evaluates the uterus and adnexal structures.

▪ It may be performed transvaginally or transabdominally, depending upon patient factors and the indication for the examination.

▪ It is imperative that the patient's human chorionic gonadotropin (hCG) state (i.e. pregnant or not) be made known to the sonologist prior to commencement of the examination. If available, quantitative serum hCG values should also be made known to the sonologist at the time of request of the study as this will determine what findings will be present at that stage of the pregnancy.

▪ Indications for transvaginal examination: It is the study of choice (over transabdominal imaging) for evaluation of female pelvic pathology.

▪ Pregnant patients (<10 weeks of gestation; after a gestational age of approximately 10 weeks, the uterus becomes an abdominal organ and fetuses are better evaluated from a transabdominal approach):

☐ Patients with pain: In early gestation, pregnant patients with pelvic pain are evaluated for ectopic gestations, threatened or missed abortion, ovarian cyst rupture, or degenerating fibroids.

☐ Patients with vaginal bleeding: Evaluation for threatened or missed abortion

- ☐ Evaluation of suspected retained products of conception
- ☐ Evaluation of suspected endometritis
- ▪ Non-pregnant patients:
  - ☐ Patients with pain: Evaluation for ovarian torsion, ovarian cyst rupture, degenerating fibroids, tubo-ovarian abscess, hydrosalpinx, endometriosis
  - ☐ Patients with vaginal bleeding: Evaluation for endometrial abnormalities (e.g. polyps, hyperplasia, tamoxifen-induced change, endometrial carcinoma [endometrial carcinoma requires pulsed Doppler interrogation]); fibroids, adenomyosis
  - ☐ Patients with adnexal masses identified on palpation or with imaging: Pulsed Doppler interrogation is required. Ultrasound may be able to distinguish benign ovarian disease from neoplasm, although this may be difficult.
  - ☐ Screening: Ovarian cancer screening is a controversial subject; however, if it is performed, it should be performed as a transvaginal examination.

INDICATIONS

- ☐ Pregnant patients: Fetal anatomic survey, fetal age determination, fetal viability assessment in the setting of vaginal bleeding or trauma, placenta previa assessment
- ☐ Non-pregnant patients: Evaluation of pelvic pain, vaginal bleeding, or adnexal masses in patients unable to tolerate transvaginal imaging

CONTRAINDICATIONS

- ☐ It is controversial whether or not transvaginal imaging should be performed in pregnant patients with a suspicion of endometritis. There is a theoretic risk of spreading infection through the probe as it is not sterile.

LIMITATIONS

- ☐ Patient factors: Patients may not be able to tolerate transvaginal imaging, thus necessitating transabdominal imaging, which may limit evaluation of pathology. Obese patients may be suboptimally evaluated due to limitations of ultrasound beam penetration.
- ☐ Operator factors: Image quality is dependent upon the sonologist.
- ☐ Technical factors: Due to the limitations of sector width of the transducers, it may be difficult to obtain a precise measurement of large masses.

11

Nuclear Medicine

General Considerations

■ There are multiple and varied uses for nuclear medicine imaging.

■ It allows both anatomic/pathologic and functional imaging.

■ It requires the administration of radioactive material (administration routes vary and include IV, intrathecal, and subcutaneous around cutaneous lesions).

■ It has poor anatomic resolution, making precise localization of disease difficult.

■ The advent of PET/PET CT allows evaluation of metabolism and perfusion with the added benefit of correlation with anatomic detail (PET CT).

IMAGING LIMITATIONS

☐ Patient factors:
- Body habitus: Patients >350 lbs cannot be imaged on conventional tables.
- Patient positioning: Patients with contractures or inability to remain stationary are difficult to image.
- Patient stability: Due to the relatively long length of some studies, patients may not be candidates for nuclear medicine studies if they require monitoring or intensive care therapy.

☐ Technologic factors:
- Different isotopes (radiotracers) have different energies and different decay times. This limits which studies can be performed in close temporal proximity to each other and dictates the order in which studies can be performed.

This is particularly important in cardiac imaging where rest and stress studies may require 2 days of imaging.

- Radioactive material decays at specific rates (half-life). Due to the variable half-lives of the agents used for clinically applied nuclear medicine, only a certain number of studies may be performed on a daily basis. Additionally, the agents that are used for the study (e.g. diseida for HIDA scans) are often scarce, limiting the number of studies that may be performed at any given time. There are strict quality-control measures in place for the agents used in nuclear imaging. If an agent does not pass quality control, its production may be halted for a significant amount of time, thus rendering it impossible to perform studies using that agent.

- Due to the rate at which different isotopes decay and the extended periods of time that are often required for the agent to be taken up by the tissues, there are limitations on when studies can be performed. For example, it takes approximately 2–4 hours for technetium-99m (^{99m}Tc) methylene diphosphonate (MDP) (the agent used for bone scans) to be cleared from the background tissues and to bind to the bones. This requires injection of the agent early in the morning so that image acquisition can be performed in the afternoon (after a 4-hour delay). Other agents, such as gallium (which is most often used for lymphoma imaging) may require as many as 2–6 days to clear background and bowel activity to an acceptable level that allows pathology to be recognized.

- Nuclear studies often require multiple days of imaging; patients must return on multiple consecutive days for completion of the imaging (this is particularly true for gallium studies).

- With all nuclear imaging studies, metallic devices in or on a patient will attenuate (stop) the radiation from reaching the detector and cause an artifact, which can obscure disease.

- Safety issues:
  - The agents used for nuclear medicine imaging are radioactive and often have long half-lives or decay to isotopes with long half-lives. This poses safety and

disposal concerns. Strict guidelines are in effect for the handling and disposal of radionuclides. Conversely, the agents used for PET imaging have extremely short half-lives, requiring rapid imaging. Some PET isotopes have such short half-lives that on-site cyclotrons are required to produce the isotopes and allow for imaging.

- Certain types of nuclear medicine studies (e.g. white blood cell [WBC] and tagged red blood cell [RBC] studies) require ex vivo (i.e. outside the patient) labeling of blood with the agent. This requires blood to be withdrawn from the patient and manually mixed with the tracer to enable binding. This has obvious drawbacks, which place technologists and patients at risk for blood-borne pathogens.

CNS Imaging

■ Nuclear medicine studies allow for physiologic and anatomic imaging. So-called ictal (injection during seizure activity) and interictal (between seizure) studies are performed to evaluate the seizure focus. Due to its properties, rapid injection of tracer is required during seizures in patients undergoing ictal SPECT imaging. Therefore, patients must be on a ward floor where isotopes and technicians are rapidly available to inject the agent once a seizure occurs.

■ Physiologic imaging may be performed in different ways in the CNS, depending upon the information that is required. Perfusion imaging may be performed, as may imaging to evaluate metabolism. The tracer is different for both types of study.

Technetium-99m Hexamethylpropyleneamine Oxime CNS Imaging

■ This is an agent used for perfusion imaging in the brain. It does not provide information about brain metabolism.

■ Imaging is performed on a typical nuclear medicine gamma camera (it is NOT a PET agent).

■ It may be used as an ictal or interictal agent (i.e. injecting while the patient is actively seizing or between seizures).

■ The radiotracer has a 6-hour half-life; however, in brain imaging, rapid imaging after tracer injection is required (within 2–6 hours).

INDICATIONS

☐ Evaluation of patients with seizures with the intent being to identify the seizure focus. It is often interpreted in conjunction with a concurrent MRI of the brain.

☐ Evaluation of brain death

CONTRAINDICATIONS: None

LIMITATIONS

☐ False-negative results can occur for the evaluation of seizures with this technique.

☐ As with all nuclear medicine imaging studies, there is poor spatial resolution of this technique; therefore, it is difficult to precisely localize the area of abnormal uptake.

F-18 Fluorodeoxyglucose CNS Imaging

■ This is an agent used for evaluation of brain metabolism. It also evaluates brain perfusion.

■ Imaging is performed on a dedicated PET camera, a modified gamma camera, or a dedicated combined PET CT camera.

■ Due to the short half-life (approximately 90 minutes) and the often remote location of a PET camera, it is typically used for interictal (between seizures) imaging.

■ As with all fluorodeoxyglucose (FDG) imaging, tracer uptake is dependent upon serum glucose levels and insulin levels. Patients should be fasting for the studies in order for uptake to occur in the brain.

INDICATIONS

☐ Evaluation of patients with seizures to identify the seizure focus. It is often interpreted in conjunction with MRIs and perfusion imaging (^{99m}Tc hexamethylpropyleneamine oxime [HMPAO]).

☐ Evaluation of patients with suspected Parkinson's, Pick's disease

☐ Evaluation of patients with cerebrovascular accident to evaluate for potential residual function

CONTRAINDICATIONS

☐ Patients actively seizing

☐ Unstable patients (Long imaging times are required and the camera is often remote from immediate medical assistance.)

LIMITATIONS

☐ The short half-life of the tracer limits the locations of patient injection and imaging.

☐ Brain uptake is dependent upon factors such as the serum glucose and insulin levels. If the serum levels are not appropriate, uptake will occur in structures outside the brain.

☐ Skeletal muscle activity at the time of tracer injection will result in uptake in the skeletal muscles, which can complicate image interpretation.

Cerebrospinal Fluid Leak

▪ This is an invasive procedure that involves a multidisciplinary approach. The procedure involves nuclear medicine technologists and physicians, ear nose throat (ENT) specialists, and neuroradiologists.

▪ It is performed as follows. Pledgets are placed into the nasal cavity (near the cribriform plate) by ENT. The patient is then transferred to the fluoroscopy suite where a neuroradiologist performs a lumbar puncture. In conjunction with the nuclear medicine technologist, the neuroradiologist administers intrathecal radiotracer. The pledgets are subsequently removed by ENT after approximately 24 hours and radioactivity assessed with a Geiger counter. If there is radioactivity on the pledgets, a cerebrospinal fluid (CSF) leak is present.

INDICATIONS

☐ Assessment of clinically suspected CSF leak (e.g. following intracranial surgery, trauma)

CONTRAINDICATIONS: None

LIMITATIONS

☐ If the pledgets are not appropriately positioned, a leak may not be identified.

☐ Small leaks that allow only minimal leakage of radiotracer may not be detectable.

Obstructive Hydrocephalus

▪ It may be necessary clinically to differentiate between communicating and noncommunicating hydrocephalus in order to appropriately treat the condition. This may not always be possible with conventional imaging such as CT and MRI.

▪ In certain cases, nuclear medicine studies may be helpful in differentiating between communicating and noncommunicating hydrocephalus.

▪ The study is performed with the intrathecal administration (i.e. into the spinal canal) of a radiotracer. Delayed imaging is then performed at intervals up to 48 hours in order to determine the type of hydrocephalus present and at what level.

INDICATION
☐ Determination of the type of hydrocephalus present and the level of obstruction

CONTRAINDICATIONS: None

LIMITATION
☐ If the lumbar puncture is difficult to perform, it may not be possible to administer the tracer into the appropriate location, thus making diagnosis impossible.

Vascular/Lymphatic

SVC/IVC Obstruction

▪ In patients in whom there is concern for superior or inferior vena cava obstruction (either from thrombosis or extrinsic compression), diagnosis may not be possible with conventional imaging methods. This is typically secondary to body habitus and inability to undergo an IV contrast-enhanced CT (e.g. due to poor renal function) or MR (e.g. pacemaker).

▪ By injecting the upper (SVC) or lower extremity (IVC) veins bilaterally simultaneously, complete occlusion or sluggish flow may be identified.

▪ The imaging agent is usually ^{99m}Tc-labeled sulfur colloid.

INDICATIONS
☐ Evaluation of patients with suspected thrombosis of the superior or inferior vena cava
☐ Evaluation of suspected extrinsic compression of the SVC or IVC

CONTRAINDICATIONS
☐ Partial vessel thrombosis: Nuclear medicine imaging does not have adequate spatial resolution to identify non-occlusive thrombus; however, sluggish flow may be identified as a secondary sign of partial thrombosis.

☐ The study can identify a location of occlusion or extrinsic compression; however, due to the fact that only vascular structures are directly visualized, the cause of the compression cannot be directly identified.

LIMITATIONS

☐ Poor spatial resolution: It may not be possible to precisely localize a site of thrombus.

☐ Non-occlusive thrombus cannot be excluded.

☐ If venous access cannot be obtained, the study cannot be performed.

☐ Very sluggish flow may be difficult to differentiate from thrombus.

Lymphatic Stasis

■ Patients may have lymphatic stasis for a variety of reasons, including nodal disease obstructing lymphatic drainage, extrinsic mass effect upon lymphatics, infections (e.g. filiariasis), and others. Lymphedema may be clinically difficult to differentiate from other causes of extremity swelling such as DVT.

■ In the past, lymphangiography was performed with iodinated contrast and x-rays. Currently, these studies may be performed with intralymphatic injection of a radiotracer (^{99m}Tc sulfur colloid). Immediate and delayed images of the lymphatics are then obtained. Obstructed or sluggish lymphatic drainage can be identified along with the level of obstruction.

INDICATION

☐ Evaluation of suspected or known lymphatic obstruction or lymphedema

CONTRAINDICATIONS: None

LIMITATIONS

☐ If there is complete lymphatic obstruction, the tracer may remain localized to the injection site.

☐ Due to the poor spatial resolution of nuclear imaging, the precise level of lymphatic obstruction may be difficult to determine.

☐ The study will only evaluate the lymphatic drainage from a region; it cannot determine the etiology of lymphatic obstruction. MR (with the appropriately tailored sequences) may be a more useful examination as the lymphatics can be evaluated if obstructed and the cause of lymphatic obstruction may be identified.

Lymphoscintigraphy/Sentinel Node Sampling

■ It involves subdermal injection of radiotracer around a lesion (usually a malignant lesion) to evaluate lymphatic involvement by tumor.

■ A total of six or more separate injections are made around a skin lesion with deposition of ^{99m}Tc-labeled sulfur colloid. Imaging is then performed immediately and following a delay of 6 hours. Both local lymphatics and whole body imaging are performed. This allows the entire lymphatic drainage pattern to be identified.

INDICATIONS

☐ Evaluation of lymphatic involvement by localized malignant skin lesions, typically melanoma

☐ Breast carcinoma, particularly to assess for sentinel node involvement. Sentinel lymph nodes are the first lymph node involved by the spread of the carcinoma. The skin is injected and imaging performed. The patient is then transferred to the operating room and a Geiger counter is used to identify the radioactive lymph node so that it may be sampled.

CONTRAINDICATIONS: None

LIMITATIONS

☐ If imaging is not performed in the appropriate timeframe, false-negative results may occur.

☐ If the injections are not appropriately placed, tracer may accumulate around the lesion and not travel into the lymphatics.

Bone Scan

■ It is performed for a variety of indications and is one of the most commonly performed nuclear medicine imaging studies.

■ The patient is administered a radiolabeled agent that binds to bone (^{99m}Tc-labeled MDP) and imaging is performed after a delay to allow adequate time for the tracer to bind to bone. Depending upon the indication for the study, imaging may be performed immediately following the administration of the

Nuclear Medicine

agent (i.e. angiographic phase images) in addition to the delayed images.

■ Due to the physical characteristics of the tracer and the physiologic uptake time of the MDP, imaging is typically performed 4 hours following the tracer administration to allow for adequate time for the agent to be taken up by the bones and to allow adequate time for the agent to be cleared from the soft tissues (to decrease background noise). For this reason, patients undergoing bone scans are administered the tracer early in the morning and are imaged in the afternoon. Due to the required delay, patients cannot be injected in the afternoon and imaged the same day in most clinical practices due to limitations of personnel and equipment.

INDICATIONS

☐ Evaluation of patients with suspected osteomyelitis. For these patients, angiographic phase (i.e. immediately after tracer administration) images are obtained as well as delayed images.

☐ Evaluation of patients with suspected reflex sympathetic dystrophy (RSD). This entity is often the consequence of prior trauma and is a cause of persistent osseous pain and bone demineralization. It too requires angiographic and delayed images of the area in question.

☐ Evaluation of patients with suspected osseous metastatic disease. Whole body bone scanning is an effective, rapid screening modality for patients with known or suspected osseous metastatic disease. The entire body can be imaged rapidly with a single injection of the bone scan agent. MRI is very sensitive and specific for metastatic disease; however, due to the lengthy imaging times required and the inability to image the whole body with MR, bone scan is the study of choice for screening patients for metastatic disease. MR is typically reserved for problem-solving specific lesions or for evaluating for complication of metastatic disease such as spinal cord compression.

☐ Metabolic bone disease may be suggested or diagnosed on the basis of bone scan results. Certain metabolic bone diseases such as hyperparathyroidism may produce what is termed a *superscan*. This is a characteristic appearance on a whole body bone scan, whereby the normally visualized renal activity is not present and the appendicular skeleton

contrast material. If the patient is to undergo thyroid imaging, a contrast-enhanced CT should not be performed within 12 weeks of the study as the uptake of the radiotracer will be affected by the contrast. The converse is not true (i.e. the patient may undergo a contrast-enhanced CT following a thyroid uptake and scan).

▪ Patients on thyroid replacement therapy (e.g. synthroid) should discontinue medication or be switched to a T3 preparation for at least 4–6 weeks prior to the examination to prevent competitive binding with the tracer for uptake. This can result in poor uptake of the radiotracer by the gland.

▪ The study allows for identification of abnormal thyroid function (i.e. uptake for hypo/hyperthyroidism) and for morphologic abnormalities including gland size, positioning, and presence (i.e. congenital absence or residual tissues). It allows identification of hyperfunctioning nodules (i.e. "hot nodules") and areas of decreased function, which may represent malignancy (i.e. "cold nodules").

INDICATIONS

☐ Evaluation of patients with known or suspected hypo/hyperthyroid states as a baseline or following therapy

☐ Evaluation of infants with suspected thyroid agenesis, dysgenesis, or lingual thyroid

☐ Evaluation of patients with palpable thyroid nodules or suspected thyroid masses/nodules. This is often performed in conjunction with ultrasound to determine if nodules identified on ultrasound are nonmalignant lesions, such as colloid cysts, or if they may represent areas of malignancy. This correlation of studies will often allow for tissue sampling (i.e. biopsy) of a single lesion (which is typically a "cold nodule") in the setting of multiple thyroid nodules.

☐ Evaluation of thyroiditis

CONTRAINDICATIONS

☐ Pregnancy: Fetuses <12 weeks of gestation have not yet fully formed the thyroid gland; therefore, iodinated agents administered to the mother may have an adverse affect on the fetal thyroid and should not be performed for routine purposes.

☐ Hyperthyroid patients may undergo thyroid storm precipitated by the administration of iodine for diagnostic or therapeutic purposes. This is a relative risk and does not preclude the patient from nuclear medicine imaging; however, if there

Nuclear Medicine

is clinical concern that the patient is at risk for thyroid storm, consultation with a nuclear medicine physician is suggested.

☐ Breastfeeding must be discontinued for several days due to excretion of the tracer into breast milk. Adequate time must be allowed for complete decay of the radiotracer. The radioactive iodine will be taken up by the infant's thyroid gland and can damage it.

LIMITATIONS

☐ Patient factors:
- As with all imaging, patient body habitus has an impact on thyroid imaging, although this is less of a factor than with whole body imaging.
- The camera used for thyroid images closely approaches the patient's head, which may be difficult for anxious patients to tolerate, thus limiting the study.
- As noted earlier, patients who have undergone recent contrast-enhanced CT imaging are not candidates for thyroid uptake and scan within 12 weeks due to the relative suppression of uptake due to the iodinated contrast. This is also true for non-ionic IV contrast, which does still have a small amount of iodine.
- Clearance time of radioactivity is dependent upon the tracer used. ^{99m}Tc pertechnetate has the shortest half-life; therefore, it is cleared the most rapidly from the body.

Iodine-131 Thyroid Imaging

■ It is performed on patients with known thyroid malignancy for the evaluation of sites of disease (staging) and sites of recurrence.

■ The tracer is administered orally and is absorbed from the gastrointestinal (GI) tract into the blood. It then travels to the thyroid gland, where it is concentrated and organified. Initial imaging is typically performed the day following administration of the thyroid capsule in order to allow enough time for background activity to clear.

■ It is performed over several days to determine all sites of disease.

INDICATIONS

☐ Evaluation of sites of metastatic thyroid malignancy

☐ Evaluation of sites of recurrent thyroid malignancy

CONTRAINDICATIONS

☐ Breastfeeding must be discontinued for weeks after imaging due to excretion of the tracer into breast milk. The radioactive iodine will be taken up by the infant's thyroid gland and can damage it.

☐ Pregnancy: Radioactive iodine will cross the placenta and can damage the developing fetal thyroid. This can result in congenital hypothyroidism.

☐ Hyperthyroid patients may undergo thyroid storm, precipitated by the administration of iodine for diagnostic or therapeutic purposes. This is a relative risk and does not preclude the patient from nuclear medicine imaging; however, if there is clinical concern that the patient is at risk for thyroid storm, consultation with a nuclear medicine physician is suggested.

LIMITATIONS

☐ The study is low resolution due to the imaging properties of the agent used; therefore, precise localization of sites of disease may be difficult.

☐ Local disease at the thyroid/surgical bed may be difficult to identify due to the concentration of agent uptake by the gland.

☐ The high energy of the radioisotope requires that a lower dose be administered due to the radiation risks.

☐ The higher energy of the tracer results in penetration of the gamma rays (radiation) through the partitions in the camera (collimator), which results in poorer resolution of the image. This may cause sites of disease to be obscured.

☐ The long half-life (i.e. decay time) of the agent leads to longer duration of radiation exposure in the body.

Radioactive Thyroid Ablation

▪ It is performed by the oral administration of radioactive iodine (I-131) following calculation of the dose required. The dose required is based on a number of factors, including the thyroid gland uptake determined by a preceding nuclear medicine thyroid uptake and scan.

▪ It is an alternative to surgical or long-term medical treatment of hyperthyroidism. The majority of nuclear medicine physicians currently attempt to completely ablate the thyroid gland, thus rendering the patient hypothyroid. The patient then requires lifelong supplemental thyroid hormone.

■ It requires an inpatient stay and isolation of the patient from children until the radioactivity that is administered diminishes to a safe level for patient contacts.

INDICATIONS
☐ Treatment of hyperthyroidism
☐ Treatment of local metastatic thyroid cancer (differentiated type only)

CONTRAINDICATIONS
☐ Pregnancy

LIMITATIONS
☐ Although the majority of patients attain complete thyroid ablation from a single dose, some patients require additional treatments.
☐ The patients uniformly require lifelong supplemental thyroid hormone.

Parathyroid Imaging

■ It may be performed with different agents, depending upon the preferences of the nuclear medicine department and the referring physicians. It may be performed with sestamibi (most commonly) or as a subtraction technique using pertechnetate and thallium.

■ It is performed as a 1-day imaging study.

■ It may be performed in conjunction with ultrasound evaluation to localize the position of parathyroid glands/adenoma.

INDICATIONS
☐ Evaluation of patients with hyperparathyroidism
☐ Evaluation of patients with known parathyroid disease to localize the position of the parathyroid glands (preoperative planning as the parathyroid glands are variably located)
☐ Evaluation of patients with recurrent parathyroid adenoma (postoperative patients)

CONTRAINDICATIONS: None

LIMITATIONS
☐ Lesion/gland size: Due to the limited spatial resolution of nuclear medicine imaging, small lesions/glands may not be identified.

□ If the patient moves between the two components of the examination, misregistration can occur, leading to difficulties with interpretation.

□ In patients with underlying thyroid abnormality, uptake in the thyroid gland may not be uniform, complicating interpretation.

□ Alternate processes such as metastases can take up thallium and mimic a parathyroid adenoma. A cancer history (if present) should be provided to the physician interpreting the examination.

Metaiodobenzylguanidine Imaging

■ It is typically labeled with I-123 or I-131.

■ It is usually performed to evaluate patients with neuroendocrine tumors.

■ Scanning is performed 1–3 days after administration of the radiotracer to allow adequate uptake of the tracer.

■ Patients are preloaded (prior to tracer injection) with potassium iodide or Lugol's solution.

■ A number of drugs will interfere with uptake of the tracer including tricyclic antidepressants, cocaine, certain antipsychotic agents, and labetalol.

■ It is particularly used to evaluate pediatric patients with neuroblastoma; it may be positive for osseous metastatic disease in the setting of a negative bone scan.

INDICATIONS

□ Evaluation of patients with known or suspected neuroendocrine tumors

□ Evaluation of suspected pheochromocytoma

□ Evaluation of neuroblastoma

CONTRAINDICATIONS: None

LIMITATIONS

□ As noted previously, certain drugs can interfere with the study.

□ There is poor resolution for small tumors.

Gallium Imaging

■ The study is performed with gallium citrate-67 (Ga-67), which has a long half-life and four imaging energies.

- The long half-life allows for delayed imaging, which is often necessary to allow for identification of all sites of disease.
- The agent may be used to evaluate for tumor or for infection. It also plays role in the evaluation of granulomatous disease (sarcoidosis) and inflammatory bowel disease.
- The patient is administered IV Ga-67, and imaging is performed initially at 24 hours. At that time, if background activity has cleared from the lungs, SPECT imaging of the chest may be performed. Typically, GI tract (i.e. bowel) activity is present at 24 hours, thus limiting evaluation of abdominal disease. If bowel activity is present, the patient returns to the nuclear medicine department at 48 hours following injection for further imaging. If there is no bowel activity, SPECT imaging of the abdomen may be performed and the study terminated. However, if there is persistent bowel activity, the patient must return on a daily basis until sufficient bowel activity has cleared to allow completion of the study. Thus, imaging may be required on a daily basis up to 6 days following injection.
- The indication for the study determines the dose of agent that is administered to the patient. A higher dose is used for tumor imaging than for imaging of suspected infections. Therefore, it is important to clarify to the imager the indication for the study so that an appropriate dose of radiotracer is administered.

INDICATIONS

☐ Evaluation of patients with suspected infection. This application is of particular importance in patients who cannot undergo CT imaging (e.g. patients with renal insufficiency or contrast allergy). Due to the relative simplicity of the study in comparison to WBC studies (discussed later; blood must be taken from and reinjected into the patient), gallium imaging is increasing in popularity for the evaluation of suspected infection.

☐ Evaluation of osteomyelitis (osteomyelitis may be evaluated with bone scan or with gallium imaging)

☐ Evaluation of patients with neoplasm: The most common application is in the evaluation of patients with lymphoma. PET CT has largely replaced gallium imaging for the evaluation of patients with lymphoma.

☐ Evaluation of lung disease: Although non-specific and now nearly completely superceded by CT, lung activity with gallium can be an indicator of underlying pulmonary

abnormalities such as infection or lung fibrosis. In patients with sarcoidosis, the degree of lung disease may be determined by generating a ratio of lung to liver activity.
□ Evaluation of sarcoidosis: In patients with known or suspected sarcoidosis, gallium may be used to evaluate for the presence of activity of the disease.

CONTRAINDICATIONS
□ Pregnancy
□ Breastfeeding (for several days) as gallium is excreted in breast milk

LIMITATIONS
□ Long imaging times over multiple days are often required, limiting usefulness for rapid diagnosis.
□ Poor spatial resolution limits the ability to localize or diagnose sites of disease.
□ Findings may be non-specific, and it may be difficult to differentiate between sites of tumor and infection.
□ In some patients with lymphoma (which is typically very active on gallium studies), the tumor is not gallium avid, meaning that the tumor does not take up the agent and thus sites of disease are not recognized. In these patients, gallium imaging cannot be used to follow tumor response to therapy.
□ Chemotherapy can alter the uptake patterns of gallium; therefore, it is recommended that gallium imaging not be performed within 3–6 weeks of chemotherapy completion.
□ There is normal uptake of gallium in the liver and spleen. Metastatic foci in these organs may be masked by the normal organ uptake, leading to false-negative results.
□ Persistent colonic activity can complicate interpretation and may not be cleared even with delayed (>96 hours) imaging.

White Blood Cell Imaging

▓ The study involves drawing a sample 30–50 cc of the patient's blood, which is then treated to separate the WBCs from the remainder of the cells and the serum. The WBCs are then labeled with indium-111 (In-111) and reinjected into the patient. The labeling process takes up to 2 hours. Imaging is then performed at both 4 hours and 24 hours following IV injection of the labeled WBCs.

- Labeling can be performed with ^{99m}Tc (^{99m}Tc labeled HMPAO). Due to its properties, imaging with ^{99m}Tc HMPAO can be performed more rapidly than In-111, often within 2 hours of injection.

INDICATIONS
- ☐ Evaluation of patients with fever of unknown origin to evaluate for occult infection
- ☐ Evaluation of inflammatory bowel disease. In some patients, early imaging at 4–6 hours following the IV administration of the labeled WBCs may identify sites of active inflammation.

CONTRAINDICATIONS: None

LIMITATIONS
- ☐ Due to the inherent risk of exposure to blood products (and the need to send blood to off-site facilities for labeling at some institutions), there is a significant risk of exposure to blood-borne pathogens. This is true not only for the technologists handling the blood but also for the patient (as the labeled blood is reinjected into the patient).
- ☐ Labeling requires a relatively large volume of blood to be withdrawn from the patient. In children, this is a relatively larger volume of blood than in adults, due to the smaller total blood volume of children. For this reason, WBC studies are not often performed in children.
- ☐ Neutropenic patients or patients with WBC dysfunction may have false-negative studies, limiting the usefulness of the study.
- ☐ Due to the physiologic uptake of the WBCs by the reticuloendothelial system (particularly the liver and spleen), infection within or adjacent to these organs may not be identified. This is also true for pulmonary infections.
- ☐ It may be difficult to differentiate inflammation from infection.

Tagged Red Blood Cell Study

- The study involves first injecting a patient with stannous pyrophosphate to prepare the RBCs for labeling. Approximately 20 minutes later, 5–10 cc of blood are drawn and centrifuged to separate the RBCs. The cells are then "tinned" and reinjected into the patient. (There are alternative methods of labeling RBCs that are not discussed here.)

▓ Tagged RBC studies are the most sensitive methods to evaluate for the site and presence of a GI bleed. Bleeds with rates as slow as 0.1 mL/min can be identified (in comparison with 1.0 mL/min with conventional angiography). However, due to the relative difficulty and increased time of labeling, sulfur colloid studies are often performed to evaluate for GI bleeds.

▓ Images are obtained over a duration of 90 minutes while the patient is positioned on the imaging table under the gamma camera. If, at the end of 90 minutes, no areas of active bleeding are identified, the patient is reimaged for 30 minutes at 2 and 4 hours following injection or at any time within 24 hours of injection if re-bleeding is suspected. For sulfur colloid imaging, imaging is performed over 20 minutes, thus it is a more rapid study than a tagged RBC study. However, delayed imaging cannot be performed due to its more rapid clearance. If patients with initially negative sulfur colloid studies re-bleed, they will require reinjection of tracer.

▓ The tracer may also be used for evaluation of an indeterminate liver mass seen on an alternate imaging study. This nuclear study is performed if there is suspicion of cavernous hepatic hemangioma. This is a benign liver mass that is typically of no clinical significance unless it is large and/or multiple. In this instance, it can cause a consumptive coagulopathy.

▓ Tagged RBC studies are performed to differentiate hemangiomas from other liver masses such as fibrous nodular hyperplasia, adenoma, and hepatoma (sulfur colloid imaging is the study of choice for these masses; see later). Currently, contrast-enhanced MR is the study of choice for the characterization of hepatic masses.

INDICATIONS

☐ Evaluation of patients with GI bleed. This study is typically performed prior to angiography to localize the vascular territory involved by the bleed.

☐ Evaluation of suspected cavernous hemangioma of the liver

CONTRAINDICATIONS: None

LIMITATIONS

☐ Small bowel bleeds may be difficult to identify and localize.

☐ Free pertechnetate (the agent used to label the RBCs) may be taken up by the gastric mucosa, leading to a false-positive study. This may be recognized by imaging to identify characteristic sites of free pertechnetate uptake such as the thyroid gland.

☐ False-negative results may occur with very slow bleeds or in patients in whom bleeding has stopped or is intermittent.

☐ Tagged RBC studies require a higher radiation dose than sulfur colloid studies and require a longer imaging time. However, they are superior to sulfur colloid studies in that delayed imaging can be performed if required without re-injection of tracer.

☐ Hemangiomas <2 cm are often below the resolution of nuclear imaging; MR is the study of choice for the characterization of small liver masses.

Meckel's Scan

■ A Meckel's diverticulum is a congenital abnormality of the GI tract in which a diverticulum arises from the bowel. This is due to failure of regression/closure of the omphalomesenteric duct.

■ Up to 30% of Meckel's diverticula contain gastric mucosa, which may produce symptoms of GI bleeding.

■ Meckel's diverticula can lead to a GI bleed from the ectopic gastric mucosa located in the diverticulum. They may cause intussusceptions (particularly in the pediatric population) and may become obstructed and present in a manner mimicking appendicitis.

■ They follow the "rule of 2's": are located 2 feet from the ileocecal valve, are present in 2% of the population, appear in children age <2 years.

■ The agent used for imaging is ^{99m}Tc-labeled pertechnetate, which is taken up by the gastric mucosa.

■ Due to normal uptake in the bladder and stomach, patients should fast for 3–4 hours prior to the study and void prior to and during the study.

■ Barium studies should not be performed within several days prior to the examination as the barium may lead to attenuation artifacts.

■ Images are acquired every 5–10 minutes for a duration of 1 hour.

INDICATIONS
- ☐ Evaluation of suspected Meckel's diverticulum

CONTRAINDICATIONS
- ☐ Acutely ill patients who may require emergent surgery for perforation

LIMITATIONS
- ☐ False-negative results can result if there is no gastric mucosa in the diverticulum.
- ☐ False negatives can also result from intussusceptions, volvulus, or infarction involving the diverticulum.
- ☐ False positives can occur due to a variety of processes such as tumors, arteriovenous malformations, and ectopic kidney.

Sulfur Colloid Imaging

- There are a variety of uses for ^{99m}Tc-labeled sulfur colloid due to its uptake in the reticuloendothelial system as well as its use for intravascular and GI bleeding abnormalities.

INDICATIONS
- ☐ GI bleeding study: Sulfur colloid imaging is frequently used to identify and localize sites of GI tract bleeding.
- ☐ Liver-spleen scan: Normally, the liver takes up the majority of the radiotracer with spleen and bone marrow demonstrating lesser amounts of uptake. In conditions where there is hepatocellular dysfunction, there is a relative "shift" of tracer uptake such that the spleen and bone marrow take up relatively more tracer and the liver relatively less. This is an indicator of liver disease and is often used to assess for signs of cirrhosis and portal hypertension.
- ☐ Evaluation of hepatic tumors: Focal nodular hyperplasia will demonstrate normal or increased tracer uptake; adenomas will appear as defects.
- ☐ Evaluation of Budd-Chiari syndrome: Due to the separate drainage of venous blood from the caudate lobe, the caudate will appear relatively "hot" or hypervascular on sulfur colloid imaging in patients with hepatic vein occlusion (Budd-Chiari).
- ☐ Intravascular uses: These are noted previously in the section, SVC/IVC obstruction.

☐ Evaluation of splenic abnormalities: Sulfur colloid imaging can detect splenic infarcts, splenic remnants (important in the setting of idiopathic thrombocytopenic purpura [ITP]), and splenosis.

CONTRAINDICATIONS

☐ Patients with allergies to products containing human serum albumin should not be administered microcolloid preparations.

☐ Sulfur colloid imaging should not be performed immediately following a barium study as the barium may produce artifacts that can affect interpretation of the images.

LIMITATIONS

☐ There is decreased sensitivity to GI bleeds in comparison to tagged RBCs.

☐ There is a decreased length of imaging time available for evaluation of GI bleeds in comparison to tagged RBCs. Unlike labeled RBCs, there is no exposure to blood products. However, unlike labeled RBCs, which continue to circulate in the blood pool for the lifetime of the cell, sulfur colloid has a limited timeframe during which imaging can be performed. If the patient were to begin to bleed a day following injection, the patient would require reinjection (unlike labeled RBCs). Sulfur colloid studies have a reported sensitivity of 0.5–1.0 mL/min bleeds.

☐ GI bleeds in the region of the splenic or hepatic flexure may be difficult to identify due to the normal hepatic and splenic uptake of the radiotracer.

☐ In severe liver disease, there may be little or no uptake of tracer.

☐ Subtle colloid shift may not be detectible.

☐ As with all nuclear imaging studies, metallic devices in or on a patient will attenuate (stop) the radiation from reaching the detector and cause an artifact, which can obscure disease.

HIDA Study

■ It is one of the most commonly requested nuclear medicine imaging studies. Currently, it is often performed as a problem-solving tool for patients with equivocal ultrasound examinations for acute cholecystitis.

- It uses ^{99m}Tc-labeled diseida, which is excreted through the biliary tree into the small bowel. It has physiologic properties similar to bilirubin.
- Patients must be NPO for at least 4 hours prior to the study. The patient is injected with the agent and imaging is performed for up to 1 hour or until the gallbladder is demonstrated to fill with the tracer. If the gallbladder is identified and small bowel activity is demonstrated, the study is negative and cholecystitis/cystic duct obstruction is not present. However, if the gallbladder is not demonstrated at 40–50 minutes following injection in the presence of small bowel activity, morphine is administered intravenously to attempt to relax the sphincter of Oddi in order to allow the gallbladder to fill. If the gallbladder is still not visualized, the patient may be returned for delayed imaging at 24 hours after injection to evaluate for delayed gallbladder filling (a sign of chronic cholecystitis).
- Cholecystokinin (CCK) may be administered during a HIDA study to promote gallbladder contraction. This is not routinely performed for several reasons, including increased study cost and limited availability of CCK. CCK also may be administered to patients in whom chronic cholecystitis is of clinical concern. A gallbladder ejection fraction can be calculated and, if decreased, it may suggest the presence of chronic cholecystitis. CCK may be administered prior to a HIDA study if the patient has fasted for >24 hours.

INDICATIONS
- ☐ Evaluation of patients with clinically suspected acute or acalculous cholecystitis in whom ultrasound is limited (e.g. by large body habitus) or is equivocal
- ☐ Evaluation of chronic cholecystitis
- ☐ Evaluation of suspected bile leak (e.g. post-cholecystectomy). CT, MR, and ultrasound can confirm the presence of a fluid collection within the gallbladder bed following recent cholecystectomy; however, as bile has fluid characteristics, it is not possible to differentiate the collection from a postoperative seroma. HIDA scans are the study of choice to identify the presence of a bile leak as the tracer will be excreted into the biliary system. Over the course of delayed imaging (up to 24 hours), if a bile leak is present, activity in the abdomen and gallbladder fossa will increase and confirm the diagnosis.

Nuclear Medicine

☐ Evaluation of infants with suspected biliary atresia. Hepatic activity will be identified; however, small bowel and gallbladder activity will not (although the gallbladder is present in up to 10% of patients with biliary atresia). Patients should be pretreated with phenobarbital to stimulate liver excretory enzymes.

CONTRAINDICATIONS

☐ Recent morphine administration. The study must be deferred for 4–6 hours if the patient has been administered morphine as the morphine will interfere with study interpretation.

☐ Recent meal. A recent meal will cause gallbladder contraction and will not allow the radiotracer to be taken up by the gallbladder, thus yielding inaccurate results. (It may result in false-positive results as the tracer cannot enter the gallbladder while it is contracting due to a recent meal.)

LIMITATIONS

☐ Limited availability of the HIDA agent limits availability of the study.

☐ Patients with hepatic dysfunction have poor hepatic uptake of the agent, limiting the amount of excretion of the tracer, thus limiting study interpretation.

☐ Because the agent competes for the same pathways as bilirubin, it may not be excreted into the gallbladder in patients with markedly elevated serum bilirubin levels (usually >5 mg/dL).

☐ False-positive results can occur in patients fasting <4 hours or >24 hours.

☐ False-positive results can be seen in chronic cholecystitis.

Gastric Emptying Study

■ It is performed to evaluate for gastroparesis, typically in diabetic patients.

■ The patients are administered a meal in which a defined amount of radiotracer is present. Imaging is then performed over a period of time to determine the length of time required for the stomach to empty. A graph is generated and gastric emptying time is determined.

INDICATIONS

☐ Evaluation of patients with suspected gastroparesis

CONTRAINDICATIONS: None

LIMITATIONS

☐ If the patient does not consume an adequate amount of the tracer, the study may be limited.

Renal Imaging

▪ There are a variety of indications for nuclear medicine renal imaging, which are discussed later. The main advantage of nuclear medicine imaging in patients with known or suspected renal disease is the lack of nephrotoxic contrast material administration. In a significant majority of the patients imaged with nuclear medicine renal studies, underlying renal dysfunction is present, thus intravenously administered nephrotoxic contrast material is contraindicated.

▪ Nuclear medicine renal imaging includes the following:
☐ Renal artery stenosis studies (captopril studies)
☐ Diuretic renograms
☐ Dimercaptosuccinic acid (DMSA) studies for evaluation of parenchymal scarring
☐ Quantification of differential glomerular filtration rate (GFR)
☐ Evaluation of vesicoureteral reflux (nuclear medicine cystography)

▪ The agent used (i.e. DMSA, diethylene triamine pentaacetic acid [DTPA], or MAG-3) depends on the study indication. For example, for renal cortical imaging (i.e. renal parenchymal scarring), DMSA is used, whereas MAG-3 and DTPA are used for both cortical and tubular function assessment. For all renal studies, the patient must be well hydrated prior to the examination, and typically, a Foley catheter is placed.

INDICATIONS

☐ DMSA: For patients with a question of renal scarring (often children with known vesicoureteral reflux/reflux nephropathy), DMSA is the study of choice.

☐ DTPA/MAG-3: Either agent may be used for diuretic renograms (i.e. furosemid [Lasix] studies), captopril studies (for renovascular hypertension), or evaluation of the GFR. MAG-3 has relatively superior physiologic characteristic, thus it is the preferred imaging agent. However, the relatively increased cost of MAG-3 decreases its use.

Captopril Studies

■ These studies are performed on patients with suspected renovascular hypertension. They involve the IV administration
of a radiotracer with immediate and delayed imaging to gen-
erate curves of renal activity such that renal perfusion may
be assessed. The patient is administered an oral angiotensin-
converting enzyme [ACE]-inhibitor (usually captopril) for the
study to determine the effect on the renal arteries and thus
determine if renal artery stenosis is present.

■ The GFR of each kidney may be determined with this study.

INDICATIONS

☐ Evaluation of patients with known or suspected renovascular hypertension

CONTRAINDICATIONS

☐ Patients with ACE-inhibitor allergies are not candidates
for the study. Additionally, patients on long-term ACE
inhibitors may not have a response to the relatively small
dose of captopril that is administered for the study.

LIMITATIONS

☐ If patients are on long-term ACE inhibitors, they may
demonstrate an inadequate response to the small dose of
captopril that is administered for the study, thus yielding
potentially false-negative results.

☐ If bilateral renal artery stenosis is present, it may be difficult
to determine the presence of a stenosis, thus leading to a
false-negative study.

Diuretic Renogram (Lasix Study)

■ It is performed for patients in whom there is a question of
obstructive uropathy (i.e. hydronephrosis) versus a capacious,
dilated but non-obstructed system (e.g. primary megaureter).
This study is often performed in children with a question of
obstruction versus megaureter.

■ The patient is administered an IV tracer, and continuous imaging is performed until activity is seen in the renal collecting
systems and renal pelvis. The patient is then administered an
IV dose of Lasix, and imaging is continued. Graphs are generated and interpretation may be performed to determine if there
is ureteral obstruction.

INDICATIONS

☐ Differentiation of lower ureteric obstruction from primary megaureter

☐ Differentiation of a capacious, dilated renal collecting system from an obstructed system (e.g. ureteropelvic junction obstruction)

CONTRAINDICATIONS

☐ Patients with a contraindication to Lasix administration should not undergo diuretic renography.

LIMITATIONS

☐ Patients on continuous diuretic therapy may not respond to the relatively small dose of Lasix administered for the study.

☐ Motion artifacts can limit interpretation of the study.

Radionuclide Cystography

▪ The study is performed to evaluate for the presence of vesicoureteral reflux, typically in the pediatric population.

▪ The study may be performed as a direct or indirect study. Direct cystography is performed in much the same way as fluoroscopically performed voiding cystourethrograms (VCUGs); that is, a Foley catheter is placed and the bladder is filled with the tracer under imaging guidance. The patient then voids under visualization and the presence of vesicoureteral reflux can be assessed. With indirect cystography, the study is performed following the IV administration of MAG-3 or DTPA. The bladder is allowed to fill by renal filtration, and imaging is performed prior to and during patient voiding. Indirect cystography is uncommonly performed.

INDICATION

☐ Evaluation of patients with suspected or known vesicoureteral reflux

CONTRAINDICATIONS

☐ Like fluoroscopic VCUGs, the study should not be performed in patients with active urinary tract infection. There is a risk of spreading a lower urinary tract infection to the kidneys in patients with vesicoureteral reflux who are undergoing the study while actively infected.

LIMITATIONS

☐ The study has largely been superceded by fluoroscopically performed VCUGs, which use a similar amount of radiation.

Nuclear Medicine

Ventilation/Perfusion Imaging

- It is performed for the evaluation of patients with suspected pulmonary thromboembolic disease.
- It is the study of choice in a large number of institutions for the evaluation of pulmonary embolism in patients with normal CXRs. However, in recent times, it has been superseded by CT pulmonary angiography.
- Patients require a recent (within 24 hours) CXR prior to the ventilation/perfusion (V/Q) scan to determine if they are candidates for V/Q or if they must undergo CT angiography. Additionally, a CXR is required to allow for interpretation of the V/Q.
- Patients must be able to cooperate with the breathing instructions for the ventilation portion of the study. If the patient is ventilated, the ventilation portion of the study cannot be performed; therefore, a "probability" for pulmonary embolism cannot be assessed although a "likelihood" can be assessed.
- It may be performed in pregnancy after discussion with the nuclear medicine physician and with the patient.
- The patient is required to breathe xenon-133 through a special mask, and first breath, equilibrium, and washout ventilation images are obtained. Subsequently, the patient is administered ^{99m}Tc labeled microaggregated albumin intravenously and perfusion imaging of the lungs is performed. The two sets of images are then evaluated in conjunction with the CXR and a probability for pulmonary embolism can be assessed.

INDICATIONS

- ☐ Evaluation of patients with suspected acute pulmonary embolism
- ☐ Evaluation of shunts

CONTRAINDICATION

- ☐ Patients with known intracardiac or extracardiac shunts should not undergo V/Q scanning as the microaggregated albumin particles may traverse the shunt and lodge in small blood vessels in end organs (e.g. brain).

LIMITATIONS

- ☐ Patients with abnormal CXRs may have "intermediate probability" V/Q scans, which often do not provide adequate clinical direction. For patients with significantly abnormal CXRs, CT angiography of the pulmonary arteries is typically performed unless there is significant contraindication to IV contrast.

☐ Patients on ventilators cannot undergo the ventilation portion of the study; thus, a probability of pulmonary embolism cannot be assessed. Based on the perfusion study, a "likelihood" of pulmonary embolus may be assigned.

☐ Obese patients and patients with significant respiratory compromise may be difficult to image.

PET CT (for Attenuation Correction)

■ PET CT is an exciting advance in the nuclear imaging arena. It provides physiologic information such as tumor viability while allowing for localization of sites of disease with the accompanying CT.

■ The resolution of PET CT is significantly higher than that of conventional nuclear imaging. This improves image quality and allows detection of smaller foci of disease than conventional nuclear studies. Because the study is performed on a combined machine that has a PET camera and a CT scanner, the images from each study can be fused with the other. Through complex physics and data manipulation, it is possible to use the CT to "attenuation correct" artifacts that might be present on the PET images due to a variety of causes such as pannus and breast attenuation, for example.

■ The study is performed with 18-FDG glucose, which has a short half-life.

■ The fused images allow for sites of disease (e.g. tumor masses, liver and lymph node metastases) to be evaluated for tumor cell viability. For example, in patients with known lymphoma, lymphadenopathy may persist on CT even when the disease is physiologically inactive. The CT alone will not be able to determine disease activity in lymph nodes that have not changed in size or are enlarged by CT size criteria (because CT is an anatomic not a functional study). However, with the PET CT, lymph nodes that contain tumor will (usually) demonstrate uptake of the PET radiotracer (18-FDG). A significant advantage of PET CT over gallium scanning in these lymphoma patients is that, unlike gallium, which requires multiple days of imaging, PET CT is completed in as few as 2 hours.

- PET CT has a variety of indications, including tumor diagnosis and staging.
- Due to the properties of the agent, patients must be appropriately prepped for the study. Patient preparation for a whole body PET CT is as follows (preparation for cardiac PET CT is different and is discussed in Chapter 9):
  - ☐ No food or drinks containing sugar, no candy, and no gum for 6 hours prior to the study (patients should be fasting to control serum glucose levels, which will determine uptake of the tracer).
  - ☐ Patients may take daily medication the day of the study (with water).
  - ☐ Avoid strenuous/physical exercise for 24 hours prior to the study (to avoid muscle uptake of the tracer, which can affect study interpretation).
  - ☐ For diabetics, insulin should be adjusted to achieve a serum glucose level of <200 mg/dL.
  - ☐ Avoid clothing with metal and jewelry (as it can attenuate the PET photons and cause artifacts).
  - ☐ Following injection of FDG, patients must remain sedentary in a dim room for 45–60 minutes (to allow uptake of the tracer).

INDICATIONS
  - ☐ Evaluation of solitary pulmonary nodules/masses to determine if they represent benign or malignant disease
  - ☐ Staging of metastatic disease (currently, PET CT is approved only for specific malignancies, including breast, lymphoma, lung)
  - ☐ Restaging of metastatic disease following treatment
  - ☐ Evaluation of inflammatory disease (e.g. sarcoid)
  - ☐ Evaluation of seizures

CONTRAINDICATIONS
  - ☐ Uncontrolled serum glucose levels
  - ☐ Recent meal
  - ☐ Unstable patient (due to relatively long imaging time)

LIMITATIONS
  - ☐ Uptake in soft tissue and muscles caused by exercise, talking, and auditory or visual stimulation following injection of the tracer can cause difficulty with interpretation.
  - ☐ Small masses, nodules, and lymph nodes (<1 cm) may be below the resolution of PET CT.

☐ Normal, physiologic bowel activity and liver or spleen activity can mask sites of disease.

☐ Cardiac (myocardial) abnormalities are not optimally detected with whole body imaging as the patient preparation and scanning methods differ. If there is concern for myocardial viability or perfusion abnormality, dedicated cardiac PET CT should be performed (see Chapter 9 for further details).

12

Angiography/Interventional Radiology

General Considerations

■ Interventional radiology is just that . . . interventional! There are great risks associated with invasive procedures performed by interventionalists; therefore, carefully consider the indications for a procedure and weigh the risks and benefits for the patient.

■ Patient factors:

☐ Patient stability: Is the patient stable enough for the procedure? Can the procedure be delayed until the patient's condition improves?

☐ Patient size: Angiography tables can accommodate patients up to 350–400 lbs. Some procedures are higher risk to obese patients than to lower weight patients because the larger body habitus increases the difficulty of visualizing vessels and organs.

☐ Patient medication: Patients on warfarin (Coumadin) or heparin must discontinue this medication and the anticoagulation needs to be reversed or partially reversed prior to the study. Aspirin, Ginkgo biloba, St. John's wort, and NSAIDs should be discontinued 5–7 days prior to the procedure in order to decrease the risk of procedure-related bleeding.

☐ Patient laboratory results: A significant number of patients undergoing interventional procedures have derangement of their coagulation parameters, renal function, and hematocrit. The degree of derangement that is safe for a procedure depends on a number of factors:

• Type of procedure: Minimally invasive procedures such as superficial lesion biopsy or PICC placement may not require complete correction of laboratory abnormalities, whereas procedures such as transjugular intrahepatic portosystemic shunt (TIPS) placement require near complete correction given the high risks of the procedure.

- Patient stability: For patients in whom an emergent interventional procedure is necessary for survival, correction of laboratory derangement may not be possible prior to the procedure. In these patients, attempts to correct metabolic abnormalities may be made during the procedure. Coordination with the interventional suite is required to attempt to correct laboratory derangements.
- Renal function: Unlike general diagnostic imaging procedures, more leeway is given for elevated renal function in cases in which a procedure is required for improved patient outcome. In general, creatinine (Cr) >1.5 mg/dL is considered impaired and discussions must ensue between the interventionalist and clinician as to the risk: benefit ratio for the procedure. In specific vascular procedures, carbon dioxide (CO_2) may be used to decrease the contrast load administered. Patients with diabetes who are on oral hypoglycemic agents such as metformin (Glucophage) must discontinue this hypoglycemic agent for 48 hours after receiving IV contrast. Additionally, these patients require that a repeat Cr level be drawn 24–48 hours following the administration of contrast to evaluate for potential nephrotoxicity.
- Contrast allergy: As with all procedures requiring IV or intra-arterial contrast administration, careful attention must be paid to a history of or risk factors for contrast allergy. If allergy history is present or the patient is at risk, a premedication regimen must be performed. The need for premedication should be communicated to the scheduler at the time of the imaging request so that the examination may be scheduled for a time when the premedication regimen has been completed. For inpatients requiring premedication, it is suggested that the housestaff stay in communication with the technologists/schedulers to ensure completion of the regimen.
- The following regimens are suggested:

Regimen 1
- Medication: Prednisone
- Route: Oral

Angiography/Interventional Radiology

- Dose: 50 mg
- Schedule: 13, 7, and 1 hour prior to procedure
- Benadryl 50 mg oral or IV is also administered 1 hour prior to procedure

Regimen 2
- Medication: Methylprednisolone (Solu-Medrol)
- Route: IV
- Dose: 125 mg
- Schedule: 6 and 1 hour prior to procedure
- Benadryl 50 mg oral or IV is also administered 1 hour prior to procedure

▪ Patient preparation: Prior to an interventional procedure, the following patient conditions must be satisfied:
  ☐ Consent for the procedure must be obtained prior to the study. This may be performed by the interventional service, with consent obtained directly from the patient or from a legally responsible proxy.
  ☐ Review of laboratory data as listed earlier with correction of deranged values
  ☐ The patient must be NPO for at least 4–6 hours prior to the procedure (due to the risk of aspiration while sedated for the procedure).

▪ Interventional procedures may be considered in two broad categories: vascular and nonvascular.

Vascular Procedures

▪ Venous access:
  ☐ PICC
    - It may be placed by interventional radiology or by a dedicated PICC nursing service.
    - There are a variety of brands of PICC lines currently available for use. PICCs may have single or double lumens. The decision for the placement of a single versus double lumen is dependent upon the access needs of the patient and should be discussed with the nurse or interventionalist at the time of request for PICC placement.
    - There are PICC lines that may be used for IV contrast injection; these are termed "power PICCs." Not all hospitals carry these "power" PICC catheters and discussion should ensue with the interventionalist to determine if a power PICC is available and required. No other (standard)

PICC line can be used for "power injection" of IV contrast material.

- PICC line placement is NOT an emergency procedure. It is not typically performed outside of standard office hours.
- It may stay in situ for up to 1 year.

INDICATIONS

☐ Prolonged venous access required (e.g. outpatient antibiotic therapy for 6 weeks)

☐ Additional access required but central venous catheter (cordis) not required

☐ Peripheral access cannot be procured but central line is not desired (PICCs are generally placed under ultrasound guidance)

CONTRAINDICATIONS

☐ Bacteremia/septicemia (relative)

☐ Patients unable to care for the catheter

- Central lines:

  ☐ Depending upon the institution, central lines may be placed by interventional radiologists only after failed attempts by the floor teams.

  ☐ Line placement may be emergent depending upon the clinical condition of the patient.

  ☐ Typically, triple lumen catheters are placed. All lumens must be tested prior to placement of the catheter. Often, one port is reserved for total parenteral nutrition (TPN), and it cannot be used for anything other than TPN.

  ☐ Note that central lines cannot be used for contrast administration for studies such as CT (due to the theoretic risk of shearing off the tip and causing embolic events).

INDICATIONS

☐ Short-term central venous access for fluid resuscitation, medications, TPN, and blood products.

☐ It is often used for very ill patients. Patients with central lines must be monitored in the ICU or stepdown unit.

CONTRAINDICATIONS

☐ Bacteremia/septicemia

- Port-a-cath/Hickman catheter:

  ☐ It is a tunneled catheter (i.e. a portion of the catheter is placed in a subcutaneous location prior to the venous entry site by dissecting through the tissues to create a tunnel).

  ☐ Tunneling theoretically decreases the risk of infection.

- It is used for long-term venous access; it is not for short-term uses (because it is tunneled under the skin).
- It may be a single or dual lumen catheter, depending upon the indication.

INDICATIONS: HICKMAN CATHETER
- Chemotherapy
- Medication such as long-term pressors

INDICATIONS: PORT-A-CATH
- Typically, there are 2 reservoirs.
- It is often used for chemotherapy in lieu of PICC lines in order to decrease the risk of line-related venous occlusions or stenosis.
- Administration of medication such as long-term pressors

CONTRAINDICATIONS: HICKMAN AND PORT-A-CATH
- Bacteremia or septicemia. Each catheter may act as a nidus for continued infection.
- Relatively short patient life expectancy. Placement of tunneled catheters requires conscious sedation and is invasive. If the patient's life expectancy is short, the risks of the procedure may far outweigh the benefits.

- Dialysis catheter:
  - These are tunneled catheters for long-term hemodialysis.
  - All are dual lumen and large bore to allow for high flow rates.
  - In order to allow for the high rates of blood flow required in dialysis, the catheters are large bore and must be positioned in large vessels (e.g. the SVC and right atrium).
  - They are typically placed by an upper extremity approach (this yields increased long-term patency rates). If there is no upper extremity access, dialysis catheters may be placed in an alternate location such as the lower extremity (although catheters in these locations have lower patency rates).

INDICATIONS
- Hemodialysis

CONTRAINDICATIONS
- Bacteremia/septicemia

LIMITATIONS
- Patients on hemodialysis often have poor venous access due to sclerosed veins caused by repeated IV use and central line placement; therefore, it may be difficult to obtain access for catheter placement.

- Patients with dialysis catheters are at risk of line infection, line occlusion (e.g. from fibrin sheaths), and peri-catheter thrombosis.
- There is a risk of pneumothorax during line placement; however, this risk is less significant than that for lines placed without ultrasound or fluoroscopic guidance.
- There is a risk of vessel perforation during dialysis catheter placement or from erosion of surrounding vessel caused by long-standing catheters.

■ Quinton catheters:
  - These are non-tunneled catheters, meaning that they enter the skin and go directly into the vein.
  - They may be placed by non-interventionalists without ultrasound.
  - These are usually single lumen, large bore catheters for short-intermediate term use.

  INDICATIONS
  - Plasmaphoresis
  - Short-term dialysis when renal function is expected to recover
  - Administration of blood products
  - Large bore venous access required for fluid resuscitation

  CONTRAINDICATIONS
  - Long-term venous access is required; tunneled catheters are more appropriate.
  - Active sepsis/bacteremia: Indwelling lines should not be placed (unless absolutely vital for patient survival) in these patients as the line will act as a nidus for persistent infection.

  LIMITATIONS
  - If line infection occurs, the line must be removed and treatment of the infection must occur prior to new line placement.

VENOUS INTERVENTIONS

Inferior Vena Cava Filter

■ The inferior vena cava filter (IVC) is a percutaneously placed device (usually titanium), typically inserted using a femoral venous approach. Filters can be placed in the SVC, although this is seldom done.

- The purpose of the IVC filter is to prevent pulmonary emboli (PE) in patients with or at risk for lower extremity or IVC DVT. Certain types of IVC filters can now be placed for temporary use (approximately 2–4 weeks' duration) as prophylaxis in patients with significant acute illness (e.g. trauma) who are at risk for DVT due to immobility. The expectation is that these patients will recover well or fully following treatment of the acute event and will return to a mobile lifestyle. These patients will then no longer require a filter as the risk of DVT will return to the level of the general population and the filter can be removed.

- The procedure is not without significant risks, which include filter migration, renal vein and mesenteric vein occlusion, IVC perforation, and IVC occlusion (this is expected when a filter is placed).

- The filter is placed below the level of the renal veins in order to prevent propagation of clot from the filter into a renal vein or occlusion of the renal vein ostium. Renal vein thrombosis can lead to loss of renal function in that kidney if not treated.

INDICATIONS

☐ Patients with PE or DVT in whom anticoagulation is contraindicated (e.g. recent surgery)

☐ Patients with DVT in whom anticoagulation has failed

☐ Patients with prolonged hospitalizations and immobility (e.g. trauma patients). In these patients, retrievable filters (i.e. temporary filters) may be used.

☐ Patients with underlying malignancy who are hypercoagulable and who have DVT

☐ Patients with DVT who have limited cardiopulmonary reserve in whom a PE would be fatal

CONTRAINDICATIONS

☐ Short life expectancy (risks of the procedure outweigh the benefits)

☐ Patients eligible for anticoagulation

☐ Patients responsive to anticoagulation

LIMITATIONS

☐ Venous access may be difficult, particularly if bilateral lower extremity DVT is present. In these patients, an upper extremity approach to the IVC (with catheter passage through the right atrium and ventricle) may be required. This approach obviously increases risks to the patient: increased procedure time, increased radiation exposure, increased contrast dose, and risk of arrhythmia from passage of the wire through the heart.

☐ It may be difficult to deploy the filter; malpositioning of the IVC filter or failure of it to fully open may occur.

☐ There is a known risk of acute venous perforation when placing the filter. Veins are lower pressure systems than arteries, thus, the risk of hypovolemic shock is less than if arterial rupture occurred. In the long-term, perforation of the IVC by a prong of the filter can occur, although this is often of little or no clinical significance.

☐ There is a known complication in the intermediate and long-term of IVC occlusion due to thrombosis. Due to the relatively long course of the process, collateral veins have adequate time to develop.

☐ IVC filter failure can occur; clots (particularly if small) can pass through the filter and cause small PE.

Thrombolysis/Thrombectomy (PE, DVT)

■ The procedure involves mechanical (thrombectomy) or chemical (thrombolysis) removal of venous clot.

■ It may be performed in deep or superficial veins or arteries (e.g. for treatment of PE)

INDICATIONS

☐ Superficial veins: Patients with clot (often related to PICC lines) who develop compartment syndrome

☐ Deep veins: Patients with DVT who are ineligible to use anticoagulation to decrease the risk of post-phlebitic syndrome and thereby decrease the risk of future varicose veins or DVT

☐ Pulmonary arteries: Patients with large PEs who are unresponsive to or ineligible for systemic anticoagulation; patients with limited cardiopulmonary reserve in whom an embolus could be fatal

CONTRAINDICATIONS

☐ Patients responsive to anticoagulation

☐ Patients with underlying cardiovascular disease; thrombectomy causes release of bradykinins, which can have adverse cardiovascular effects

☐ Patients with contraindications to heparin or tissue plas-
minogen activator (tPA) (thrombolysis) (e.g. GI bleed, thrombocytopenia, recent surgery)

TIPS

▪ TIPS is performed in patients with hepatocellular dysfunction,
typically as the result of cirrhosis.
▪ It is a percutaneously performed procedure with high risk. It is
often performed only in tertiary referral centers due to the high
risk of the procedure and of the patient population.
▪ It may be performed as an elective or emergent procedure
depending upon the indication for the procedure.
▪ Due to the inherent hepatic dysfunction, correction of underlying metabolic and hematologic derangement is required before
TIPS can be performed. This correction should be coordinated
with the interventional suite. Occasionally, patients are too
acutely ill to allow time for complete correction of underlying coagulation abnormalities; these patients may require the
procedure to commence while their coagulation abnormality is
being corrected.
▪ TIPS artificially creates a shunt between the portal and hepatic
veins to allow hepatic perfusion and decreased portal venous
pressures. Ultrasound is often required prior to the procedure
to determine which vessels are patent.

INDICATIONS
☐ Emergent: Variceal bleeding not responsive to sclerotherapy
or banding
☐ Emergent: Treatment of hepatic venous occlusion such as
portal vein or hepatic vein occlusion (Budd-Chiari)
☐ Emergent: TIPS revision in patients with recurrent GI bleeds
☐ Elective: Treatment of intractable ascites related to hepatic
dysfunction and portal hypertension
☐ Elective: Treatment of pleural effusion related to hepatic
dysfunction and portal hypertension

CONTRAINDICATIONS
☐ Portal vein occlusion
☐ Liver failure

LIMITATIONS
☐ Patients who require emergent TIPS are often gravely ill and
may not survive the procedure.

□ Procedure complications can occur and include liver capsule perforation with bleeding; vessel dissection, which can lead to occlusion; procedure failure; or biliary fistulas.

□ TIPS can occlude or stenose over time and stenting or revision may be required.

□ Liver dysfunction may continue with ultimate failure of the TIPS.

DIALYSIS DECLOT

□ Dialysis declotting is performed on patients with thrombosed arteriovenous dialysis fistulas or arteriovenous dialysis grafts.

□ It involves accessing the venous and arterial aspects of the fistula/graft and mechanically removing the clot. It also requires evaluation of the draining veins and feeding artery for stenosis. Areas of stenosis require angioplasty. If the procedure is not successful, surgical revision may be required.

□ It is typically NOT an emergency (if emergent dialysis is required, a temporary percutaneous catheter can be placed; see earlier).

INDICATIONS

□ Decreased flow rates demonstrated at the time of dialysis

□ Arteriovenous graft/fistula thrombosis

CONTRAINDICATIONS

□ Long-standing graft/fistula occlusion

□ Recurrent graft/fistula thrombosis. It often requires surgical revision or new fistula/graft formation.

LIMITATIONS

□ Procedure failure is not an uncommon complication of the procedure and may require temporary venous access (e.g. Quinton catheter placement) until a surgical revision of the graft can be performed.

□ Due to the heparin administration required for the procedure, patients with clotting abnormalities may not be candidates or should be carefully monitored to decrease the risk of procedure-related hemorrhage.

Venograms

■ This is a diagnostic study typically of the upper extremity veins.

■ It was formerly the study of choice for evaluation of patients with suspected DVT. This has now been replaced by Doppler ultrasound, which is non-invasive. In rare cases, venography may be performed for evaluation of patients with suspected DVT in cases in which ultrasound or MRI cannot be performed or results are inadequate or equivocal.

■ It requires placement of large bore peripheral venous IVs.

INDICATIONS

☐ It is typically performed as a roadmap for planning of dialysis fistulas/grafts.

☐ It is performed rarely as a diagnostic study for DVT (as indicated earlier).

CONTRAINDICATIONS

☐ Patients with IV contrast allergies or anaphylaxis are not candidates for the study.

☐ Patients in whom venous access cannot be obtained in the extremity in question are not candidates for the study.

LIMITATIONS

☐ Very small vessels may be below the resolution of imaging (although angiography is the most sensitive imaging modality for this purpose).

☐ Thrombosed vessels will not fill with contrast material, thus cannot be evaluated. Vessels beyond the level of occlusion will not be evaluated, thus the extent of occlusion or proximal stenosis cannot be evaluated with this technique. Ultrasound or MR may be required to evaluate these other vessels.

Arterial Procedures

■ These are invasive procedures, which may be performed as diagnostic studies or as definitive treatments of underlying arterial conditions.

■ Patients must be screened to determine if they are candidates for angiography.

■ Patients with IV contrast allergies or anaphylaxis are not candidates for the study unless premedication is administered.

■ Patients with poor renal function are not candidates for the examination due to the risk of contrast-induced nephropathy. In some cases, CO_2 angiography with small doses of iodinated contrast may be performed. These cases should be discussed with the interventionalist.

■ Abnormalities of coagulation, including those affecting platelets, international normalized ratio, and prothrombin time/

partial thromboplastin time, should be corrected prior to the procedure (particularly if elective).

Aortography with and without Lower Extremity Run-Off

- It involves an arterial puncture, usually of the femoral artery. A wire is then advanced under fluoroscopic guidance into the aorta and directed toward the vessel of interest. A catheter is then advanced over the wire and is connected to a contrast-containing power injector. Under fluoroscopy, contrast is injected and images of the arteries are obtained.

- Currently, CT angiography (CTA) and MR angiography (MRA) are the imaging studies of choice for the diagnosis of vascular disease. CTA and MRA are non-invasive techniques that allow for the identification of vascular abnormalities in patients who are candidates for the procedure (see Chapters 6 and 7). The other advantage of non-invasive imaging techniques with CTA and MRA is the ability to evaluation adjacent structures, which may cause compression of the vessels or other abnormality. These techniques also allow the vessel walls to be evaluated for early disease, unlike conventional catheter angiography.

- The study may be diagnostic to determine the presence or absence of disease or disease extent. If the abnormality is not amenable to percutaneous treatment, the study is terminated; however, if the lesion is amenable to catheter therapy, the procedure may continue and definitive therapy may be performed (see later).

INDICATIONS

☐ Trauma: Although CT has largely supplanted catheter angiography in the evaluation of trauma patients with suspected aortic injury, angiography may be required to confirm the diagnosis or to initiate treatment.

☐ Peripheral arterial occlusive disease: In patients with ongoing claudication, angiography may be performed to evaluate for the presence and extent of disease. If the lesion is amenable, angioplasty or stent placement may be performed (see later). As noted, in some institutions, CTA or MRA is replacing catheter angiography for diagnosis.

☐ Evaluation of mesenteric ischemia (acute and chronic)

☐ Evaluation of acute GI bleed (this is undertaken after the vascular territory is localized by a nuclear medicine GI bleeding study to allow directed evaluation)

CONTRAINDICATIONS

☐ Contrast allergy (relative): Patients should be premedicated for the procedure.

☐ Renal dysfunction: If a patient's renal function is elevated, he or she may not be eligible for angiography. If renal function is borderline, hydration with or without Mucomyst (acetylcysteine) may be administered. Alternatively, CO_2 angiography can be performed to decrease the contrast load administered (this requires direct discussion with the interventionalist to determine if this is a feasible option).

LIMITATIONS

☐ In rare patients, arterial access cannot be obtained. In these patients, the study cannot be performed.

Angioplasty

■ It involves percutaneous positioning of an inflatable balloon, which is mounted on a catheter.

■ Under fluoroscopic guidance, the balloon is placed across an area of vessel narrowing (stenosis) and inflated to a specific pressure.

■ The success or failure of the procedure is determined with additional contrast administration under fluoroscopy.

INDICATIONS

☐ Short segment arterial stenosis

CONTRAINDICATIONS

☐ Long segment stenosis

☐ Positioning of the stenosis or vessel not accessible

LIMITATIONS

☐ Some lesions are not amenable to stenting; this may not be determined until the time of the diagnostic portion of the study.

☐ Lesions that are long-standing or highly stenotic may not respond to angioplasty and stenting. This leads to procedure failure.

☐ If the lesion is highly stenotic, it may not be possible to cross it with a wire. In this case, angioplasty cannot be performed.

☐ Restenosis following angioplasty or stenting may occur.

Stent Placement

■ If a vessel is stenotic, it may require the placement of a stent to maintain or establish patency.

■ The stent is placed into the vessel over a catheter during angiography. The stenosis may be angioplastied prior to stent placement, or the stent may be deployed across the stenosis without prior angioplasty.

INDICATIONS

☐ Restenosis of a vessel segment

☐ Iliac artery stenosis

☐ Long segment stenosis

CONTRAINDICATIONS

☐ Small vessels: Stents are not custom made and may not fit in all vessels.

LIMITATIONS

☐ Some lesions are not amenable to stenting; this may not be determined until the time of the diagnostic portion of the study.

☐ Lesions that are long-standing or highly stenotic may not respond to angioplasty and stenting; this leads to procedure failure.

☐ If the lesion is highly stenotic, it may not be possible to cross it with a wire; in this case, angioplasty cannot be performed.

☐ Restenosis following angioplasty or stenting may occur.

Thrombolysis

■ It involves a diagnostic angiogram as described earlier. Once vessel (or vascular graft) thrombosis is confirmed, catheter-directed infusion of a thrombolytic can be performed with heparin, urokinase, or tPA.

■ Catheter infusion of a thrombolytic is performed with a catheter that has multiple side holes. The catheter is placed across the thrombosed vessel (or graft), and the agent is infused in both a pulsed (large bolus dose) and a continuous infusion (typically overnight). The patient is then reimaged with a contrast injection through the catheter (usually the next day) to determine the success of the procedure. Depending upon the follow-up imaging, the infusion may be stopped (if successful), continued (if incomplete but decreased clot burden), or terminated (due to failure; patients then go to surgery).

INDICATIONS

☐ Arterial graft occlusion (e.g. lower extremity bypass graft)
☐ Cerebral vessel occlusion
☐ Subacute arterial thrombosis (acute native vessel occlusion requires thrombectomy or surgery)

CONTRAINDICATIONS

☐ Contrast allergy (relative): Patients should be premedicated for the procedure.
☐ Renal dysfunction: If a patient's renal function is elevated, he or she may not be eligible for angiography. If renal function is borderline, hydration with or without Mucomyst may be administered. Alternatively, CO_2 angiography can be performed to decrease the contrast load administered (this requires direct discussion with the interventionalist to determine if this is a feasible option).

CONTRAINDICATIONS TO THROMBOLYSIS/ANTICOAGULATION

☐ Recent surgery
☐ Thrombocytopenia
☐ Recent GI bleed
☐ Pregnancy
☐ Heparin-induced thrombocytopenia

LIMITATIONS

☐ Patients may develop hemorrhage in the retroperitoneum, in the rectus sheath, at the arterial puncture site, and in other places due to the thrombolytic agent. These patients should be routinely monitored with repeat lab tests.
☐ If the procedure is unsuccessful, the graft or vessel can occlude, leading to a surgical emergency for limb salvage.
☐ There is a risk of showering emboli distal to the site of vessel or graft occlusion, which can lead to embolic small vessel occlusion (e.g. of the digital arteries leading to the "blue toe syndrome"). If severe, long-standing, or untreated, digital amputations may be required.

Embolization (Emergent [e.g. GI bleeding], Elective [e.g. Uterine Artery Embolization])

■ Embolization involves an initial angiogram to identify the site and cause of bleeding. In the case of GI bleeding, a nuclear medicine bleeding study must be performed prior to angiography to identify the vascular distribution of the bleed. Nuclear medicine sulfur colloid and tagged–red blood cell studies (see Chapter 11) are more sensitive than angiography for slow bleeds and help direct vessel-specific angiography (e.g. celiac axis, superior mesenteric artery, inferior mesenteric artery).

- The site and cause of bleeding determine the material and method of embolization (e.g. for temporary occlusion, Gelfoam is used [e.g. in GI bleeds], whereas coils are used for permanent vessel occlusion (e.g. cerebral aneurysms).

INDICATIONS

- ☐ Embolization may be performed on an emergent basis (e.g. GI bleed) or as an elective procedure (e.g. uterine artery embolization).
- ☐ Emergent:
  - Trauma: Splenic or hepatic lacerations
  - Trauma: Acute vessel injury (e.g. vessel injury in pelvic fractures)
  - GI bleeds due to a specific vascular abnormality (e.g. a diverticular bleed, aneurysm)
  - Pseudoaneurysm formation related to a major vessel
  - Aneurysm formation related to a major vessel
- ☐ Elective:
  - Vascular malformations (e.g. pulmonary or hepatic arteriovenous malformations, as part of hereditary hemorrhagic telangiectasia) or cutaneous vascular malformations
  - Uterine artery embolization for fibroids: Contrast-enhanced MR is often performed prior to embolization to determine if the patient is a candidate for the procedure.

CONTRAINDICATIONS

- ☐ Contrast allergy (relative): Patients should be premedicated for the procedure.
- ☐ Renal dysfunction: If a patient's renal function is elevated, they may not be eligible for angiography. If renal function is borderline, hydration with or without Mucomyst may be administered.
- ☐ Vessel is not amenable to embolization.

LIMITATIONS

- ☐ Embolization may not be adequate for treatment of the site of bleeding; surgical intervention may be required in certain circumstances (e.g. brisk GI bleeding leading to hemodynamic compromise).

□ Embolization may not be possible based upon the location of the abnormality (e.g. if embolization of a bleeding vessel will require occlusion or partial occlusion of a vital artery, it may not be possible to embolize safely without risk to the vital artery). This is particularly true in abnormalities of the liver (e.g. vascular malformations) in which the main hepatic vessels cannot be embolized without risk to the main hepatic blood supply.

Thrombin Injection for Pseudoaneurysm

■ It involves percutaneous injection of a thrombogenic agent (thrombin) for the purposes of clotting the lumen of a pseudoaneurysm.

■ It is now the procedure of choice for treatment of pseudoaneurysm formation related to femoral vessel injury (from catheterization) or to arteriovenous fistula/arteriovenous grafts. It has replaced ultrasound-guided compression of the neck of a pseudoaneurysm.

■ The diagnosis is made by ultrasound, which is performed prior to intervention.

INDICATIONS

□ Treatment of ultrasound-proven pseudoaneurysm

CONTRAINDICATIONS

□ Rarely, a pseudoaneurysm is not amenable to thrombin injection due to its position in relation to the vessel. This is due to the risk of propagation of thrombogenic material into the main vessel, which can lead to main vessel arterial occlusion.

LIMITATIONS

□ Failure of thrombin injections to completely thrombose the pseudoaneurysm may occur. This requires a second injection of thrombin.

□ Small pseudoaneurysms may spontaneously thrombose; therefore, they do not require the added risk of the procedure.

Aortic Stent Grafts

■ This is emerging as a leading treatment for aortic aneurysm repair.

■ This type of graft is less invasive and carries a lower mortality and morbidity rate than surgery alone for abdominal aortic aneurysm repair.

■ It is performed in the operating room by both vascular surgeons and interventionalists.

■ Patients are first evaluated with a dedicated "stent graft protocol" CTA to determine if they are candidates for the procedure. A series of measurements is made from the CT to determine if the patient is a candidate for stent graft repair and, if so, measurements for graft sizing are made based upon the CT.

INDICATION
☐ Treatment of abdominal aortic aneurysm

CONTRAINDICATIONS
☐ Contrast allergy (relative): Patients should be premedicated for the procedure.
☐ Renal dysfunction: If a patient's renal function is elevated, they may not be eligible for angiography. If renal function is borderline, hydration with or without Mucomyst may be administered.
☐ Aneurysm configuration is not amenable to the procedure.
☐ Emergent therapy is required (e.g. aneurysm rupture). The components of the stent graft must be preordered and are not available for emergent procedures.

LIMITATIONS
☐ Patients who are treated with endografts require follow-up imaging, typically with CT. This follow-up is required to evaluate for complications from or failure of endograft placement. One of the most significant complications seen with endograft placement is the "endoleak." There are four grades of endoleak, the majority of which require treatment. These are typically identified with CT imaging.
☐ Local complications can occur at the site of entry of the endograft and may require treatment.

Pulmonary Artery Angiography

■ It involves catheterization of the femoral vein. A wire and catheter are then advanced from the femoral vein, up the IVC, and across the right atrium and right ventricle into the pulmonary arteries.

Angiography/Interventional Radiology

■ It is an invasive procedure with significant risks, which include vessel injury, cardiac chamber perforation (rare), and arrhythmia (as the catheter crosses the right ventricle).

■ Diagnostic pulmonary angiography for the purposes of identification of PE has been largely been replaced by CTA, which is a non-invasive imaging modality.

INDICATIONS

☐ Identification of PE in cases in which CTA is contraindicated or inconclusive

☐ Treatment of PE (thrombectomy or thrombolysis)

☐ Measurement of pulmonary artery pressures (e.g. for diagnosis of pulmonary arterial hypertension)

☐ Diagnosis with or without treatment of pulmonary arteriovenous malformations

CONTRAINDICATIONS

☐ Patients who have started anticoagulation based on a clinical diagnosis of PE. The anticoagulation must be discontinued and clotting parameters returned to normal so that a pulmonary angiogram can be performed safely.

☐ If the patient has presumptively been treated for PE for some time (e.g. 24 hours) prior to a request for a pulmonary angiogram to confirm the diagnosis, the risk of a false-negative study is high. There is a high likelihood that the clot burden would have resolved (particularly if small) or resolved following anticoagulation therapy.

LIMITATIONS

☐ CT pulmonary angiography has largely replaced conventional catheter angiography due to the relative safety of CT in comparison to catheter angiography.

☐ Patients with IVC filters require an upper extremity approach for a pulmonary arteriogram due to the inability to pass a catheter through the filter and the risk of showering emboli from the filter into the pulmonary circulation.

☐ Lower extremity venous access may be difficult in patients with known lower extremity DVT. There is also a risk of embolic phenomena to the pulmonary circulation from venous thrombus while attempting access for a pulmonary angiogram. A lower extremity Doppler (DVT) study is often requested prior to catheterization in order to evaluate for the presence and extent of venous clot.

NONVASCULAR PROCEDURES

Biliary

- Cholecystostomy tube:
  - ☐ It is a drainage catheter placed percutaneously to drain the gallbladder in patients with cholecystitis who are too unstable to undergo surgical cholecystectomy.
  - ☐ It may be performed at the bedside with ultrasound guidance if the patient is too unstable to be moved to the interventional radiology suite.
  - ☐ It is associated with a high mortality (up to 40%) due to the underlying clinical state of the patient.

  INDICATION
  - ☐ Temporary treatment of acute acalculous cholecystitis

  CONTRAINDICATIONS
  - ☐ Metabolic derangement such as coagulopathy must be corrected prior to the procedure.

  LIMITATIONS
  - ☐ If the gallbladder is located very superficially, it may not be safe to perform the procedure as there is not adequate liver to place the catheter through to tamponade the gallbladder for bile leaks and bleeding.
  - ☐ The procedure may be very difficult to perform in obese patients as it may be difficult to visualize the gallbladder with ultrasound (the procedure is performed with ultrasound guidance).

Percutaneous Cholangiogram

- It is similar to endoscopic retrograde cholangiopancreatography (ERCP) in that the bile ducts are opacified with contrast in order to identify a site of disease.
- Unlike ERCP, the bile ducts are accessed percutaneously (i.e. through the skin) in a blind fashion. This allows access to peripherally located bile ducts and for internal/external drainage catheters to be placed, whereas ERCP-placed drainage catheters and stents can be placed internally only and do not drain to the skin.
- It is a difficult procedure to perform, particularly if the bile ducts are not dilated. It may require a preprocedure MR

cholangiopancreatography (MRCP) or ERCP to create a "road-map" of the biliary tree so that an approach for percutaneous puncture can be planned.

INDICATIONS

- ☐ Evaluation of suspected bile duct pathology in patients who are not candidates for ERCP or in whom ERCP has failed
- ☐ Drainage of obstructed bile ducts, which may be palliative in the case of patients with tumors such as cholangiocarcinoma (Klatskin tumor)
- ☐ Drainage of infected bile ducts (remember that cholangitis is NOT an imaging diagnosis but rather is made via direct visualization of pus in the biliary tree)
- ☐ Possible stenting of bile duct stenosis
- ☐ Access for placement of drainage catheters

CONTRAINDICATIONS

- ☐ Unstable patients
- ☐ Patients who are candidates for ERCP with stenting

LIMITATIONS

- ☐ Patients with non-dilated ducts, in whom a diagnostic study is requested for evaluation of duct pathology (e.g. sclerosing cholangititis), percutaneous cholangiography may be difficult. This is due to the small size of the ducts that must be accessed in a blind manner. In these patients, percutaneous transhepatic cholangiography (PTC) is reserved for patients who fail ERCP or MRCP.

Gastric

Gastric (G-tube)

- ■ It is a catheter placed through the anterior gastric wall to the skin surface for the purpose of administering medication and feedings to patients who are unable to take oral material but in whom enteral nutrition is desired.
- ■ It may be placed in a number of ways by a number of services including operatively (by surgeons), endoscopically (by gastroenterologists), or percutaneously (by interventionalists).
- ■ Patients should be NPO after midnight the night before the procedure. A nasogastric tube should also be in place prior to the procedure as this will provide a landmark for the procedure.

■ The stomach is distended with air during the examination, placing the patient at aspiration risk; therefore, the NPO order is essential for the procedure.

■ Some interventionalists will administer oral contrast (e.g. barium) the day prior to the procedure in order to outline the colon and thus decrease the risk of inadvertent colonic injury during the tube placement.

INDICATIONS

☐ Patients unable to take oral medications or nutrition for any reason (e.g. stroke, malignancy, dementia)

☐ Patients with recently performed fundoplications in order to feed and decompress the stomach temporarily

☐ Drainage: For patients with chronic hypersecretion or bowel obstruction, the G-tube may function as a method to drain gastric secretions.

CONTRAINDICATIONS

☐ Patients unable to care for the catheter

☐ Local infection

☐ Gastroesophageal reflux: In patients at risk of or with documented gastroesophageal reflux, there is a risk of aspiration. In these patients, a gastro-jejunostomy tube is often placed so that the gastric tube functions for drainage while the jejunal tube is used to administer feeds and medications.

LIMITATIONS

☐ If patients are near the end of life (near comfort care), parenteral nutrition (via IV) and fluids may be administered without the risk of the procedure.

☐ There is risk of procedure failure.

☐ The tube may not obtain an adequate seal with the stomach or may not be adequately fixed to the anterior abdominal wall. This can result in a G-tube leak, which can cause peritonitis or an abscess.

☐ G-tubes do occasionally occlude (clog) due to the consistency of administered materials and thick gastric secretions. The occlusion often can be treated by injecting material such as ginger ale through the tube. If this conservative measure fails or if the tube falls out, it may need to be replaced. If the tube has been in place for an extended period of time and a mature track to the skin surface has developed, it is often possible to simply place a new tube through the track and confirm the positioning by KUB immediately following injection of 30–60 cc of Gastrografin (sodium amidotrizoate) through the tube. If the tube is new, it may require replacement under fluoroscopy by the interventionalist.

☐ Infection with abscess formation or skin necrosis can occur.

Gastrojejunal Tube

■ It is similar to a gastric tube with the addition of a separate catheter whose tip terminates in the jejunum. The jejunal catheter is placed through the same entry site as the gastrostomy port.

■ Patients should be NPO from midnight the night before the procedure.

INDICATION

☐ In patients at risk of or with documented gastroesophageal reflux, there is a risk of aspiration. In these patients, a gastrojejunostomy tube is often placed so that the gastric tube functions for drainage while the jejunal tube is used to administer feeds and medications.

CONTRAINDICATIONS

☐ Patients unable to care for the catheter
☐ Local infection

LIMITATIONS

☐ Similar to gastrostomy tube

Jejunal (J) Tube

■ This is a catheter placed from the skin surface into the proximal jejunum, bypassing the stomach.

■ It may be placed surgically or by interventionalists.

INDICATIONS

☐ Patients with gastric outlet obstruction from any cause (e.g. diabetic gastroparesis, malignancy) who require parenteral nutrition or medications
☐ Patients in whom long-term parenteral nutrition is required

CONTRAINDICATIONS

☐ Patients unable to care for the catheter
☐ Local infection

LIMITATIONS

☐ Similar to gastrostomy tube

Biopsies

■ These may be performed by diagnostic radiologists or interventionalists. The type of biopsy and the modality used for the biopsy are case-specific and should be discussed with the radiologist prior to examination scheduling.

- Certain lesions are not amenable to percutaneous biopsy and may require surgical biopsy.
- Certain lesions are readily visible with one imaging modality (e.g. CT) but cannot be seen with a second modality (e.g. ultrasound).
- The golden rule of biopsies is as follows: If the lesions cannot be adequately visualized at the time of the procedure or cannot be safely sampled, a biopsy SHOULD NOT be performed.

INDICATIONS
- ☐ Tissue diagnosis is required for a lesion.

CONTRAINDICATIONS
- ☐ Patient medication: Patients on Coumadin or heparin must discontinue this medication and the anticoagulation must be reversed or partially reversed prior to the study. Aspirin, Ginkgo biloba, St. John's wort, and NSAIDs should be discontinued 5–7 days prior to the procedure.
- ☐ Patient laboratory results: A significant number of patients undergoing interventional procedures have derangement of their coagulation parameters, renal function, and hematocrit.

LIMITATIONS
- ☐ Lesions may not be visible at the time of biopsy (e.g. due to decreased size in response to treatment).
- ☐ Lesions may not be visible without IV contrast on CT or MR; therefore, these lesions may not be amenable to biopsy with these modalities even if they are clearly visible on a diagnostic contrast-enhanced study. If a biopsy can be performed safely in the expected location of the lesion (after review of the diagnostic CT), an attempt can be made to perform a percutaneous biopsy with the knowledge that a false-negative result may occur, requiring repeat biopsy or surgical biopsy.
- ☐ If there is inadequate tissue surrounding the lesion (e.g. superficial lesions in the liver), there is a significantly increased risk of the development of uncontrolled bleeding from the biopsy as there is not enough tissue to tamponade a site of bleeding.
- ☐ Some lesions are too close to vital organs for safe percutaneous biopsy to be performed (e.g. the aorta in retroperitoneal masses).

Abscess Drainage

■ It is performed for patients with mature, walled-off fluid collections (abscesses) in whom antibiotic therapy alone is not sufficient for treatment.

■ An abscess must be documented by an imaging study (typically CT) prior to request for drainage.

■ The abscess must be large enough and accessible enough for the procedure to be performed safely.

INDICATIONS

☐ Patients who are persistently febrile despite adequate antibiotic treatment

☐ Patients who are septicemic

☐ Recurrent abscess formation in a given location

CONTRAINDICATIONS

☐ The collection is small or not easily accessible.

☐ The patient is unstable.

LIMITATIONS

☐ A drain is left in place if the collection is large enough to require continued drainage and cannot be aspirated at the time of the initial procedure.

☐ Loculated collections (i.e. collections with many septations) may not be amenable to drainage as there are many locules of fluid that are not continuous with one another due to the septations. In these cases, attempts may be made to disrupt the septations at the time of the intervention (with a wire) or the catheter may be placed and tPA flushed at intervals through the catheter in an attempt to break up the septations.

Tumor Ablation/Chemoembolization

■ For patients with solitary or <3 malignant hepatic lesions (hepatocellular carcinoma or metastatic disease), chemoablation or radiofrequency (RF) ablation may be performed to treat local disease.

■ The lesions must be identified, localized, and characterized prior to the procedure.

■ The procedure involves percutaneous placement of a catheter into the tumor (RF ablation) with delivery of radio waves to disrupt the tumor cells. Chemoablation is performed with a catheter placed through the hepatic artery (from a femoral artery approach) and instillation of chemotherapeutic agents and toxins to the vessels supplying the tumor.

INDICATIONS
☐ Solitary or ≤3 hepatocellular carcinomas or metastatic lesions

CONTRAINDICATIONS
☐ Lesion inaccessible to catheter placement
☐ Widely metastatic disease
☐ ± Tumor recurrence

LIMITATIONS
☐ Patients with small lesions or lesions in locations such as the hepatic dome or a superficial location are often not amenable to percutaneous RF or cryoablation.
☐ If the entire tumor is not ablated, local recurrence may occur.
☐ Follow-up imaging may be difficult to interpret for recurrence due to the material used in the procedures. These materials produce artifacts that can make it difficult to evaluate the periphery of the lesions.

Renal

Nephrostomy Tube

▣ This is a drainage catheter percutaneously placed for the treatment of hydronephrosis.
▣ An obstructed renal collecting system or ongoing pyelonephritis should be confirmed with imaging (typically CT or ultrasound) prior to the procedure.
▣ The catheter is placed into the dilated renal pelvis under ultrasound guidance with one portion of the catheter in the renal pelvis and the other end coursing to the skin surface and draining into a bag taped to the patient's skin.

INDICATIONS
☐ Chronically or acutely obstructed collecting systems
☐ Palliative for patients with pelvic malignancy with resultant obstructive uropathy
☐ Hydronephrosis with a superinfected collecting system

CONTRAINDICATIONS
☐ Inability to access system
☐ Short life expectancy

LIMITATIONS
☐ Percutaneous access to the collecting system may be difficult, particularly if the patient is obese or kyphotic.

- [ ] Occlusion of the nephrostomy tube may occur if the drainage is thick and viscous.

Nephroureteral Stent

▪ These are similar to nephrostomy tubes with the notable exception of the second end of the catheter traversing the ureter and not extending to the skin surface. This portion of the catheter is coiled and anchored within the bladder.

INDICATIONS

- [ ] They are the same as listed previously for nephrostomy tube plus known obstruction to the ureter.
- [ ] It is also performed for patients unable to tolerate or care for a catheter extending to the skin surface.

CONTRAINDICATIONS

- [ ] Inability to access system
- [ ] Short life expectancy

LIMITATIONS

- [ ] Percutaneous access to the collecting system may be difficult, particularly if the patient is obese or kyphotic.

Thorax

▪ Chest tube (Denver catheter):
  - [ ] This is a small caliber chest tube placed into the pleural cavity for long-term pleural fluid drainage.

INDICATION

- [ ] Long-standing or rapidly reaccumulating pleural effusion (e.g. malignant)

CONTRAINDICATIONS

- [ ] Bacteremia/septicemia
- [ ] Patient unable to tolerate or care for catheter
- [ ] Small pleural effusion
- [ ] Bleeding diathesis

LIMITATIONS

- [ ] If a diagnostic tap is required, a catheter is not required.
- [ ] If patients have liver disease or hypoalbuminemic states, the albumin must be replaced if large volumes of fluid are to be removed (this is more often the case in therapeutic paracentesis).
- [ ] If there are a large number of loculations (septations), it may be difficult to remove fluid as the pockets do not

freely communicate. In these cases, attempts can be made to break up the loculations with a wire at the time of catheter placement or with tPA instillation following catheter placement.

Pleurodesis

■ This involves placement of a foreign material (e.g. erythromycin) to cause an inflammatory reaction in the pleural space. This causes the lung to "stick" to the pleural surface, thus decreasing the risk of spontaneous or recurrent pneumothorax.

INDICATIONS

☐ Recurrent pneumothorax/chylothorax/hydropneumothorax

CONTRAINDICATIONS

☐ Patients with risk of allergy to the material

LIMITATIONS

☐ Procedure failure may occur

☐ There can be a marked inflammatory response to the material, which can produce reactive pleural effusions.

Peritoneal

■ Ascites drainage catheter:

☐ This is a drainage catheter placed into the peritoneal cavity for long-term drainage of recurrent or refractory ascites.

INDICATIONS

☐ Patients requiring frequent or recurrent paracentesis for rapid accumulation of ascites (e.g. malignancy, cirrhosis)

CONTRAINDICATIONS

☐ There is increased risk of infection from an indwelling line; therefore, immunosuppressed patients are at increased risk of infection.

☐ Short life expectancy

LIMITATIONS

☐ Small amounts of ascites do not require catheter placement for drainage; aspiration is typically sufficient.

☐ Loculated ascites may be difficult to drain due to septations, which prevent free communication of the ascites; a wire or tPA may be required to disrupt some of the loculations.

13

Pediatric Radiography

Chest Imaging

Chest Radiography (PA, lateral)

■ It is the initial step in imaging acute cardiopulmonary disease.

■ It may be performed on a stationary or portable radiography unit.

■ It involves frontal (AP) and lateral views of the chest if the patient is cooperative with the examination. If the patient is unstable or if the technologist is unable to position the patient for the study, only a frontal view is obtained. Lateral radiographs are not typically obtained with a portable unit for patients in intensive care units due to the limits of the technology and the severity of the patient's clinical condition. The patient's condition often will limit the ability of the technologist and the support staff to position the child for the radiographs. In certain circumstances, a cross-table lateral view may be obtained (i.e. a film is placed on one side of the patient and the x-ray beam is exposed across the supine patient to reach the film, giving a lateral projection of the chest). This is most often performed to evaluate chest tube positioning or other support apparatus. Loculated pneumothorax can be demonstrated on a lateral or cross-table lateral CXR.

■ Daily "routine" radiographs are only truly indicated in patients with indwelling catheters (e.g. endotracheal tubes) to assess for line positioning. Patients with acute changes in cardiopulmonary status may also require repeat examinations at short intervals.

■ For patients with pneumonia, CXRs should be obtained only at the completion of antibiotic therapy or if the patient fails to improve with appropriate antibiotic coverage.

INDICATIONS
- ☐ Increased work of breathing
- ☐ Shortness of breath
- ☐ Chest pain (e.g. to evaluate for pneumonia, pneumothorax, rib fracture)
- ☐ Desaturation (e.g. to evaluate for pneumonia, pulmonary edema)
- ☐ Cyanosis
- ☐ Fever/sepsis
- ☐ Pleural effusion
- ☐ Line placement
- ☐ Evaluation of patients with known malignancy to evaluate for thoracic metastatic disease (surveillance)

CONTRAINDICATIONS
- ☐ Repeated films increase the patient's radiation exposure.

LIMITATIONS
- ☐ Patient positioning: If a patient cannot be appropriately positioned for the study, subtle abnormalities such as pulmonary nodules or pneumothoraces may not be identified.
- ☐ Small pulmonary nodules, pleural effusions, or fungal disease may not be detected with routine radiography.
- ☐ Radiographic findings often lag behind clinical signs by as much as 48 hours.

Decubitus Radiographs

- ▪ It is the radiographic imaging study of choice to evaluate layering versus loculated pleural effusions; it evaluates for air trapping.
- ▪ Bilateral decubitus images are obtained to evaluate right and left pleural abnormalities.

INDICATIONS
- ☐ Suspected foreign body aspiration: For children in whom an aspirated foreign body is suspected, bilateral decubitus images may be obtained. If a foreign body is present, the affected side will demonstrate air trapping on decubitus imaging, thus confirming the diagnosis.
- ☐ It may allow for evaluation of underlying pulmonary parenchymal abnormalities by allowing pleural fluid to move into the now dependent lateral hemithorax. This will allow the parenchyma at the lung bases, which were obscured by the pleural fluid, to be evaluated.

☐ It may occasionally be useful to evaluate for subtle pneumothorax, particularly in premature infants (a lateral view is more commonly obtained for this indication).

☐ It may allow for identification of loculated pleural fluid. CT should be performed only to evaluate for loculated pleural effusions if the patient is too unstable or immobile for decubitus positioning.

CONTRAINDICATIONS

☐ Unstable patients may not be stable enough for positioning.

LIMITATIONS

☐ Patient positioning: If a patient cannot be appropriately positioned for the study, the study may not be diagnostic.

☐ With large amounts of pleural fluid, the underlying lung parenchyma cannot be identified.

Rib Films

▪ Most rib series include a frontal view of the chest and bone algorithm (i.e. higher radiation dose) views of the ribs. Multiple projections are obtained.

▪ The films are often unnecessary as the main complication of rib fracture is pneumothorax, which is best assessed on frontal views of the chest. Displaced rib fractures are often visualized on conventional CXRs. Non-displaced rib fractures are often not visualized on CXR or rib films; these non-displaced fractures typically do not alter patient management.

▪ CT is not an appropriate method to evaluate for rib fractures as the images are obtained in the axial plane, thus fractures oriented in this plane are often not visualized.

INDICATIONS

☐ There are limited indications unless a non-displaced rib fracture in the absence of a pneumothorax will have a clinical impact. Even in cases of suspected child abuse, rib films are not typically obtained.

CONTRAINDICATIONS

☐ Radiation dose is high, particularly in the pediatric population.

LIMITATIONS

☐ High radiation exposure for limited diagnostic value

Musculoskeletal Imaging

Conventional Radiographs

▦ These films are the first step in evaluation of musculoskeletal abnormalities.

▦ The films may be performed on a stationary unit or portably.

INDICATIONS FOR PORTABLE IMAGING

☐ There are few true indications for portable musculoskeletal radiographs. Portable radiographs tend to be limited by technique and patients' clinical conditions. They may be performed in unstable patients for evaluation of suspected acute fractures.

▦ Optimal radiographs include a minimum of two projections at 90 degrees to each other (i.e. frontal and lateral views). In children, two orthogonal views (i.e. 90 degrees to each other) are typically obtained. Additional views may be obtained as warranted for evaluation of specific clinical questions.

▦ Radiographs are of little use in evaluation of suspected muscular, cartilage, or ligament injury.

▦ Radiographs are of little use in the evaluation of suspected early osteomyelitis as there is often a 10–14 day lag in radiographic manifestations of osteomyelitis. Even at 14 days, it may not be possible to identify changes of osteomyelitis (i.e. a false-negative study). The sensitivity of radiographs is low for osteomyelitis until late stages of the process when often irreversible bone changes are present.

▦ In patients with acute traumatic injury who do not have radiographically apparent fractures at the time of initial radiography, follow-up radiographs in 7–10 days may be obtained to evaluate for radiographically occult fractures. This will allow time for bone resorption around the fracture site to occur, making the fracture line visible; it also allows time for the development of callus, which may allow for identification of the site of injury.

INDICATIONS

☐ Trauma (evaluation for fractures)

☐ Clinical deformity with suspected underlying osseous abnormality (e.g. short limb, bony protrusion)

☐ Evaluation of suspected metabolic or congenital bone disease such as dwarfism or eosinophilic granulomatosis (a skeletal survey is often performed for this purpose). The survey consists of frontal and lateral views of the skull; frontal CXR; frontal abdominal x-ray; frontal views of the arms, legs, hands, and feet; and a lateral view of the cervical, thoracic, and lumbar spine).

☐ Evaluation of suspected child abuse (typically performed as part of a skeletal survey in patients with a high clinical suspicion of abuse)

☐ Osteomyelitis: Limited usefulness in the acute setting

☐ Evaluation of suspected or known scoliosis: Measurements of the degree of scoliosis can be obtained from radiographs obtained for this purpose, which can determine the need for medical or surgical management.

CONTRAINDICATIONS

☐ Repeat films should be limited due to risks of radiation exposure, particularly in the pediatric population.

LIMITATIONS

☐ Patient positioning: This is of particular importance in the pediatric population given that a significant number of fractures (particularly of the elbow) are identified by indirect signs. These indirect signs include malalignment of the bones and the presence of a joint effusion. If the radiographs are not well positioned, these indirect signs of injury may be obscured.

☐ In children with open physes, fractures may be difficult to identify, particularly Salter-Harris type I fractures. In these cases, repeat radiographs in 7–10 days may be useful. Children are often empirically treated with splinting if there is a clinical suspicion of fracture, even in the absence of radiologic findings.

☐ Osteomyelitis: Radiographs are often not positive in the setting of acute infection. This is particularly true for joint space infection (i.e. septic joint). By the time there are radiographic findings of a septic joint, the damage has been incurred; septic joints must be identified early (usually by tapping the joint), thus, radiographs are of limited use in this setting. Findings of osteomyelitis are often not detectable on x-ray for at least 10–14 days after the onset of infection, thus radiography plays a limited role in the identification of osteomyelitis prior to this time period. Additionally, radiographs may not be diagnostic for infection even in patients with known osteomyelitis as it is a process that occurs in the medullary (bone marrow) space of the bone. The medullary space is difficult to evaluate with x-rays; however, it is well evaluated with MR imaging. The studies of choice for patients with suspected osteomyelitis are bone scan and contrast-enhanced MRI.

Neuroradiology

Conventional Radiographs

- Conventional radiographs have little role in current modern-day neuroimaging.
- Skull radiographs are often obtained with CXRs and abdominal radiographs as part of a shunt series to evaluate for possible shunt disruption as an etiology for shunt dysfunction.

INDICATIONS
- ☐ Shunt series to evaluate for ventriculoperitoneal or ventricu-loatrial shunt disruption
- ☐ Evaluation of acute osseous injury to the cervical spine in the setting of trauma

CONTRAINDICATION
- ☐ If CT is considered for evaluation of bony abnormalities of the head and neck or facial bones, conventional radiographs should not be obtained as the additional radiation exposure is unnecessary.

LIMITATIONS
- ☐ Conventional radiographs have low sensitivity for non-displaced fractures of the facial bones, sinus disease, and others. CT is more sensitive and involves a radiation dose similar to that of the number of films that would be required for full evaluation with conventional radiography.

Gastrointestinal Imaging

Conventional Radiographs

- These are often the first imaging evaluations of abdominal pathology.
- A complete abdominal series includes an erect frontal view of the chest and erect (decubitus if the patient cannot be maintained in the erect position) and supine views of the abdomen/pelvis.

- The erect CXR is obtained to evaluate for acute cardiopulmonary disease, such as pneumonia, which may mimic abdominal pain. Additionally, it allows for evaluation of subdiaphragmatic pneumoperitoneum.
- Erect and supine views of the abdomen/pelvis are preferred in order to evaluate for bowel loop dilation and air-fluid levels, which may indicate an obstruction or ileus, as well as to evaluate for pneumoperitoneum. However, if erect radiography is not possible due to the patient's clinical status, tangential beam imaging (i.e. right side up decubitus imaging) may be performed.
- Cholelithiasis or nephrolithiasis may be visible radiographically; however, radiography is of little or no value in the evaluation of acute cholecystitis or renal obstruction. Radiographs are, however, useful in the uncommon conditions of gangrenous cholecystitis or emphysematous pyelitis.

INDICATIONS
- ☐ Evaluation of patients with abdominal pain
- ☐ Evaluation of patients with suspected or known bowel obstruction
- ☐ Evaluation of patients with suspected bowel perforation
- ☐ Evaluation of infants with suspected necrotizing enterocolitis; for this indication, a supine view is typically obtained. If there is a suspicion for a bowel perforation in the setting of necrotizing enterocolitis, a decubitus view of the abdomen is obtained.
- ☐ Initial evaluation of suspected bowel atresia
- ☐ Evaluation of line positioning (e.g. nasogastric, nasojejunal, umbilical arterial catheter, umbilical venous catheter)

CONTRAINDICATIONS
- ☐ If a patient is already scheduled to undergo diagnostic abdominopelvic CT, there is no additional value in conventional radiographs. They simply add additional radiation dose to the patient for no additional diagnostic yield.

LIMITATIONS
- ☐ Patient positioning:
  - • If portions of the abdomen are not included on the radiograph, areas of potential pathology cannot be evaluated.
  - • If patients are not placed in an erect position for the CXR, subdiaphragmatic pneumoperitoneum may not be identified.

- If the patient is not placed in the right side up decubitus position for a long enough period of time, free air may not be identified as there is not adequate time for the air to mobilize into a non-dependent position over the liver contour. Patients should be kept in the right side up position for at least 3 minutes prior to obtaining the image to allow the free air to mobilize.
□ Small bowel obstruction: In patients with small bowel obstruction in whom all of the bowel loops are filled with fluid and not air, the obstruction may not be identified on x-rays. Fluid cannot be readily identified on x-ray, thus, the presence of dilated bowel loops may not be identified. The diagnosis may be suggested by secondary signs of a near complete absence of bowel gas on the x-ray.
□ Non–bowel-related pathologies such as abscesses are typically radiographically occult. CT is required for diagnosis of these entities.
□ If patients are not appropriately positioned for examinations or left in the upright or decubitus positions for adequate amounts of time, small to moderate amounts of pneumoperitoneum may not be recognized.
□ Obese patients are difficult to image as they often exceed the size of the imaging plate, thus portions of the bowel/soft tissues may not be included on the examination.
□ Many gallstones are radiographically occult.
□ Acute inflammatory processes (e.g. acute cholecystitis and appendicitis) are radiographically occult. The only true indication for abdominal radiographs in patients with suspected cholecystitis or pyelonephritis who have been imaged previously with ultrasound is the evaluation of emphysematous cholecystitis or emphysematous pyelonephritis in which air is present in the gallbladder wall (cholecystitis) or kidney (pyelonephritis/pyelitis). The air may be difficult to identify on ultrasound (see Chapter 10); however, it is readily visible on CT.

Genitourinary Imaging

Conventional Radiographs
▪ They are of limited value in the evaluation of genitourinary pathology.

- They may be useful to evaluate the presence of renal/ureteral or bladder calculi, to grossly evaluate stone burden, to evaluate for stone passage or morphologic changes following nephroureteral stent placement or lithotripsy.
- They may be useful to detect air in cases of emphysematous pyelitis or cystitis.

INDICATIONS
- ☐ Evaluation of suspected renal, ureteral. or bladder calculi

CONTRAINDICATIONS
- ☐ If patients are already scheduled to undergo a CT for the evaluation of nephroureterolithiasis, there is no indication for the additional radiation exposure of an abdominal radiograph (KUB).
- ☐ Morbid obesity: If a KUB is being requested for the evaluation of the presence and location of a stone in an obese patient, there is little role for the film. The limitations of the film (due to underpenetration of the body by the x-ray beam) will render it useless for identification of a stone; CT should be performed in these patients.

LIMITATIONS
- ☐ Overlying bowel gas will often obscure the renal contours, limiting evaluation for small stones.
- ☐ Ingested material within the bowel may mimic a calculus.
- ☐ Not all calculi are dense on conventional radiographs. If there is a high clinical suspicion for a renal, ureteral, or bladder calculus, a non-contrast CT of the abdomen and pelvis (flank pain protocol) CT may be obtained.

14

Pediatric Fluoroscopy

▦ Fluoroscopy is mainly used in the evaluation of GI and genitourinary abnormalities in the pediatric population. It is occasionally used in airway evaluation, in diaphragmatic excursion (motion), and as procedure guidance.

▦ Always minimize the radiation dose to the child; either by alternative imaging modalities that do not require ionizing radiation or by careful fluoroscopic practice to minimize the dose per study.

GI Fluoroscopy

▦ Proximal GI tract:
  ☐ Modified barium swallow:
    • The study is typically performed in conjunction with a speech pathologist.
    • It evaluates the oral phase of digestion and the swallowing mechanism, and it allows visualization of aspiration during the course of the examination.
    • The study involves the administration of barium mixed with liquids and solids of varying consistency. The patient is monitored dynamically using fluoroscopic images while he or she is chewing and swallowing.
    • The study does not evaluate the esophagus distal to the pharynx.
    INDICATIONS
  ☐ Evaluation of patients with swallowing difficulties and suspected aspiration

CONTRAINDICATIONS

☐ Children with known aspiration should be reimaged only if there is clinical evidence to suggest resolution or improvement of the aspiration. In patients with known aspiration, repeated barium studies increase the risk of aspiration pneumonia/pneumonitis.

LIMITATIONS

☐ If the child refuses to ingest the barium/barium-coated food, the study cannot be performed. Unlike esophagrams and upper GI series for which it is possible to pass a nasogastric (NG) tube to administer barium, this is not possible with a modified barium swallow. For a modified swallow study, the patient must be able to ingest the material so that oromotor skills/coordination and largyngeal penetration/aspiration can be assessed.

☐ Due to the rapidity of the swallowing mechanism, multiple swallows may be necessary to allow for adequate evaluation of the oropharyngeal mechanism.

Esophagram (Barium Swallow)

■ The study is performed by a radiologist without the assistance of a speech pathologist.

■ The patient is administered liquid barium orally and is monitored by fluoroscopy. Occasionally, the child will refuse to drink the barium, at which time an NG tube may be placed and the barium administered through the tube.

■ The study evaluates the entire esophagus including the cervical esophagus. It does not evaluate for aspiration, although this may occasionally be noted during the course of the examination, at which time the study is typically terminated due to the risk of aspiration pneumonitis.

■ The examination allows for identification of intrinsic masses/lesions (i.e. those arising from the esophagus itself) or extrinsic masses (arising from outside of the esophagus and causing mass effect upon the esophagus (e.g. vascular rings/slings, lymphadenopathy).

■ It allows for evaluation of esophageal motility in a gross manner (i.e. allows for identification of grossly abnormal esophageal peristalsis). Motility may be abnormal in cases of achalasia or chronic disorders such as long-standing reflux esophagitis.

■ The study allows for evaluation of gastroesophageal reflux. Although reflux may be identified with a barium examination, if reflux is not demonstrated, it does not mean that it is not present. Gastroesophageal reflux may not be detected at the time of a barium study, even if it is documented to occur (e.g. with pH probes).

■ Esophagrams do not evaluate the stomach!

■ The study is never an emergency unless there is a suspected obstructing foreign body, and gastroenterologists are not immediately available for endoscopy. In certain cases, foreign body retrieval can be attempted with a catheter under fluoroscopic guidance.

INDICATIONS

☐ Evaluation of patients with dysphagia
☐ Evaluation of suspected gastroesophageal reflux
☐ Evaluation of patients who are vomiting (e.g. due to gastroesophageal reflux)
☐ Evaluation of patients with stridor
☐ Evaluation of suspected esophageal foreign body
☐ Evaluation of suspected tracheoesophageal fistula

CONTRAINDICATIONS

☐ Known aspiration
☐ Unstable patients (e.g. hypoxic, intubated)

LIMITATIONS

☐ The study uses ionizing radiation; therefore, imaging time and radiation (fluoroscopy) use should be kept to a minimum.
☐ If patients refuse to ingest the liquid barium, an NG tube may be required to instill barium into the GI tract.
☐ Gastroesophageal reflux may not be elicited even if present, thus leading to a false-negative study.
☐ If an NG tube has to be placed to instill barium (i.e. in patients who refuse to drink the contrast), motility cannot be assessed as no oral contrast passes spontaneously through the esophagus.
☐ As only barium is given without an effervescent agent (e.g. Alka-Seltzer), the lining of the esophagus (i.e. the mucosa) cannot be assessed for erosions or ulcers. These, however, are uncommon in the pediatric population.
☐ In patients with esophageal strictures (e.g. post-ingestion of caustic material, following tracheoesophageal fistula

repair), the stricture may be so tight that no contrast can be passed beyond the stricture in order to evaluate the remainder of the esophagus.

☐ In patients with pure esophageal atresia, only a blind ending proximal pouch is present. If contrast is placed into this pouch, there is a high risk of aspiration into the lungs. If there is concern for pure esophageal atresia, an attempt should be made to gently pass an NG tube under fluoroscopy in order to confirm the diagnosis.

☐ The location of the extrinsic compression is readily identified; however, the precise etiology of the compression may not. The patient likely will require additional investigative studies such as CT angiography or MRI if vascular abnormalities are the question.

☐ The study may be falsely negative for gastroesophageal reflux as it is intermittent and imaging is performed for a finite time period.

☐ If an inadequate volume of contrast is present in the gastric fundus, a false-negative study may occur as there is insufficient barium to detect the reflux.

☐ Small tracheoesophageal fistulas may be below the resolution of imaging.

☐ If the radiologist performing the study is unaware of the concern for a tracheoesophageal fistula, the diagnosis may not be made. This is due to the manner in which the study is performed for the diagnosis of a fistula; it is performed slightly differently than a routine esophagram.

Upper GI Series (Upper GI/Barium Swallow with Upper GI)

■ The patient is administered liquid barium orally (or through an NG tube) and is monitored by fluoroscopy.

■ The study includes evaluation of the distal esophagus, stomach, and duodenum. It does not evaluate the small bowel.

■ The study is an emergency only if there is a question of malrotation causing midgut volvulus.

INDICATIONS

☐ Upper GI is a functional and anatomic study. It allows for evaluation of gastroesophageal reflux (functional) as well as evaluation of malrotation (anatomic).

☐ Evaluation of persistent vomiting

☐ Evaluation of weight loss (often performed in conjunction with a small bowel series to evaluate for diseases such as Crohn's)

☐ Evaluation of abdominal pain (i.e. midgut volvulus)

☐ Evaluation for malrotation

CONTRAINDICATIONS

☐ Known aspiration

☐ Unstable patient (i.e. hypoxia, intubated)

LIMITATIONS

☐ The study uses ionizing radiation; therefore, imaging time and radiation (fluoroscopy) use should be kept to a minimum.

☐ If patients refuse to ingest the liquid barium, an NG tube may be required to instill barium into the GI tract.

☐ Gastroesophageal reflux may not be elicited even if present, thus leading to a false-negative study.

☐ If an inadequate amount of barium is instilled, gastroesophageal reflux may be inadequately assessed.

☐ If too much barium is placed into the stomach, it may obscure identification of the exact location of the duodenal-jejunal (D-J) junction, thus limiting evaluation for malrotation.

☐ If the child is not positioned appropriately, the position of the D-J junction may be obscured.

Small Bowel Follow-Through

▪ The patient is administered liquid barium orally (or through an NG tube) and is monitored by fluoroscopy and abdominal radiographs (KUBs).

▪ The study may be combined with an upper GI to evaluate the distal esophagus, stomach, and duodenum in addition to the small bowel.

▪ It allows for evaluation of small bowel loops to the level of the ileocecal valve and cecum. It does NOT evaluate the colon.

▪ Small bowel follow-through (SBFT) is a functional and anatomic study. It allows for evaluation of transit time, which may be increased in malabsorptive states or decreased in patients on medications, for example. It allows for evaluation of small bowel loop caliber, transition points in small bowel obstruction, and abnormalities of small bowel folds. Small bowel folds may be abnormal in morphology and thickness in a variety of systemic disorders including celiac sprue, malabsorption states, and inflammatory bowel disease, to name a few.

■ It has limited usefulness in evaluation of intraluminal masses (enteroclysis is preferred; see later).

■ Due to the variability in transit times, the study typically is scheduled as the first case of the day. This is particularly true for patients with known or suspected small bowel obstruction as transit is often markedly prolonged and off-shift monitoring is difficult.

■ It is almost never an emergency study.

INDICATIONS

☐ Evaluation of suspected small bowel pathology

☐ Obstruction (allows for identification of the site of obstruction and the degree e.g. high- or low-grade or partial)

☐ Inflammation/infection: It allows for identification of abnormal small bowel loops, which may indicate infection or inflammatory processes such as Crohn's disease/ulcerative colitis (in backwash ileitis). The location of the abnormality is often critical in determining the infectious agent as infections such as giardiasis tend to affect the duodenum, whereas agents such as tuberculosis, *Yersinia*, and *Salmonella* tend to affect the terminal ileum. The terminal ileum is also the earliest site of disease in Crohn's and may be the only small bowel manifestation of ulcerative colitis (which tends to be a colonic disease process).

☐ Malabsorption: In malabsorptive states, transit times of the contrast are often increased and the barium becomes dilute due to the large volume of fluid that is in the lumen of the bowel.

CONTRAINDICATIONS

☐ If abdominopelvic CT is to be performed for the evaluation of acute small bowel pathology (e.g. small bowel obstruction), SBFT should not be performed. The oral contrast material administered for the SBFT is very dense, which is necessary for visualization on fluoroscopy. However, the contrast is too dense for CT imaging and causes significant image artifact. This can render the CT uninterpretable. If CT is being considered, it should be performed prior to SBFT.

LIMITATIONS

☐ The study uses ionizing radiation; therefore, imaging time and radiation (fluoroscopy) use should be kept to a minimum.

☐ If patients refuse to ingest the liquid barium, an NG tube may be required to instill barium into the GI tract.

☐ The study often is not performed dynamically (i.e. the patient is not monitored with fluoroscopy while drinking). Therefore, the D-J flexure is often not identified and is not routinely evaluated on this examination. If malrotation is of concern, the study may be combined with an upper GI.

☐ The terminal ileum may be difficult to separate from adjacent bowel loops; therefore, it may not always be easy to evaluate.

☐ In patients with known or suspected small bowel obstruction, effort should be made to schedule the study as the first examination of the day as motility is often markedly delayed and the study may extend over a long period of time. As the purpose of the study is to determine the point of obstruction and to attempt to identify the cause of obstruction (e.g. adhesions), intermittent fluoroscopy should be performed with attempts to separate bowel loops in an effort to identify the obstruction. If the study is performed during off hours, it is difficult to carefully monitor these cases.

☐ In high-grade obstructions, the contrast may remain immobile for prolonged periods of time without reaching the site of obstruction. In these cases, the study may be terminated prior to completion in favor of operative intervention.

☐ If close monitoring is not performed, focally abnormal bowel loops may not be identified; therefore, it is important that the study be scheduled early in the day to allow dedicated monitoring.

☐ Contrast may become very dilute due to the presence of intraluminal fluid. This may limit the sensitivity of the study.

Enteroclysis

▪ A large caliber, long NG catheter is placed beyond the ligament of Trietz at the beginning of the examination. Barium and methylcellulose are then (alternately) injected by hand through the catheter to distend the small bowel. This is performed under fluoroscopy.

■ The study cannot be combined with upper GI or imaging of the colon.

■ The examination allows for evaluation of the lumen of the small bowel, thus masses can be more readily detected than with conventional SBFT. It allows for better characterization of small bowel fold abnormalities. It does NOT allow for true evaluation of small bowel motility.

■ The contrast (diluted by the methylcellulose) allows for evaluation of the mucosal surface (i.e. the lining) of the small bowel. This allows for identification of masses.

■ The study is not routinely performed for evaluation of small bowel pathology.

INDICATIONS

☐ Evaluation of known or suspected intraluminal mass

☐ Evaluation of previously demonstrated (SBFT) small bowel fold abnormality

☐ Evaluation of unexplained GI bleed in patients with negative workup (to include upper GI/SBFT/BE/endoscopy)

☐ Evaluation for possible lead point in recurrent (i.e. >3) intussusceptions

CONTRAINDICATIONS

☐ Acute esophageal disease: There is a theoretic risk of esophageal perforation due to the placement of the large bore enteric tube.

☐ Patients with acute small bowel pathology/inflammation are at risk of bowel perforation due to the increased pressure in the bowel lumen from the contrast and methylcellulose instillation.

LIMITATIONS

☐ The study may not be well tolerated by children, thus it may not always be possible.

☐ Small masses may be below the resolution of imaging.

■ If there is a significant time interval between the abnormal SBFT and the enteroclysis, the acute abnormality may have resolved, thus diagnosis may not be possible.

■ If the abnormality affected a single or a few loops of small bowel on the SBFT, these loops may be difficult to isolate on the enteroclysis.

Hypaque Enema

- A Foley catheter is placed in the rectum and taped in place. The balloon is NOT inflated due to the risk of damage to/perforation of the rectum. Hypaque is instilled into the colon via gravity or may be hand injected.
- The patient is rolled into different positions on the imaging table during the study to opacify the entire colon.
- It allows for evaluation of strictures, masses, intussusception (air enema is the study of choice), obstruction.
- It does not require a bowel preparation.

  INDICATIONS
  - [ ] Failure to pass meconium within the first 48 hours of life
  - [ ] Suspected distal intestinal obstruction
  - [ ] Evaluation of suspected colonic fistulas
  - [ ] Suspected strictures (e.g. after necrotizing enterocolytis [NEC])
  - [ ] Therapeutic (patients with meconium ileus/meconium ileus equivalent)

  CONTRAINDICATIONS
  - [ ] Acute abdomen: If there is concern of bowel perforation, the study should not be performed. Surgical intervention is required in these patients.

  LIMITATIONS
  - [ ] If an inadequate seal is produced with the tape, contrast will leak out around the catheter and inadequate filling of the colon will occur.
  - [ ] If a stricture is present, it may be difficult to instill contrast beyond this level to evaluate for additional sites of stricture.
  - [ ] If the level of obstruction is in the distal ileum, it may not be possible to reflux contrast into the small bowel in order to make the diagnosis.

Air Enema

- A Foley catheter is placed in the rectum and taped in place. Air is then insufflated to a maximum pressure of 120 mm Hg.
- It is performed only for the diagnosis and treatment of intussusception.
- The patient should be evaluated by the surgical service prior to request for air enema to ensure that it is safe to proceed with the

pneumatic reduction. The procedure is contraindicated if the patient exhibits peritoneal signs (treated with surgery) or if the patient has had three prior intussusceptions (as there is likely a lead point, which will cause recurrent intussusceptions).

- Air reduction is preferred over barium as it provides a cleaner surgical field should attempts at radiologic reduction fail.

INDICATIONS

☐ Intussusception reduction in patients with positive plain film or ultrasound findings of intussusception

☐ If ultrasound is negative but clinical suspicion is high for intussusception, air enema may be performed for evaluation.

CONTRAINDICATIONS

☐ Peritoneal signs: If there is clinical suspicion or radiographic findings that suggest bowel perforation, air reduction should not be performed and the patient should be managed surgically.

LIMITATIONS

☐ Air enema may be unsuccessful to reduce the intussusception, thus requiring surgical intervention. The likelihood of success decreases if symptoms have been present for several days (suggesting the presence of intussusception with bowel edema for several days) or if a lead point is present.

☐ If an inadequate seal is achieved, air pressure may be inadequate to reduce the intussusception.

☐ Careful attention must be paid to the air pressure generated as a pressure >120 mm Hg increases the risk of perforating the colon.

Airway Fluoroscopy

- It is performed under fluoroscopy with the patient awake.
- The study evaluates the airway, including the hypopharynx, trachea, and main bronchi.
- It allows for evaluation of tracheomalacia, intraluminal masses (CT or bronchoscopy are the optimal studies), strictures.
- It is often performed in conjunction with an esophagram for patients with recurrent pneumonia.
- Airway fluoroscopy alone does not require patient preparation prior to the study. If performed in conjunction with an esophagram, the patient should be NPO for 4 hours prior to the study.

INDICATIONS

☐ Evaluation of patients with stridor

☐ Evaluation of patients with aspiration in whom there is concern for an airway abnormality

CONTRAINDICATIONS

☐ Intubated patients cannot be adequately evaluated; the study should be postponed until the patient is extubated.

LIMITATIONS

☐ The study uses ionizing radiation, therefore, imaging time and radiation (fluoroscopy) use should be kept to a minimum.

15

Pediatric CT

General Considerations

- Remember radiation! Carefully consider the indications for the examination and determine if imaging is required or if alternative imaging modalities are available.

- Contrast: Unless there is known or suspected underlying renal disease, a serum creatinine (Cr) is not required prior to IV contrast administration in the pediatric population.

- Sedation: CT has a relatively short imaging time in comparison to MRI; however, patients must be immobile during the CT study in order for adequate imaging to be performed. In some children, this may require sedation. Two types of sedation are employed for CT and MRI: conscious sedation and general anesthesia.

  - ☐ Conscious sedation: This requires the presence of a trained nurse and physician to monitor the patient and administer the sedation. The patient is administered short-acting agents with both amnestic and sedative properties. A functioning IV is required, as is cardiovascular monitoring equipment.

  - ☐ General anesthesia: This requires the presence of an anesthesiologist or nurse anesthetist. The patient is completely sedated for the study. This requires both pre-sedation screening and post-sedation monitoring by the anesthesiology service.

- IV access: Given the relative difficulty of acquiring IV access in children, in inpatients, when possible, a functioning IV should be in place prior to the patient's transfer to the CT scanner. For CT angiography (CTA) studies (e.g. CTA of the chest for vascular rings), a relatively large bore IV should be in place.

The size of the IV should be appropriate to the patient's age and size. The larger the IV, the higher the rate of contrast injection, thus the better the imaging study.

■ IV contrast: For abdominal/pelvic imaging, IV contrast is frequently administered. Chest and brain imaging may not require the administration of IV contrast. The specific indications for contrast-enhanced CT (CECT) are considered later.

■ Oral contrast: In general, for abdominal/pelvic imaging, oral contrast is beneficial for evaluation of bowel pathology. This is particularly the case in young children who lack intra-abdominal fat and may be difficult to evaluate.

CT of the Thorax

There are four main categories of chest CT: routine non-contrast CT, CECT, CTA for pulmonary embolism (PE), and high-resolution chest CT.

Non-Contrast CT of the Thorax

■ It is the most common protocol used.
■ Images are obtained through the thorax, from the thoracic inlet through the upper abdomen.
■ No IV contrast is administered.
■ It is most often employed to evaluate findings identified on conventional radiographs (e.g. pulmonary nodules, cystic lung lesions).

INDICATIONS
☐ Evaluation or follow-up of pulmonary nodules and masses
☐ Evaluation of suspected or known cystic lung lesions (e.g. congenital cystic adenomatoid malformation or congenital lobar emphysema)
☐ Staging/restaging of lymphoma (with the exception of hilar lymphadenopathy). It is more commonly performed in conjunction with CT of the abdomen and pelvis, in which case IV contrast is administered.
☐ Evaluation of thoracic metastatic disease in patients with osteosarcoma (tends to metastasize to the lung)
☐ Evaluation of aortic size/follow-up of aneurysms (for patients with aortic valvular disease or collagen vascular disease)

Pediatric CT

☐ Evaluation of patients with suspected anomalies of the tracheobronchial tree. (This abnormality may be evaluated with or without IV contrast. If the suspicion is of a vascular ring causing airway compromise, IV contrast is administered. If bronchial tree anomalies are suspected, IV contrast is not required [e.g. evaluation of suspected bronchiectasis].)

CONTRAINDICATIONS

☐ If there is concern that airway compromise from masses or tracheomalacia exists, it may be unsafe to proceed with the examination (i.e. with the patient supine) if an airway is not in place or if anesthesiology is not available for emergent airway protection should the patient decompensate.

LIMITATIONS

☐ There is a low sensitivity for hilar lymphadenopathy.

☐ CT is of little use in patients with acute processes such as pneumonia. If a patient demonstrates clinical findings consistent with an infectious process and conventional radiographs demonstrate an infiltrate, there is little to be gained from CT in the acute setting. The parenchyma involved by the infectious process cannot be further evaluated. If, however, radiographic findings persist following appropriate therapy for an infectious process (with expected radiographic resolution lagging behind clinical findings by several weeks), a CT may be appropriate at that time to evaluate for occult malignancy.

☐ Evaluation of the lung parenchyma is limited in young patients who are unable to breath-hold or in patients who require sedation and cannot comply with breath holding instructions.

☐ Evaluation of suspected pulmonary sequestration is better performed following the administration of IV contrast. Contrast will allow for identification of a feeding vessel (if of adequate size for resolution on CT), which may clinch the diagnosis.

Contrast-Enhanced CT of the Thorax

■ It is less commonly used than non-contrast CT.

■ The most common indication for CECT is central lesions with a question of hilar lymphadenopathy or vascular involvement or for vascular rings.

- Average contrast dose: Dependent upon patient age and weight
- Requires a large bore IV; PICC lines and central lines cannot be injected. Port-a-caths may be used for routine chest CECT but may not be used for CTA.
- Renal function: For pediatric patients, Cr levels are not typically obtained prior to IV contrast administration unless there is a clinical suspicion of underlying renal dysfunction.
- Contrast allergies: For patients with a history of contrast allergy, premedication with steroids is required. The regimen for premedication is discussed in the body CT section, later.

INDICATIONS
- ☐ Evaluation of central lesions to evaluate for hilar involvement of lymphadenopathy
- ☐ Evaluation of vascular structures, particularly vascular rings. This is usually performed as a CT angiogram (CTA) and requires a large bore IV (as large as is feasible depending upon the patient's age) and size.
- ☐ Evaluation of patients with known or suspected malignancy (e.g. lymphoma, neuroblastoma, Wilms tumor). This is often performed in conjunction with CECT of the abdomen and pelvis.

CONTRAINDICATIONS
- ☐ IV contrast allergy
- ☐ Impaired renal function

LIMITATIONS
- ☐ Limited evaluation of the lung parenchyma in young children and patients unable to comply with breath holding instructions
- ☐ Due to the relatively small IVs that can be placed in pediatric patients, longer injection times are required for IV contrast administration, limiting the density of the bolus. This limited density limits vessel enhancement and may render interpretation difficult.
- ☐ Motion artifact may severely degrade the images, particularly in very young infants who are "wrapped and fed" and imaged without sedation.

CT Angiography for Pulmonary Embolism

- There are few indications for evaluation of PE in the pediatric population.

■ This study is performed for the sole indication of evaluation of possible PE. The lung apices and bases are excluded from the study. Images through the pulmonary vasculature are obtained at intervals of 1.3 mm with overlap.

■ The study should not be performed in lieu of a CXR in a patient with an acute event as there are a variety of CXR findings that may provide an explanation for the patient's symptoms and circumvent the radiation dose and contrast load of a CTA.

■ Average contrast dose: Based upon patient weight; approximately 1 cc/kg non-ionic contrast

■ Requires at least a 20 g IV or larger for adequate bolus (depending on patient size)

■ Renal function: As earlier

■ Contrast allergies: As earlier

INDICATIONS

☐ Evaluation of acute or chronic thromboembolic events. In the pediatric population, these type of events are uncommon and typically seen in patients with malignancy or underlying hypercoagulable states.

High-Resolution CT of the Thorax

■ It is performed as a non-contrast examination. Images are obtained with a slice thickness of 1 mm at intervals of 10 mm in both inspiration and expiration. Thus, only 10% of the pulmonary parenchyma is imaged. At our institution, however, a routine non-contrast CT of the thorax is obtained prior to the high-resolution images. It is advisable to discuss the local protocol with the imaging department in order to optimize the study to answer the clinical question.

■ It is performed solely for the evaluation of interstitial lung disease.

■ It is not an appropriate study to use to evaluate for pulmonary nodules as only approximately 10% of the lungs are imaged (unless a standard chest CT is a part of the protocol; in these cases, only the standard chest CT would be required).

■ Patients must be able to breath-hold for at least 20 seconds for the study, thus, it is suggested that the study not be performed on patients hospitalized with superimposed acute pulmonary processes or in small children who cannot comply with breath holding instructions. Rather, it is suggested that the study be performed electively following resolution of the acute illness.

INDICATIONS

☐ Identification and evaluation of interstitial lung diseases such sarcoid, lymphangitic spread of tumor, and drug toxicity

☐ Evaluation of air trapping in asthma, bronchiectasis

☐ Evaluation of perfusion abnormality

☐ Evaluation of chronic lung disease

CONTRAINDICATIONS

☐ Inability to comply with breath holding instructions

☐ Acute respiratory illness

☐ Inability to lie flat

☐ Inability to breath-hold for at least 10–20 seconds

LIMITATIONS

☐ Respiratory or patient motion may render the study uninterpretable.

☐ Incomplete inspiration or expiration may make it difficult to identify areas of air trapping or abnormal perfusion. This may lead to false-negative results.

☐ Hilar and mediastinal adenopathy, which can be present in some interstitial diseases, may be difficult to recognize on the non-contrast examination, particularly if only inspiratory/expiratory high-resolution images are obtained.

CT of the Musculoskeletal System

▪ The majority of CTs performed for the evaluation of musculoskeletal pathology are performed as non-contrast imaging (i.e. without IV contrast).

▪ Images are most commonly obtained directly in the axial plane. With multislice CT technology, the axial data can be reconstructed into images in the sagittal and coronal planes.

▪ Imaging is confined to the specific region of clinical interest. CT is not an appropriate modality to screen for diffuse disease (e.g. diffuse osseous metastatic disease, for which a bone scan is a more appropriate investigation).

INDICATIONS (NON-CONTRAST CT)

☐ Identification of occult fractures not demonstrated on conventional radiography

☐ Preoperative planning of documented fractures

- □ Evaluation of congenital anomalies (e.g. tarsal coalition)
- □ Characterization of the matrix of a bone lesion identified on conventional radiography

CONTRAINDICATIONS (NON-CONTRAST CT)

- □ Evaluation of ligaments, tendons, menisci; MR is the study of choice for these structures
- □ Evaluation of suspected abscesses as IV contrast is required to evaluate for enhancing collections
- □ Evaluation of osteomyelitis; bone destruction does not occur until late in the disease. If there is concern for osteomyelitis, nuclear medicine bone scan or MR is recommended

LIMITATIONS (NON-CONTRAST CT)

- □ Patient factors: If the patient cannot be properly positioned (e.g. in patients with contractures or fractures), it may be difficult to image the fracture in a useful plane.
- □ Images may be degraded by streak artifact if an external fixator or internal fixation is present.
- □ Collections such as hematomas can be identified without the administration of IV contrast. However, infected hematomas (unless they contain air) and abscesses cannot be identified without IV contrast.
- □ Soft tissue masses such as liposarcomas and malignant fibrous histiocytomas cannot be characterized on non-contrast CT. MR with IV contrast is the optimal imaging modality for primary soft tissue tumors as it allows for localization of and characterization of the mass, and evaluation of the extent of tumor involvement.
- □ Primary bone tumors may be characterized on non-contrast CT; however, if there is a soft tissue component to the tumor, this may not be recognized or characterized on a non-contrast CT examination. CECT or, preferably, MR should be performed for the evaluation of known or suspected soft tissue components.

INDICATIONS (CONTRAST-ENHANCED CT)

- □ Evaluation of suspected abscesses
- □ Evaluations of vascular compromise by the presence of a soft tissue or osseous mass

CONTRAINDICATIONS (CONTRAST-ENHANCED CT)

- □ Poor renal function or contrast allergy

LIMITATIONS (CONTRAST-ENHANCED CT)

- □ Small abscess collections may be below the resolution of CT.

□ Intraosseous abscesses (i.e. an abscess in the bone marrow or cortex) are not typically visualized on CT. Contrast-enhanced MR is the imaging study of choice for this indication.

□ Infected joint prosthesis cannot be definitively determined on CT; nuclear medicine imaging or contrast-enhanced MR are the studies of choice.

□ Streak artifact from metal prosthesis can mask collections, particularly if small.

□ Obese patients may be difficult to image, particularly if the area of interest is small, if the patient is too large and touches the sides of the CT scanner gantry (causing artifact), or if the collection is small.

General Considerations in Body CT Imaging

■ There should be a valid indication for the examination, particularly given the risks of IV contrast and the significant radiation doses attained. Radiation dose is of even greater concern in the era of multirow detector CT imaging. If a diagnosis may be made on clinical grounds only, a CT scan may be circumvented if it is deemed unnecessary. Consideration should also be given to potential imaging studies, which require lower doses of or no radiation (e.g. can the question be answered with conventional radiographs or ultrasound?).

■ Weight limits: Patients >350 lbs in weight cannot be imaged on standard CT tables. CT scanners do exist to image patients exceeding standard table weight limits; however, these are typically found at veterinary hospitals and are often not readily available for clinical imaging. Weight limits usually are not an issue in the pediatric population unless the patient's girth exceeds the diameter of the CT scanner aperture (52 inches).

■ IV contrast:

□ It is often required in the evaluation of suspected abdominopelvic pathology. The indications for IV contrast are discussed later.

□ For all inpatients, it is recommended that peripheral IV access be obtained on the floor prior to the examination. PICC lines cannot be used for the administration of IV contrast agents, particularly for arterial phase imaging as rapid infusions are not possible through the small lumens. Additionally, there is a risk of PICC line disruption with high rates of contrast injection. There is a subset of PICC lines ("power PICCS") that is designed to accommodate higher pressure/volume injections. These PICC lines currently cost more, however, and not all institutions use them. Discussion with the local PICC service and interventional and diagnostic radiologists is recommended to determine if these PICC lines are available at the institution and if they can be used for CT examination.

☐ Institutions vary as to the limit of renal function at which they may safely administer IV contrast. The nephrotoxic effects of IV contrast are well recognized. In the pediatric population without risk of or known renal dysfunction serum Cr levels are not routinely obtained prior to IV contrast administration.

☐ If patients are on dialysis (either hemodialysis or peritoneal dialysis), attention should be paid to the schedule of dialysis. It is advisable that patients undergoing CECT examinations be dialysed within 24 hours following the contrast dose. This is mainly related to volume and osmotic effects of the IV contrast agents.

☐ Patients with diabetes who are on oral hypoglycemic agents (e.g. Glucophage [metformin hydrochloride]) require that the agent be discontinued for 48 hours following the administration of IV contrast. Additionally, they require that a repeat Cr level be drawn 24–48 hours following the administration of contrast to evaluate for potential contrast-induced nephropathy.

☐ Consideration should be given to the necessity of IV contrast in patients with a history of thyroid carcinoma. If possible, IV contrast should be avoided in these patients as it has effects upon thyroid tissue and thus may affect the uptake of nuclear medicine radiotracers. This in turn may have an impact on the restaging and treatment of these patients with radioactive iodine. The iodinated IV contrast will compete for binding sites in the thyroid and sites of thyroid disease, which may lead to a false-negative result due to lack of radiotracer uptake.

☐ A history of prior contrast reaction should be obtained prior to a request for a contrast-enhanced imaging study. Contrast reactions can range from minimal reactions such as hives to full anaphylactoid-type reactions requiring cardiopulmonary resuscitation efforts. The severity of a prior contrast reaction is not a predictor of the severity of a future contrast reaction. Patients with hives from a past CECT may go on to manifest a much more severe reaction. If a risk of contrast reaction exists, or if there is a documented reaction, pre-medication regimens should be implemented prior to the examination.

Premedication for Patients with IV Contrast Allergies

▥ A variety of regimens are in clinical use for the premedication of patients with known or suspected contrast reaction.

▥ The need for premedication should be communicated to the scheduler at the time of the imaging request so that the exam-ination may be scheduled for a time when the premedication regimen has been completed. For inpatients requiring premedi-cation, it is suggested that the housestaff stay in communication with the technologists/schedulers to ensure completion of the regimen.

▥ There are a variety of protocols in use for premedication. The two most common for adults are as follows; these regimens should be converted to a pediatric dose (most hospital pharma-cies can perform the conversion):

  ☐ Regimen 1
    • Medication: Prednisone
    • Route: Oral
    • Dose: 50 mg
    • Schedule: 13, 7, and 1 hour prior to CECT
    • Benadryl 50 mg oral or IV is also administered 1 hour prior to CECT.

  ☐ Regimen 2
    • Medication: Solu-Medrol (methylprednisolone sodium succinate)
    • Route: IV
    • Dose: 125 mg
    • Schedule: 6 and 1 hour prior to CECT
    • Benadryl 50 mg oral or IV is also administered 1 hour prior to CECT.

CT of Hepatic Abnormalities

▥ Hepatic lesions are commonly identified on routine abdomi-nal imaging. Most of these lesions are below the resolution of

CT and thus cannot be further characterized. Typically, these lesions do not require further follow-up.

■ Hepatic imaging requires the administration of IV contrast in order to identify lesions.

■ If hepatic lesions are suspected on a clinical basis or have been identified on other imaging studies and require further evaluation, a CT may be obtained. Three-phase hepatic imaging is typically performed in order to characterize lesions. Three-phase hepatic imaging consists of the following:

☐ Non-contrast 5-mm thick images through the liver

☐ Thin section (2.5 mm) axial images through the liver in the arterial, portovenous, and delayed phases of IV contrast enhancement

☐ Oral contrast is not required for the examination.

■ Three-phase contrast imaging is not required for all hepatic lesions. For patients in whom hepatic lesions have previously been documented, routine abdominopelvic CT may be performed with single phase imaging after IV contrast administration. This is particularly of use in the follow-up of known hepatic metastatic disease.

INDICATIONS

☐ There are few indications for dedicated hepatic imaging (i.e. hepatic mass protocol imaging) in the pediatric population. Dedicated imaging should be performed if there is a high clinical suspicion for hepatic metastatic disease in the setting of a "normal" routine CECT of the abdomen and pelvis.

CONTRAINDICATIONS

☐ Patients who cannot receive IV contrast because they have poor renal function, they lack IV access, or they have an allergy to it are not candidates for this examination.

☐ Young patients with hepatitis or cirrhosis who are at increased lifetime risk of developing hepatoma may be better screened with MRI as it does not involve the use of ionizing radiation. Repeated use of CT increases the lifetime risk of radiation-induced malignancy.

LIMITATIONS

☐ Due to the small IV size that is obtainable in the pediatric population, true arterial phase imaging is difficult to obtain. This limits the identification and characterization of hepatic masses.

Pediatric CT

□ Minimal difference in timing of IV contrast material between follow-up examinations may make it difficult to evaluate for interval change in size or presence of some hepatic lesions. This may make it difficult to determine if the lesion is still present, if it represented a vascular shunt, or if it has increased in size (and is therefore suspicious for a hepatocellular carcinoma).

Imaging of the Biliary Tree

▪ CT may be helpful in the evaluation of suspected biliary tree obstruction, particularly when evaluating for associated obstructing masses such as metastatic disease or extrinsic masses compressing the biliary tree (e.g. duodenal duplication cysts, choledochal cysts).

▪ Ultrasound is often the investigation of choice to evaluate the biliary tree for several reasons, including lack of ionizing radiation, increased sensitivity to early biliary dilatation (often prior to CT manifestations of ductal dilation), and more reliable characterization of gallbladder pathology.

▪ CT is not sensitive for the detection of cholelithiasis or early cholecystitis; however, CECT is superior to ultrasound in the evaluation of suspected common bile duct stones.

INDICATIONS

□ Evaluation of suspected common bile duct stones
□ Evaluation of suspected mass obstructing the intra- or extrahepatic bile ducts
□ Evaluation of suspected choledochal cysts (MR is the study of choice)

CONTRAINDICATIONS

□ Patients who cannot receive IV contrast are not candidates for CECT.
□ CT cholangiography cannot be performed on patients who cannot undergo percutaneous cholangiograms.

LIMITATIONS

□ The lack of intra-abdominal fat limits evaluation of the porta hepatis in children, thus extrinsic masses compressing the extrahepatic biliary tree may be difficult to identify.
□ Biliary tract pathology is better identified and characterized with ultrasound.

☐ CT is not sensitive for the detection of subtle biliary obstruction; CECT is required as it allows differentiation of vascular structures and periportal edema from ductal dilation.

☐ CT has relatively low sensitivity for the detection of choledocholithiasis, although it is more sensitive than ultrasound for this indication.

☐ CT is of limited usefulness in the evaluation of acute cholecystitis. The diagnosis may be suggested based on gallbladder wall enhancement, gallbladder wall thickening, and mesenteric fat inflammation centered on the gallbladder.

☐ CT has poor resolution for the identification of cholelithiasis. Although some stones may be dense and therefore can be seen on CT, not all stones are visible and it is often not possible to differentiate sludge from small stones. Ultrasound is the imaging modality of choice for this indication.

☐ CECT may not detect infiltrating masses, such as cholangiocarcinoma, which tend to enhance late (8–10 minutes following IV contrast enhancement). MR is a more sensitive modality for the evaluation of these late enhancing masses.

☐ Some pancreatic masses cannot be readily identified on CT or MRI. If there is high clinical suspicion for the presence of a pancreatic mass in the setting of a negative CT or MR, endoscopic ultrasound may be performed for further evaluation. Endoscopic ultrasound involves passage of an ultrasound-mounted endoscope into the stomach. The stomach serves as a good window for high-resolution evaluation of the adjacent pancreas. Transgastric biopsies also may be performed via this route if a mass is identified.

Imaging of the Spleen

■ There are few specific indications for dedicated splenic imaging with CT.

■ Splenic lesions are often identified incidentally on routine CT studies.

■ CT often cannot characterize splenic lesions.

INDICATIONS
☐ Suspected splenic trauma
☐ Suspected splenic infarction
☐ Suspected splenic abscess formation
☐ Suspected autosplenectomy in sickle cell patients

☐ CT may be useful in the identification or confirmation of residual splenic tissue in patients with idiopathic thrombocytic purpura.

☐ IV contrast is required for all of these diagnoses with the exception of suspected autosplenectomy and residual splenic tissue.

CONTRAINDICATIONS

☐ Patents who cannot receive IV contrast

LIMITATIONS

☐ Inability to characterize splenic lesions

☐ In children, due to the relatively late phase of imaging that is related to the small size of peripheral IV lines, splenic lesions are often not identified as the lesions equilibrate with normal splenic tissue and cannot be identified.

☐ Splenic imaging is notoriously difficult. No single imaging modality currently exists that can characterize the majority of splenic lesions. CT is no exception. Although splenic masses can be readily identified on CT, there are no accurate imaging characteristics that will allow for lesion identification. Splenic biopsy is not routinely performed given the highly vascular nature of the organ.

☐ Non-contrast examinations are of limited benefit as splenic infarctions or abscesses cannot be readily detected without IV contrast administration.

☐ Infiltrating splenic processes such as lymphoma, sarcoid, and amyloid cannot be readily distinguished from other splenic abnormalities.

Imaging of the Pancreas

▨ CT is frequently requested for the evaluation of suspected pancreatitis. CT is often unnecessary to confirm a biochemically documented episode of acute pancreatitis as the imaging findings may be minimal or absent.

▨ Ultrasound is the imaging study of choice in the evaluation of cholelithiasis as a potential cause of pancreatitis.

INDICATIONS

☐ Diagnosis of pancreatitis in patients with midline abdominal pain of unknown etiology

☐ CT is useful in the follow-up of patients with documented pancreatitis in whom symptoms persist or worsen. Oral contrast is recommended for the study in order to separate the pancreatic parenchyma from surrounding duodenum. Additionally, because pancreatic inflammation can cause secondary colonic inflammation, oral contrast is required for adequate bowel distension. IV contrast is necessary to evaluate for pancreatic necrosis, which is manifest by regions of decreased or absent pancreatic enhancement.

☐ CT may also be used to evaluate suspected or known pancreatic masses. Typically, the CT is performed with non-contrast and contrast-enhanced images in multiple phases of IV contrast enhancement. Oral contrast may be useful for the study to allow separation of the duodenum from the pancreas as well as to evaluate for possible duodenal involvement by tumor.

CONTRAINDICATIONS

☐ Patients who cannot receive IV contrast are not candidates for the study.

LIMITATIONS

☐ Patients with pancreatitis may manifest minimal or no CT findings in early or mild cases; therefore, CT is of limited or no value in these patients and the radiation dose in quite high and unnecessary.

☐ The etiology of pancreatitis is often not discernable on CT. For example, neither cholelithiasis nor pancreas divisum is routinely identifiable on CT.

☐ Small pancreatic tumors may not be identifiable on CT or MRI. Endoscopic ultrasound is the imaging study of choice for the evaluation of suspected pancreatic masses that are occult on CT or MRI.

☐ Resectability of pancreatic tumors can be difficult to determine with certainty on imaging studies. Features that determine resectability include degree of involvement of the SMA and SMV, local lymph node involvement, and distant disease (e.g. liver metastases). The degree of vessel involvement can be underestimated with current imaging modalities.

Imaging of the Adrenal Gland

■ Small adrenal lesions are commonly identified incidentally on CTs obtained for a variety of clinical indications. These lesions are often benign entities such as myelolipomas and adenomas, which then do not require further imaging or follow-up.

■ If an adrenal lesion is identified that does not demonstrate CT characteristics of a benign lesion on CECT, further evaluation may be warranted if there are no prior studies to document stability. This is particularly important in patients with known neoplasms in whom an adrenal metastatic deposit would change staging and management.

■ Indeterminate adrenal lesions may be evaluated by CT or MRI. CT is a more cost-effective method of evaluating these lesions and involves both non-contrast and IV contrast-enhanced imaging. IV contrast is required for the evaluation of adrenal lesions as it is the percentage rate of washout of IV contrast from the adrenal gland, which allows characterization of the lesion.

■ CT is also helpful in the diagnosis and follow-up of adrenal hemorrhage. Non-contrast imaging is adequate to evaluate for adrenal hemorrhages.

INDICATIONS

☐ Evaluation of known or suspected adrenal neuroblastoma

☐ Differentiation of renal mass (often Wilms tumor) from adrenal mass

☐ Evaluation of previously (often incidentally) identified adrenal lesions for the purposes of lesion characterization. If an adrenal lesion measures water or fat density on CT, no additional evaluation is required as this signifies benignity. However, even benign lesions such as angiomyelolipomas can enhance. Thus, they are often indeterminate lesions when incidentally identified on CECT at the time of imaging for unrelated pathology. Adrenal washout imaging allows a lesion to be characterized as benign if there is 50% washout of contrast material from the lesion in 15 minutes.

☐ Evaluation of suspected adrenal hemorrhage. IV contrast is not required for this diagnosis; however, follow-up imaging may be necessary to evaluate for an underlying adrenal mass once the hemorrhage has resolved.

☐ Evaluation of adrenal trauma. This is often incidentally identified at the time of routine CECT of the abdomen in the setting of acute trauma.

CONTRAINDICATIONS

☐ There is debate as to whether or not it is safe to give IV contrast to patients who have known or suspected pheochromocytoma. It has been proposed that these patients should not be given IV contrast material; if they require IV contrast, they should first receive alpha-blockade. These proposals are due to the reported risk of precipitating a catecholamine storm due to IV contrast administration. It is advisable to discuss these cases with your local imaging department in order to determine the policies.

LIMITATIONS

☐ It may not be possible to fully characterize an adrenal lesion on CT. Lipid-poor adenomas (i.e. adenomas in which the amount of fat is so small that it cannot be detected on CT) may not be characterizable with this method. Non-contrast MRI may be a more sensitive study to characterize these lesions.

☐ Adrenal masses that contain hemorrhage may not be identified on initial imaging due to the presence of hemorrhage. If there is suspicion of hemorrhage into an underlying mass, a follow-up study or contrast-enhanced MRI should be considered in order to evaluate for the presence of a pathologic adrenal mass.

☐ It may be difficult to differentiate adrenal hemorrhage from congenital adrenal neuroblastoma as they may have similar imaging characteristics at initial presentation. In general, imaging is repeated at 6 weeks following initial diagnosis. At this interval, the appearance of adrenal hemorrhage will have changed, thus generally allowing diagnosis.

☐ It may be difficult to differentiate a renal from a suprarenal (i.e. adrenal) mass on CT, particularly in small, thin children. Images can be reformatted (depending upon the CT scanner and manner of acquisition) into different planes, which may assist in localizing the mass. If the mass still cannot be localized, MR may be performed as it allows direct acquisition of images in different planes.

Imaging of the Kidneys

■ There is a vast array of renal pathology, which may be identified with CT imaging. Communication of the clinical question to the radiologist conducting the examination is of key importance as different types of renal abnormalities must be imaged in different ways (i.e. IV contrast studies versus non-contrast imaging versus other imaging modalities [e.g. ultrasound]).

■ Non-contrast renal CT imaging:

☐ This type of CT study is performed without oral or IV contrast. The patient is placed in the prone position (to allow for differentiation of calculi lodged at the ureterovesical junction and thus less likely to pass versus calculi free in the bladder). The main indication for non-contrast renal imaging is for the evaluation of renal/ureteral or bladder calculi and the identification of associated renal or ureteral obstruction.

☐ Patients should be appropriately screened for the examination. Although other disease entities, such as appendicitis or diverticulitis may occasionally be identified with non-contrast imaging, the examination is suboptimal for complete evaluation of bowel pathology, abscesses, and other intra-abdominal/pelvic abnormalities.

INDICATIONS

☐ Evaluation of renal, ureteral, or bladder calculi

☐ Evaluation of retroperitoneal hemorrhage in the setting of hematocrit drops in coagulopathic patients

LIMITATIONS

☐ Due to the lack of intra-abdominal fat in the majority of pediatric patients, localization of calculi to the ureters may be difficult, limiting evaluation effectiveness.

☐ Due to the lack of oral and IV contrast, other disease processes, particularly bowel pathology, may not be identifiable.

■ Contrast-enhanced genitourinary imaging:

☐ It may be performed to diagnose acute renal/ureteral or bladder disease. It also may be performed to evaluate or follow-up suspected or known renal abnormalities.

☐ Renal abnormalities may be incidentally identified on imaging performed for an alternative diagnosis.

☐ Although a diagnosis of pyelonephritis may be suggested on the basis of a CECT, it is not an imaging diagnosis (i.e. it is a diagnosis made on clinical grounds). Imaging features of infection may be present or absent and thus are not reliable for establishing the diagnosis. Complications of urinary tract infections and pyelonephritis may be recognized on CT, ultrasound, and MR. The main complications are renal and perinephric abscesses; these may be identified on any of the modalities mentioned.

INDICATIONS

□ Evaluation of suspected traumatic renal/ureteral/bladder injury. It requires the administration of IV contrast.

□ Delayed CT imaging (at >5 minutes) to evaluate for injury to the collecting system or ureter is performed. The time delay allows for the normal filtration and excretion of contrast into the collecting system and ureter, at which time, collecting system leaks may be identified. Suspected bladder injury may require additional imaging for diagnosis and characterization. Imaging of suspected bladder injury may be performed under fluoroscopic or CT imaging. This process (cystogram/CT cystogram) requires direct instillation of contrast through a Foley catheter into the bladder.

□ Evaluation of suspected vascular injury, including trauma to the vascular pedicle. Renal infarction also may be identified by the presence of wedge-shaped areas of decreased renal perfusion. CT also may be performed in the subacute period to evaluate the sequelae of renal perfusion abnormalities.

□ CECT may be performed to grossly estimate renal function. The kidneys normally filter and excrete IV contrast agents. In normally functioning kidneys, excretion is symmetric. In patients with obstruction, excretion may be delayed or absent.

□ CECT is useful to identify suspected perinephric abscesses. It is a useful study to plan percutaneous drainage of these collections as well as to follow the collections to resolution. Ultrasound and MR are alternatives as they will often give the same information without the use of ionizing radiation.

□ CECT also may be performed as a dedicated study to evaluate renal masses identified on prior imaging studies or in at-risk patients or symptomatic patients. This type of study is commonly termed a *renal mass protocol CT* and is discussed next.

Imaging of Suspected Renal Masses (Renal Mass Protocol CT)

■ This is an abdominal CT performed for the express purpose of evaluating the renal parenchyma. For this reason, the pelvis is not imaged, and only an abdominal CT should be requested by the ordering clinician.

▪ The study is composed of non-contrast CT images through the abdomen followed by thin section images through the kidneys in multiple phases of IV contrast enhancement. No oral contrast is required for the study.

GENERAL CONSIDERATIONS

☐ As IV contrast is required for the study, renal function should be assessed shortly prior to the scheduled examination. This is of particular importance in patients with diabetes, with prior nephrectomy, with partial nephrectomy (e.g. for Wilms tumor), or with known renal insufficiency. In patients with an elevated Cr (>1.5 mg/dL), a CECT cannot safely be performed due to the renal toxic effects of IV contrast. In these patients, known or suspected masses must be evaluated by ultrasound or MRI.

INDICATIONS

☐ The study is performed to evaluate known or suspected renal masses for neoplastic lesions. A renal mass protocol is not required to follow up a previously documented benign lesion or to follow metastatic lesions or known primary renal malignancies. These patients simply require a routine CECT of the abdomen and pelvis to assess for interval change in size or morphology of the previously documented lesions.

☐ Evaluation of indeterminate renal masses demonstrated on alternative imaging studies (e.g. ultrasound, routine CECT)

☐ Follow-up of suspicious masses, which remain indeterminate

☐ Differentiation of renal from suprarenal (i.e. adrenal) masses

☐ Screening of patients with prior partial or total nephrectomy for Wilms tumor. MR may be a better modality for the long-term follow-up of these patients due to the lack of ionizing radiation and iodinated IV contrast.

☐ Surgical planning for partial nephrectomy

☐ Screening of patients with inherited syndromes (e.g. von Hippel-Lindau) who are at risk of developing renal cell carcinomas; CT or MR may be performed for this indication

CONTRAINDICATIONS

☐ As indicated for routine CECT of the genitourinary system

LIMITATIONS
□ The urothelium cannot be adequately assessed with this technique; CT urography is the imaging modality of choice.
□ A mass is deemed suspicious for malignancy if it demonstrates enhancement of >10 HU. However, there may be artifactual causes of apparent enhancement or lack of enhancement including streak artifact related to patient's arms at the side when the scan is performed and noisy images in obese patients in whom accurate attenuation values cannot be assessed.
□ Small masses may be difficult to characterize on CT.

CT Cystogram

■ A cystogram is a retrograde study performed by instilling contrast material into the bladder through a Foley catheter. The contrast is diluted in saline and is dripped into the bladder under gravity.

■ Cystograms may be performed under fluoroscopy (see Chapter 4) or under CT. CT cystography increasingly is being used due to its ability to show more superior anatomic detail than conventional cystograms, allowing accurate assessment of location of injury and intra- versus extraperitoneal bladder rupture.

■ CT cystography involves several scans of the pelvis (the abdomen is not imaged), which often include a non-contrast examination (to evaluate for hemorrhage) followed by imaging with the bladder distended. This allows for bladder wall integrity to be assessed. If there is a bladder leak/rupture, contrast will extend across the site of injury (which may be directly visible) and will extend around the bladder. The location of the contrast extravasation can be determined. If the contrast is confined to the retropubic region and perivesicular space, it is determined to be extraperitoneal. If it extends to surround loops of bowel and other structures within the peritoneum, it is deemed to be intraperitoneal bladder rupture.

■ Management of bladder rupture is dependent upon the location of bladder rupture. Extraperitoneal bladder rupture often results from trauma (e.g. pelvic fractures), whereas intraperitoneal injury most often results from injury during pelvic surgery.

▓ Extraperitoneal bladder rupture is treated conservatively with Foley catheter placement to maintain the bladder in a constant state of decompression, thus allowing the site of injury to heal.

▓ Intraperitoneal bladder rupture is treated surgically with direct repair of the site of injury. Uncommonly, it may be treated conservatively similar to extraperitoneal bladder injury.

INDICATIONS

☐ Evaluation of patients with pelvic fractures to assess for associated extraperitoneal bladder injury. It should be noted that if patients experience trauma with a distended bladder, it is possible to have intraperitoneal bladder injury or both intra- and extraperitoneal bladder injury.

☐ Assessment of uremic patients with recent trauma or surgery. In cases of intraperitoneal bladder rupture, urine leaks into the peritoneal cavity where it is absorbed back into the blood. This causes an elevation of serum blood urea nitrogen (BUN)/Cr levels and can present as acute renal failure or uremia. This does not occur in isolated extraperitoneal bladder rupture as the urine is not absorbed.

☐ Evaluation of patients with recent abdominal or pelvic surgery in whom there are symptoms or uremia, abdominal pain, hematuria, or new ascites. Intraperitoneal bladder rupture may present in this fashion.

CONTRAINDICATIONS

☐ Questionable urethral injury: In these patients, the study should be performed under fluoroscopic guidance in order to first evaluate the urethra. A retrograde urethrogram (see Chapter 4) is first performed by placing the tip of the Foley catheter into the urethral meatus and hand injecting contrast under fluoroscopy to evaluate for leak (urethral injury). If there is no leak, the Foley catheter can be advanced and a conventional cystogram can be performed at that time.

☐ Unstable patients: If a trauma patient is unstable at the time of the initial imaging, it is advisable that the patient is managed acutely and stabilized prior to CT cystography.

LIMITATIONS

☐ Small perforations in the bladder wall may not be identified at CT imaging.

☐ If the bladder is not fully distended (e.g. due to patient discomfort or blood clot within the Foley catheter or bladder), small or slow bladder leaks may not be identified. Small amounts of extravasated contrast material may be visible in the intra- or extraperitoneal space, however, thus allowing diagnosis.

☐ If patients are imaged after stabilization with an external fixation device for pelvic fracture, streak artifact from the metallic device may mask contrast extravasation and may complicate diagnosis.

CT Imaging of Gynecologic Disease

▪ CT has a limited role in the evaluation of suspected or known gynecological abnormalities. MR and transvaginal/transpelvic ultrasound are the imaging modalities of choice.

▪ CT may, on occasion, identify adnexal or uterine abnormalities. This is particularly true in the case of adnexal masses where CT may identify and occasionally characterize an adnexal mass. CT is particularly helpful in the identification of fat contained within an adnexal mass, thus (usually) providing a diagnosis of benign disease.

▪ CT is very useful in the evaluation of suspected omental disease from gynecological primaries.

INDICATIONS

☐ Characterization of fat-containing ovarian masses (e.g. dermoid): Transvaginal ultrasound and MR are the imaging modalities of choice.

☐ Evaluation of known or suspected metastatic disease in patients with known ovarian neoplasm

LIMITATIONS

☐ CT often cannot localize large masses to the ovaries or uterus. This is particularly the case in young females with little intraperitoneal fat and with large masses.

☐ CT cannot adequately characterize ovarian masses unless there is fat contained within them (e.g. dermoid).

☐ Ovarian torsion cannot be excluded on the basis of CT. Ultrasound is the imaging modality of choice for the evaluation of suspected ovarian torsion.

☐ Processes such as endometriosis are not well evaluated with CT. Ovarian masses (e.g. endometriomas) cannot be characterized on CT.

CT Imaging of Bowel Pathology

■ CT is increasingly employed in the evaluation of bowel pathology, particularly in the setting of acute abdominal pain or known bowel obstruction.

■ As bowel abnormalities may be manifest by subtle findings such as minimal bowel wall thickening, adequate distension of the bowel by oral contrast is imperative for an optimal study. Patients are required to consume a total of 8 oz of barium or Hypaque. Hypaque is used in patients with suspected acute bowel abnormality in whom the possibility of emergent/urgent surgical intervention exists; Hypaque has less risk of peritonitis and is less viscous than barium. Although oral contrast is very important for evaluation of the bowel, particularly in patients with a lack of intra-abdominal fat, it may not be possible to administer the contrast to young patients.

■ IV contrast is also of the utmost importance in the evaluation of acute bowel abnormality, particularly when there is a suspicion of intra-abdominal/pelvic abscess. In the absence of IV contrast, fluid collections may not be identified or may not be recognized as organized, walled-off collections.

INDICATIONS

☐ Acute bowel pathology:
- CT is quickly becoming the imaging study of choice in the identification of bowel obstruction, site of transition, and possible masses or extrinsic abnormalities.
- Primary diagnosis or evaluation of complications from inflammatory bowel disease. IV contrast is of particular importance in this setting in order to evaluate for walled-off or drainable abscess cavities.
- Evaluation of appendicitis
- Bowel perforation and pneumoperitoneum
- Identification of bowel ischemia. IV contrast is required in this setting, particularly to allow for possible identification of arterial or venous thrombus within the mesenteric vasculature.
- Identification of acute bowel infection (e.g. *Clostridium difficile* colitis)

CONTRAINDICATIONS

☐ Oral contrast is recommended for all studies in which bowel pathology is suspected. However, barium is not recommended if there is concern for bowel perforation due to the increased risk of peritonitis and contamination of the surgical field. In patients presenting with suspected acute bowel pathology, Hypaque is administered. Hypaque is not administered for routine abdominal imaging due to its very unpalatable taste.

☐ Rectal contrast may be unsafe in patients with toxic megacolon or severe colitis due to the increased bowel distension and pressure related to the contrast volume.

☐ Patients with known or suspected perirectal abscess may not be optimal candidates for rectal contrast for evaluation of the abscess. Although rectal contrast is clearly more rapid than oral contrast (which requires a 2-hour minimum delay for transit to the rectum in these patients), there is a risk of traumatizing the anus or rectum while placing the catheter and instilling the contrast. If rectal contrast is considered or desired in these patients, it is advisable to discuss with the radiologist.

LIMITATIONS

☐ Inadequate opacification of the bowel or underdistension of bowel may lead to false-negative results.

☐ Transition points in bowel obstruction may be difficult to identify.

☐ Lack of intra-abdominal fat in children may make identification of bowel pathology difficult.

☐ CT is not specific or sensitive for the identification of the cause of GI bleeding. Although processes such as diverticulosis/diverticulitis can be detected on CT and may be the cause of the GI bleed, causes of GI bleeding often go undetected on CT. Nuclear medicine studies (e.g. sulfur colloid or tagged red blood cell studies) or catheter angiography may be necessary to identify causes of GI bleeding.

☐ In patients with small bowel obstruction, the precise site and cause of the obstruction may be difficult or impossible to identify on CT. The majority of small bowel obstructions are the result of adhesions related to prior surgery. Adhesions cannot be directly visualized on CT, however, and they may be suggested by an angulated appearance of bowel loops with a transition point to decompressed bowel at the site of obstruction.

☐ If patients cannot tolerate oral contrast, it may be difficult to evaluate the bowel, particularly if the bowel is not distended. This may cause false-positive or false-negative results. False-positive results can be seen if the bowel is not fully distended, leading to it appear thick-walled and thus simulating disease. Alternatively, false negatives can occur if the bowel is not adequately distended to allow evaluation of the wall for masses and thickening.

☐ If there is not a long enough delay between the ingestion of oral contrast and the study performance, the entire bowel may not be opacified. This is particularly important in cases in which there is a concern for appendicitis.

☐ It may not be possible to differentiate the cause of bowel wall abnormality. For instance, it is often not possible to differentiate among wall thickening caused by infection (e.g. colitis), inflammation (e.g. inflammatory bowel disease), or neoplasm.

☐ Bowel injury in the setting of trauma is often not identified on CT examination. It is very uncommon to identify direct evidence of bowel injury (e.g. free intra-abdominal air, leakage of oral contrast, IV contrast blush). More often, there is indirect evidence, which is not specific (e.g. free pelvic fluid in the absence of a solid organ injury).

CT Imaging of the Vasculature

▪ CECT imaging is employed preoperatively to evaluate acute vascular abnormalities, known or suspected vascular anatomic variants (e.g. aberrant vessels or a duplicated aortic arch), and neoplasms, in order to allow safe and accurate resection.

CT Imaging of the Aorta

▪ It may be performed with or without IV contrast, depending upon the indication for the study.
▪ Non-contrast aortic imaging:
  ☐ It may be performed to identify or follow-up the size of an aortic aneurysm.
▪ Contrast-enhanced aortic imaging:

☐ The most frequent use of CT for aortic imaging is in the setting of suspected or known aortic dissection. Imaging includes both non-contrast and IV contrast-enhanced images. Non-enhanced images are obtained to allow for identification of a high attenuation intramural hematoma, which has prognostic importance. Intramural hematoma is masked once IV contrast is administered. Contrast administration is required to evaluate for a dissection flap, which indicates the presence of blood dissecting between the aortic intima and media. For patients who are unable to receive non-ionic IV contrast (either on the basis of renal insufficiency or contrast allergy), high-dose gadolinium may be of benefit to identify the dissection flap.

☐ Congenital vascular abnormalities can be characterized with CECT imaging.

CT of Renal Vasculature

■ Some institutions advocate the use of CECT with computer-generated reformatted images in various planes for the evaluation of renal artery stenosis. This examination cannot be performed in patients with Cr levels >1.5 mg/dL due to the risk of contrast-induced nephrotoxicity.

■ CTA also may be performed to evaluate potential renal donors. This allows for identification of the number and position of the renal arteries and veins prior to organ harvest.

■ Vasculopathy such as that seen in neurofibromatosis and fibromuscular dysplasia can be well evaluated with renal CTA.

■ CTA is performed with thin section images obtained through the abdomen following IV contrast administration. The contrast is timed for maximum enhancement as a timing bolus prior to the study.

INDICATIONS

☐ Evaluation of known or suspected renal artery stenosis in patients with renal impairment or hypertension

☐ Evaluation of the renal arteries or veins in patients with a history of trauma, prior biopsy, and vascular malformation. This allows for evaluation of the presence, size, and location of a vascular lesion such as an arterial aneurysm. The study also may assist in preprocedure (surgery or percutaneous intervention) planning for repair.

☐ CTA may be performed for evaluation of patients with known renal tumors in whom partial resection is planned. This allows for evaluation of the vascular supply to the tumor as well as assessment of the location of large vessels that may be traumatized during surgery.

CONTRAINDICATIONS

☐ Patients with borderline or elevated renal function should not receive IV contrast.

LIMITATIONS

☐ Patients previously treated for renal artery stenosis with metallic stents may be difficult to evaluate for recurrent stenosis due to streak artifact related to the presence of the stent. This is becoming less problematic with the implementation of 64-slice multidetector row CT scanners.

☐ In patients with slow flow in a vascular malformation (e.g. a venous varix), it may be difficult to characterize the abnormality as a vascular lesion and it may be difficult to determine if there is still flow in the abnormality (if it is slow flow).

☐ If the study is not appropriately timed, a true arterial phase may not be obtained; therefore, the arterial structures may not be optimally evaluated.

CT Imaging of Veins

▓ CT plays a limited role in the evaluation of venous abnormalities.

▓ Venous thrombus within the inferior vena cava or iliac/femoral venous system may be identified with scanning delays set for optimal venous opacification by contrast material.

▓ The study is performed following the administration of IV contrast. The abdomen and pelvis are scanned (unless pelvic clot only is suspected, in which case only the pelvis may be required). A delay of 90–120 seconds following IV contrast administration is required to allow time for contrast to opacify the vessels and prevent artifacts.

INDICATIONS

☐ Evaluation of thrombus within the inferior vena cava, pelvic veins, and gonadal veins

CONTRAINDICATIONS

☐ IV contrast allergy or impaired renal function

LIMITATIONS
- ☐ Mixing of contrast opacified blood with non-opacified blood can cause all or part of the vein to appear dark. This can simulate the presence of partially occlusive or occlusive venous thrombosis. It is therefore imperative to perform the scan after a delay following IV contrast administration to decrease the chance of a false-positive result.

CT of the Nervous System

Non-Contrast CT of the Brain
- It is the initial imaging study for evaluation of acute neurological abnormality.
- Routine imaging for acute events or trauma does not require the administration of IV contrast.

INDICATIONS
- ☐ Evaluation of acute stroke
- ☐ Evaluation of acute change in mental status
- ☐ Evaluation for intraparenchymal hemorrhage, subarachnoid hemorrhage (SAH), epidural or subdural hemorrhage
- ☐ Evaluation of traumatic injury
- ☐ It is commonly used in the evaluation of new or increased frequency of seizures; however, this is of low yield and MRI is the study of choice.

CONTRAINDICATIONS
- ☐ Patients who are actively seizing should be stabilized prior to the examination, if possible.
- ☐ There is an increased risk of cataract formation from the radiation used for the CT examination. The necessity and benefits of the CT should be weighted carefully against the risks of the radiation exposure before the scan is performed. Patients with a history of seizure or headache with multiple prior studies may not require a CT examination, thus decreasing the risk of radiation exposure.

LIMITATIONS
- ☐ Patient motion may produce significant artifacts, thus decreasing sensitivity for abnormalities.
- ☐ Dense vessels may mimic areas of pathology (i.e. intracranial hemorrhage). This is particularly true in children and patients with hyperviscosity syndromes such as polycythemia vera as the increased iron content of the blood renders intravascular blood more dense on CT.

☐ Patients with prior surgical or endovascular treatments for processes such as aneurysm repair may have suboptimal examinations due to the significant streak artifact related to the clips.

☐ Early ischemia (infarcts) may not be visible on CT. Areas of infarction often are not visible on CT for 12–24 hours after the onset of symptoms. The major role for CT in patients with clinical symptoms of acute stroke is to exclude intracranial hemorrhage, which would contraindicate antithrombolitic therapy.

☐ Patient motion may limit the examination as small lesions may not be well visualized through the artifact.

☐ Patient apparel (e.g. earrings, hairpins) may cause significant artifact, thus limiting evaluation of adjacent areas of the brain.

☐ For patients with seizures, MR is the imaging modality of choice as subtle lesions (e.g. heterotopic gray matter) are not detectable on CT.

☐ Masses within the brain may not be identifiable on noncontrast CT imaging unless there is associated edema or mass effect. If there is concern for the presence of a mass, CECT or MR is recommended.

Contrast-Enhanced CT of the Brain

▦ It is performed following the administration of IV contrast.
▦ IV contrast is not administered for routine cases.

INDICATIONS

☐ Evaluation of intracranial masses, suspected or known metastatic lesions

☐ Evaluation of suspected intracranial infection

☐ It may be useful to confirm the presence of isodense subdural hematomas.

☐ It may demonstrate meningeal enhancement in patients with meningitis, particularly tuberculous or fungal.

CONTRAINDICATIONS

☐ IV contrast allergy

☐ Elevated Cr

☐ Acute trauma: IV contrast may mask or mimic SAH. If there is concern for SAH, IV contrast should not be administered before a head CT is performed. This includes CECT of the neck, chest, abdomen, or pelvis. If IV contrast is administered, it will take ≥6 hours to clear the contrast from the subarachnoid space.

LIMITATIONS

☐ Patient motion may limit the examination as small lesions may not be well visualized through the artifact.

☐ Patient apparel (e.g. earrings, hairpins) may cause significant artifact, thus limiting evaluation of adjacent areas of the brain.

☐ Hemorrhagic masses that have bled acutely may not be as readily identifiable as solid/cystic masses due to the presence of blood products. Subacute imaging following evolution of the hemorrhage or MRI may prove more diagnostic.

☐ Meningeal processes (e.g. infection) may not be detected with CECT imaging. In cases of fungal or tuberculous meningitis, thick meningeal enhancement may be identified.

☐ Contrast should not be administered to patients in whom SAH is suspected as contrast within vessels may mimic or mask the hemorrhage. Similarly, as contrast may circulate within the intracranial vasculature for several hours after administration, patients with SAH should not be imaged for several hours after contrast administration for any imaging study.

CT Angiography of the Neck and Circle of Willis

■ The study is performed with a timed bolus of IV contrast.

■ The area of interest (i.e. carotid arteries or circle of Willis) must be defined prior to commencement of the examination as the images are acquired differently for the two examinations. Although it is possible to evaluate both the carotid arteries and the circle of Willis with the same contrast bolus, dedicated imaging of each is recommended to optimize image quality. This is particularly true if an older CT scanner is used (i.e. single slice scanner).

■ A large bore IV is required (≥20 gauge is required for the examination as a rapid contrast infusion is required for the examination).

■ A non-contrast CT of the brain may or may not be performed prior to the CTA depending upon the institutional protocol. In the acute setting, a preceding CT may have been performed, demonstrating the acute abnormality (i.e. SAH). In this case, if the non-contrast CT was obtained within a few hours of the CTA, a repeat non-contrast CT may not be required, thus limiting the radiation dose to the patient.

INDICATIONS

☐ Carotid CTA (CTA of the neck):
  • Evaluation of carotid injury following trauma (e.g. penetrating injury, seatbelt injury, or vertebral artery injury in the presence of a cervical vertebral fracture)
  • Evaluation of carotid stenosis
  • Follow-up of carotid dissection or stenosis
☐ CTA of the circle of Willis:
  • Evaluation of patients with suspected aneurysm (e.g. acute SAH in the absence of trauma). CTA is becoming the study of choice in these patients due to its high sensitivity and non-invasive nature.
  • Follow-up of known aneurysm: In some patients who are poor treatment risks, CTA may be performed to evaluate for interval growth of a previously demonstrated aneurysm.
  • Evaluation of known or suspected vascular malformation (e.g. arteriovenous malformation)
  • Preoperative planning: In patients with known vascular abnormalities (e.g. aneurysm or arteriovenous malformations), CTA may be performed prior to surgery or endovascular therapy (e.g. coiling, glue).
  • Postoperative evaluation: In patients treated for intracranial vascular abnormality, a postprocedural CTA may be performed to evaluate for the efficacy of treatment. Surveillance over the longer term also may be performed with CTA in order to avoid more invasive procedures (i.e. angiography).

CONTRAINDICATIONS

☐ IV contrast allergy
☐ Elevated Cr

LIMITATIONS

☐ CTA of the neck:
  • Patient motion may produce artifacts, which can obscure disease or mimic areas of stenosis.
  • Metallic objects within the neck (e.g. bullet fragments, surgical clips) may render portions of the vessel uninterpretable due to streak artifact.

- Poor timing of the contrast bolus may lead to a poor study in which areas of disease may not be identified; this is more problematic on CT scanners with fewer detectors (e.g. 4-slice or 8-slice scanners).

☐ CTA of the circle of Willis:
  - Patient motion may produce artifacts, which can obscure disease or mimic areas of stenosis.
  - Metallic objects within the cranium (e.g. clips or coils from prior vascular abnormality treatment) may render portions of the vessel uninterpretable due to artifact.
  - Poor timing of the contrast bolus may lead to a poor study in which areas of disease may not be identified; this is more problematic on CT scanners with fewer detectors (e.g. 4-slice or 8-slice scanners).
  - Difference in imaging slices or patient positioning may make direct comparison of aneurysm size and shape difficult or suboptimal.

CT of the Sinus

■ The study is performed for the evaluation of acute and chronic sinus disease.
■ The examination is typically performed without IV contrast unless there is a suspicion of fungal sinusitis or intracranial spread of infection.
■ Routine sinus imaging includes imaging of the sinuses only and does not image the entire cranium unless specifically requested.
■ There is a significant radiation dose involved with CT of the sinuses, particularly to the lens. Therefore, if sinusitis can be diagnosed on clinical grounds (which it generally can), CT should be avoided unless there is concern for complications of sinusitis. In cases of complications of sinusitis, IV contrast is typically necessary in order to evaluate for ascending infection causing an intracranial epidural abscess.

INDICATIONS
☐ Evaluation of acute or chronic sinus disease
☐ Preoperative planning for sinus surgery
☐ Evaluation of the postsurgical sinus
☐ CECT of the sinuses is performed if there is concern for invasive sinusitis (e.g. mucormycosis or aspergillus in immunosuppressed patients).

□ CECT of the sinuses and brain are performed if there is concern for extension of sinus infection into the epidural space of the brain.

CONTRAINDICATIONS

□ Radiation exposure should be avoided, if possible.

LIMITATIONS

□ Patients with multiple surgeries may have distorted anatomy, which may render interpretation of acute abnormalities difficult, particularly if prior examinations are not available for comparison.

□ Patients who cannot be appropriately positioned (e.g. with the head hanging over the gantry) may be difficult to image adequately as direct coronal imaging cannot be performed, thus, evaluation of the osteomeatal units may not be possible.

□ In the postoperative patient, it may be difficult to differentiate surgical changes from recurrent sinusitis. Comparison studies are highly useful in the interpretation of the postoperative sinus as it allows for more accurate depiction of residual/recurrent disease as opposed to postoperative change.

CT of the Facial Bones

■ The study is performed as a non-contrast examination for routine imaging.

■ The examination evaluates the osseous structures of the face, including the mandible and orbits. With multidetector CT, images are acquired in the axial plane and the data is reformatted into sagittal and coronal planes.

INDICATIONS

□ Non-contrast images are most commonly obtained for the evaluation of acute facial trauma.

□ Contrast-enhanced images may be obtained to evaluate for possible sites of infection and drainable abscess collections.

CONTRAINDICATIONS

□ IV contrast allergy

□ Elevated Cr

LIMITATIONS

□ Motion artifact will significantly degrade image quality and may obscure or mimic sites of disease.

☐ Metallic artifacts (e.g. metallic teeth fillings, tongue piercings, prior fracture fixation hardware) cause significant artifact and may obscure disease.

CT of the Orbits

■ The study may be obtained without or with IV contrast, depending upon the indication.

■ The study provides dedicated imaging of the orbits only; it does not evaluate the entire face.

■ Images are obtained in the axial plane. With multirow detector CT, the data are reformatted into sagittal and coronal images.

INDICATIONS

☐ Non-contrast CT of the orbits: The study is routinely performed for the evaluation of direct orbital trauma. Coronal reformatted images are of particular value in the assessment of orbital floor injury and possible muscle entrapment. The study does not evaluate the remainder of the facial bones; if there is concern for a second site of injury, a non-contrast CT of the facial bones should be obtained.

☐ CECT of the orbits:
  • Evaluation of ocular muscular abnormalities such as orbital pseudotumor and thyroid ophthalmopathy
  • Evaluation of orbital or facial cellulitis to evaluate for presence of and extension of abscess
  • Evaluation of known or suspected orbital or ocular masses (e.g. retinoblastoma, melanoma metastases)

CONTRAINDICATIONS

☐ IV contrast allergy

☐ Elevated Cr

LIMITATIONS

☐ Motion artifact will significantly degrade the images. This is of particular importance in the identification of orbital trauma (fractures) as a fracture may be obscured by motion or false-positive results may be obtained.

☐ Patient positioning: If patients are obliquely positioned within the CT gantry, sites of disease may be obscured.

☐ Metallic foreign bodies (e.g. bullet fragments) may produce artifact, which can render the study uninterpretable.

☐ It may be difficult to differentiate between a phlegmon and a mature walled-off orbital abscess.

CT of the Petrous/Temporal Bone

- The study may be performed without or with IV contrast–dependent upon the indication for the examination.
- There are highly specific indications to evaluate pathology of the temporal bone, vestibular system, middle and inner ear.
- Imaging is performed in thin section axial and coronal projections of the petrous apex only. This specific study does not image the entire brain.
- If the clinical indication is infection or cholesteatoma, particularly mastoiditis, the study requires the administration of IV contrast. For all other indications (e.g. evaluation of the ossicles, inner ear anatomy, fractures), IV contrast is not required.

INDICATIONS
- □ Non-contrast:
  - • Evaluation of petrous bone fracture
  - • Evaluation of hearing loss (i.e. evaluation for otosclerosis)
  - • Preprocedure planning for cochlear implants
- □ Contrast-enhanced:
  - • Evaluation of cholesteatoma
  - • Evaluation of masses
  - • Evaluation of infection (e.g. mastoiditis)

CONTRAINDICATIONS
- □ IV contrast allergy
- □ Elevated Cr

LIMITATIONS
- □ Due to the small size of the structures of the petrous bone (e.g. ossicles), volume averaging with adjacent structures may limit evaluation.
- □ Motion artifact can limit the examination.
- □ Fractures may be in the plane of the scan, thus they may not be easily evaluated; this is typically not a significant limitation as the images are reconstructed into different planes, thus the fracture line often becomes evident.

CT of the Neck

- The study may be performed with or without IV contrast. CECT is preferable to allow increased conspicuity of lymph nodes and areas of pathology.

■ The study differs from CTA in several ways. CTA requires a timed bolus of IV contrast to be administered followed by scanning at a specific timed delay. Routine CECT of the neck does not require contrast bolus timing; a scan is usually performed a few minutes after the contrast is administered. CTA is also performed as thin section axial images, which are then reformatted into different planes; CT of the neck is performed in 3–5 mm sections and is usually not reformatted into different imaging planes.

INDICATIONS

☐ Evaluation of possible infectious processes such as retropharyngeal abscess

☐ Evaluation of palpable abnormalities (e.g. extent of multinodular goiters, branchial cleft cysts, thyroglossal duct cysts). Ultrasound may be useful for the evaluation of palpable abnormalities; however, CT allows for better characterization of the anatomic relationship of the abnormality to adjacent structures, which may allow for a definitive diagnosis. Retrosternal masses cannot be adequately evaluated with ultrasound as the sternum reflects the ultrasound beam; thus, they cannot be evaluated. CT is the study of choice for these lesions.

☐ Evaluation of suspected masses such as paragangliomas. Primary head and neck neoplasms are often occult on imaging; however, associated lymphadenopathy may be identified.

☐ Evaluation of lymphadenopathy (e.g. melanoma, lymphoma)

CONTRAINDICATIONS

☐ IV contrast allergy

☐ Elevated Cr

LIMITATIONS

☐ Metallic artifact related to dental repair (e.g. fillings, bridges) or piercings cause significant artifact, thus limiting evaluation.

☐ Motion artifact may obscure or mimic disease.

☐ Patients who lack fat may be difficult to evaluate for lymphadenopathy due to lack of soft tissue contrast.

CT of the Cervical Spine

■ It is performed as a routine without IV contrast.

INDICATIONS
- ☐ It is typically performed in the setting of acute trauma. The study is performed as direct axial images with reformatted images provided in the sagittal and coronal planes.
  - In the pediatric population, in an attempt to reduce radiation exposure, it is common practice to scan C1 and C2 at the time of head CT performed for trauma. The remainder of the cervical spine is evaluated with conventional radiographs. In younger children, it is difficult to evaluate the atlanto-axial articulation and the dens with radiographs as younger patients often do not cooperate by opening their mouths for imaging of the dens.
  - It requires patient cooperation as motion artifact can render a study non-diagnostic, particularly in the setting of subtle fractures.
  - Cervical spine CT may be performed with IV contrast in a very specific setting, the evaluation of infection. CT with IV contrast is helpful in the evaluation of epidural abscess formation or soft tissue collections, particularly in postoperative patients. MR, however, is more sensitive for the evaluation of small epidural collections and is the study of choice for the evaluation of osteomyelitis/discitis.

INDICATIONS
- ☐ Non-contrast cervical spine CT:
  - Evaluation of traumatic injury: The study may be performed in the acute setting to evaluate for acute fracture, disc herniation, or epidural hematoma. The study does not evaluate for ligamentous injury.
  - Follow-up of known cervical spine fracture: This allows for assessment of the degree of healing and any changes in alignment of fracture fragments, which may require further surgical intervention or external fixation.
  - Evaluation of known or suspected congenital bony anomalies of the cervical spine
  - Evaluation of known or suspected bone lesions (e.g. aneurysmal bone cyst, lymphoma)
- ☐ CECT of the cervical spine:
  - Evaluation of discitis/osteomyelitis
  - Evaluation of epidural abscess

CONTRAINDICATIONS
- ☐ IV contrast allergy

☐ Elevated Cr

LIMITATIONS

☐ Non-contrast CT of the cervical spine:
- Motion artifact can significantly degrade images and may obscure subtle fractures or produce artifacts that mimic fracture.
- Streak artifact related to patient jewelry or cervical spine collars may degrade images.
- In patients with prior surgical fixation, artifact related to the metal hardware may render images uninterpretable.
- Patients poorly positioned within the CT gantry may be difficult to evaluate as the vertebrae may not appear aligned; this is particularly difficult in older patients with a significant kyphosis who cannot be laid flat for the study.
- Ligaments and muscles are not well delineated on CT, thus ligamentous injury cannot be assessed. MR is the study of choice to evaluate ligamentous injury.
- CT is insensitive to evaluation of the spinal cord; MR is the study of choice for the evaluation of spinal cord injury.

☐ CECT of the cervical spine:
- In patients with surgical hardware, artifact related to the hardware may render the study uninterpretable.
- Early changes of discitis/osteomyelitis may be occult on CT; MR is a more sensitive study for the early detection of these entities.

CT of the Thoracic/Lumbar Spine

INDICATIONS

▦ It is performed as a routine without IV contrast.

▦ It may be performed in the setting of acute trauma. It is performed as direct axial images with reformatted images provided in the sagittal and coronal planes.

▦ It requires patient cooperation as motion artifact can render a study non-diagnostic, particularly in the setting of subtle fracture.

▦ Thoracic/lumbar spine CT may be performed with IV contrast in a very specific setting, the evaluation of infection. CT with

IV contrast is helpful in the evaluation of epidural abscess formation or soft tissue collections, particularly in postoperative patients. MR, however, is more sensitive for the evaluation of small epidural collections and is the study of choice for the evaluation of osteomyelitis/discitis.

▪ Reconstructed images of the thoracic and lumbar spine (sagittal and coronal images) may be obtained in the trauma setting from data obtained of the chest, abdomen, and pelvis. The data are reconstructed into thinner slices and the reformats are performed.

▪ There is a high radiation dose involved in scanning the entire spine; effort should be made to localize the level of concern so that only that limited area may be scanned.

▪ Thoracic/lumbar spine CT may be performed with IV contrast in a very specific setting, the evaluation of infection. CT with IV contrast is helpful in the evaluation of epidural abscess formation or soft tissue collections, particularly in postoperative patients. MR, however, is more sensitive for the evaluation of small epidural collections and is the study of choice for the evaluation of osteomyelitis/discitis.

INDICATIONS
- ☐ Non-contrast:
  - Evaluation of acute traumatic injury
  - Evaluation of disc disease in the setting of radiculopathy
  - Evaluation of suspected or known bony masses (e.g. enchondroma, giant cell tumor, chondroblastoma). CT allows for evaluation of the extent of the tumor as well as characterization of the location and matrix, which may allow for the diagnosis to be made.
  - Contrast-enhanced:
    - Evaluation of infection (osteomyelitis)
    - Evaluation of suspected tumors involving the paraspinal soft tissues, nerve roots, or spinal cord

CONTRAINDICATIONS
- ☐ IV contrast allergy
- ☐ Elevated Cr

LIMITATIONS
- ☐ Motion artifact can significantly degrade the images.
- ☐ Metallic hardware such as spinal fusion rods and surgical clips can produce streak artifact and limit evaluation of adjacent structures.

☐ Unlike MRI, CT cannot evaluate for the presence of edema in the muscles, nerve roots, or spinal cord; edema may occur due to compression of the nerves in trauma or disc disease. MR is the imaging study of choice for these patients.

☐ CT has poor contrast resolution compared with MR; therefore, CT is not adequate to evaluate for the presence of ligamentous or muscle injury in the setting of infection.

■ CT cannot evaluate for edema in or replacement of the bone marrow in processes such as osteomyelitis or metastatic disease; therefore, changes of osteomyelitis or tumor may not become apparent until late in the disease. MR is the study of choice for these indications.

16

Pediatric MRI

General Considerations

- MRI is often used as a problem-solving tool in body imaging (e.g. lesions) identification and characterization of liver lesions.
- MR is not cost- or time-effective as a screening tool for metastatic disease in the chest/abdomen/pelvis. CT is the imaging study of choice for staging/restaging patients with known malignancies; however, MR is emerging as an alternative screening method for recurrent lymphadenopathy in patients with lymphoma and in children with malignancy in whom radiation considerations are of tantamount concern. MR is, however, increasingly requested for the evaluation of metastatic disease for a variety of primary malignancies. With improvements in MR equipment, it is becoming feasible to image patients with MR for metastatic disease.

ADVANTAGES OF MR VERSUS CT

- ☐ Absence of ionizing radiation
- ☐ Gadolinium (the MR contrast agent) is significantly less nephrotoxic than CT contrast agents (both ionic and nonionic contrast). Nephrotoxic effects have been reported with gadolinium.
- ☐ Better soft tissue resolution than CT.

DISADVANTAGES OF MR VERSUS CT

- ☐ Length of study: MR examinations can require a minimum of 20 minutes up to several hours of imaging time whereas CT often requires <2–5 minutes (particularly in the era of multislice scanners). Children may require sedation to remain immobile for the examination.

- [ ] Due to the configuration of the magnet, patients with claustrophobia may be unable to complete the examination. The majority of radiology departments do not have the staff or medications available to be able to medicate patients prior to an MR examination; therefore, it is recommended that patients with known claustrophobia be provided sedatives/anxiolytics by their primary caregivers. These should be made available to patients prior to the date of their examination. If patients are going to require conscious sedation for their examination, this should be made known to schedulers at the time of the study request so that conscious sedation can be arranged.
- [ ] Patients unable to lie completely supine are difficult to image.
- [ ] Patients with respiratory compromise may not be able to tolerate supine positioning. Patients with inability to breathhold may be unable to comply with key sequences that may result in suboptimal or uninterpretable studies.
- [ ] There are a number of contraindications to MRI, which will be detailed in the following section.

Contraindications to MR Imaging

ABSOLUTE CONTRAINDICATIONS
- [ ] Cardiac valves (now only St. Jude valve)
- [ ] Metallic foreign bodies within the orbits (patients with exposure history should be screened for metal with orbital radiographs prior to the MR examination)
- [ ] Patients with ferromagnetic surgical clips (e.g. cerebral aneurysm clips)
- [ ] Patients with pacers or automatic implantable cardioverter defibrillators (AICDs) cannot be imaged with MR due to the effect of the magnetic field upon the devices.

Relative Contraindications

- ▪ Recently placed cardiac stents (within 1–2 days)
- ▪ Obesity: The majority of MR scanners have a table limit of 350 lbs. Patients exceeding this limit cannot be imaged on conventional MR scanners. Patient girth is also a limitation; if patients exceed a certain circumference, they will not fit into the bore of the magnet.

- Claustrophobia: Many patients are unable to tolerate a complete MR examination because they are claustrophobic. If there is a preexisting history of claustrophobia, the patient may be booked to undergo the examination under sedation or the patient may require anesthesia if sedation is inadequate to allow completion of the study.
- Inability to lie supine: Patients who are unable to lie completely flat are often poor candidates for MRI. Images may be suboptimal due to patient positioning. Additionally, if patients are unable to be appropriately positioned based upon respiratory compromise when in a supine position, they often are unable to tolerate the examination. MRI of solid organs such as the liver and kidneys often requires patients to breathhold for 20–30 seconds. If patients are unable to do so, the images may be degraded to the degree of being uninterpretable.

Musculoskeletal MRI

- MR is the study of choice to evaluate ligamentous, tendinous, and cartilage injuries.
- Three types of studies may be performed: non-contrast MR, IV contrast-enhanced imaging, and MR arthrography.
- Suitability of candidates for MRI should be assessed prior to a request for a study.
  CONTRAINDICATIONS
  □ Presence of a pacer/AICD
  □ Recent cardiac stent placement
  □ Obese patients (>350 lbs)
  □ Claustrophobic patients (relative contraindication)
  □ Unstable patients

Non-Contrast Musculoskeletal MRI

- This is the study of choice for the evaluation of sports injuries (particularly of the knee).
- A non-contrast study is an efficacious way to evaluate for occult fracture without the additional radiation of CT.
- Non-contrast studies are inadequate to evaluate for labral pathology of the glenoid and acetabulum.
  INDICATIONS
  □ Evaluation of ligament, cartilage, tendon injuries

☐ Evaluation of occult fracture
☐ Evaluation of avascular necrosis (AVN), particularly of the hip
☐ Evaluation of muscle injuries

CONTRAINDICATIONS

☐ Contractures: If patients cannot be appropriately positioned the study may be suboptimal or false positives/false negatives may occur.
☐ Inability to maintain positioning: If patients cannot remain still without movement, the imaging will be suboptimal and may be of no diagnostic value.
☐ Unstable patients should not be placed in the magnet for routine, non-emergent imaging.
☐ Claustrophobia (relative): Sedation may be given as the patients are not required to comply with instructions such as breath holding.

LIMITATIONS

☐ Partial thickness ligament or cartilage tears may not be identified on non-contrast examinations.
☐ Loose bodies may be difficult to recognize in the absence of joint fluid or contrast.
☐ Labral injuries are difficult to diagnose without IV contrast.

IV Contrast-Enhanced Musculoskeletal MRI

■ The study involves the administration of IV gadolinium, which is a water-based compound that is visible with MRI.

General Considerations

■ Gadolinium is less nephrotoxic than ionic and non-ionic CT contrast. Gadolinium is generally safe for use in patients with elevated creatinine (Cr) levels up to 5.0 mg/dL.
■ Given the recent recognition of gadolinium-related nephrogenic systemic fibrosis (NSF), patients with known or suspected renal dysfunction should have a Cr level drawn prior to the examination, as per institutional guidelines.
■ Although less common than in ionic/non-ionic contrast imaging, contrast reactions can occur and may occasionally be life-threatening. Premedication protocols are the same as those for other contrast allergies.

INDICATIONS
- [ ] IV gadolinium is required for the evaluation of all suspected or documented musculoskeletal masses.
- [ ] Evaluation of osteomyelitis
- [ ] Gadolinium-enhanced MR is the study of choice for the evaluation of soft tissue tumors including location, extent, and neurovascular involvement
- [ ] Preoperative planning for possible limb-sparing procedures for treatment of musculoskeletal malignancies.
- [ ] Follow-up of resected neoplasms to evaluate for residual or recurrent disease
- [ ] Evaluation of known or suspected marrow-replacing lesions such as lymphoma, metastatic disease, infection
- [ ] Evaluation of presence and extent of osteomyelitis
- [ ] Evaluation of soft tissue vascular and lymphatic malformations (MR angiography [MRA] may be needed for evaluation of vascular malformations)

CONTRAINDICATIONS
- [ ] Renal dysfunction due to the risks of NSF
- [ ] Lack of adequate IV access

LIMITATIONS
- [ ] It may be difficult to differentiate recurrent tumor from normal postoperative appearances in cases of soft tissue tumor resection.
- [ ] Metallic hardware (e.g. intramedullary rods, hip prostheses, surgical clips) cause artifact, which may render study performance suboptimal or difficult to interpret.
- [ ] Some slow flow vascular malformations (e.g. venous malformations) may be difficult to differentiate from lymphatic malformations.
- [ ] Vessel occlusion may be difficult to differentiate from very slow flow.

MR Arthrography

- There are few indications for MR arthrography in the pediatric population.
- It involves fluoroscopically guided instillation of a gadolinium-based solution into the joint of interest in order to evaluate for pathology.
- As with the IV administration of contrast, there is a risk of contrast reaction. As with any percutaneous procedure, there

is also a minimal risk of bleeding or infection related to the procedure.

INDICATIONS
- ☐ The majority of MR arthrograms are performed in the postoperative patient to evaluate for reinjury.
- ☐ Shoulder arthrography is often performed to evaluate for rotator cuff pathology as well as labral injury.
- ☐ Hip arthrography is useful to evaluate for injury to the acetabular labrum.

CONTRAINDICATIONS
- ☐ Active joint infection
- ☐ Immediate postoperative state (relative)

LIMITATIONS
- ☐ Metallic hardware (e.g. bone anchors, prostheses) may make image acquisition and interpretation difficult.
- ☐ It may be difficult to differentiate postoperative appearances from reinjury in ligament/tendon repairs.
- ☐ It may be difficult to access a joint following surgery due to fibrous scar tissue; therefore, it may be difficult or impossible for an adequate amount of contrast to be instilled into the joint.

Body MRI

MR of the Liver
- ▪ It requires the patient to be able to breath-hold for 20–30 seconds.
- ▪ It is performed both without and with IV gadolinium (noncontrast imaging sequences are obtained prior to the administration of IV contrast).
- ▪ It is often performed based on the recommendations of another imaging study. Lesions that cannot be characterized on CT or ultrasound are often referred for MRI to characterize the lesion.

INDICATIONS
- ☐ Identification of hepatic masses in patients with a high clinical suspicion of hepatic disease. This is particularly useful in children with limited contrast-enhanced CTs (CECTs) in whom hepatic metastatic disease is of clinical concern.
- ☐ Characterization of liver masses identified on ultrasound or CT imaging

CONTRAINDICATIONS

☐ Patients with severe liver dysfunction are at increased risk of developing NSF following IV contrast administration. These patients should have a Cr drawn 24 hours prior to the MR, and if the Cr clearance (estimated glomerular filtration rate [eGFR]) is <40, IV contrast should not be administered. Local imaging center policies on gadolinium may differ; thus, it is advised that a discussion occur with the local radiology department to determine the policy.

☐ Patients with significant ascites should not be imaged on a 3-tesla scanner due to an artifact produced by the magnetic field in the presence of ascites. The artifact is called the *dielectric effect* and is seen mainly on T2-weighted sequences, rendering them limited for the evaluation of disease. The effect is present but to a much lesser extent on 1.5-tesla scanners, thus these are the preferred scanners for patients with known or suspected ascites.

LIMITATIONS

☐ Due to the long imaging times, young patients may require sedation or general anesthesia during the study. This limits the patient's ability to breath-hold and may degrade images.

☐ Respiratory motion causes artifacts, which may render the study uninterpretable.

☐ The small IVs used for pediatric patients do not allow "power injectors" to be used, which can affect the timing of the contrast bolus and limit the study.

Magnetic Resonance Cholangiopancreatography

▇ It does not require the administration of IV gadolinium.

▇ There is a relatively short imaging time (10–20 minutes).

▇ The study evaluates the intra- and extrahepatic biliary ducts.

INDICATIONS

☐ It may be performed prior to endoscopic retrograde cholangiopancreatography (ERCP) as an anatomic roadmap.

☐ Evaluation of suspected common bile duct (CBD) stones

☐ Evaluation of suspected sites of biliary obstruction

☐ It may be useful to evaluate for ductal involvement by sclerosing cholangitis.

☐ Evaluation of known or suspected choledochal cysts

CONTRAINDICATIONS

☐ Recent meal: This may contract the gallbladder and stimulate the sphincter of Oddi.

☐ Recent pain medication administration may affect the sphincter of Oddi.

LIMITATIONS

☐ It is of limited usefulness in patients with normal caliber ducts as the ducts are often below the resolution of the MRIs. The bile ducts in pediatric patients are particularly small, making evaluation for subtle ductal disease (e.g. beaded ducts in sclerosing cholangitis) even more difficult.

☐ Normal structures such as the sphincter of Oddi may mimic disease (i.e. CBD stones).

☐ In patients with prior cholecystectomy, metallic clips within the surgical bed may produce artifact significant enough to distort the MR cholangiopancreatography (MRCP) images, thus rendering them uninterpretable.

☐ Pneumobilia (e.g. in patients with prior papillotomy for choledocholithiasis), may mimic a CBD stone.

☐ As with all MRI, motion and respiratory artifact will substantially degrade image quality and may render studies uninterpretable.

☐ Without IV contrast, masses and neoplastic strictures (i.e. cholangiocarcinoma) may not be identified.

MR of the Pancreas

■ It requires the administration of IV contrast following non-contrast imaging. It is often imaged as part of an abdominal MR study (see earlier).

■ It is often performed to evaluate for occult pancreatic lesions or to evaluate pancreatic findings identified on other imaging modalities such as endoscopic ultrasound, CT, or ultrasound.

■ As with other imaging modalities, MR often cannot differentiate between focal pancreatitis and malignancy.

■ It may be performed for preoperative planning to determine if a pancreatic mass is resectable.

INDICATIONS

☐ Identification of suspected pancreatic mass: MR is less sensitive than CT and endoscopic ultrasound for the identification of small pancreatic masses. If an MR fails to demonstrate a pancreatic mass in a patient in whom there is a high clinical suspicion (e.g. in hormone-producing tumors [e.g. insulinomas]), additional evaluation with a pancreatic mass CT (see Chapter 15) or endoscopic ultrasound may be performed.

☐ Staging/restaging of known pancreatic malignancy: MR may be performed for this indication; however, CT also may be performed and is often the imaging modality of choice. This is particularly true in patients with a newly diagnosed pancreatic neoplasm who require a determination of resectability. In these patients, adjacent vascular involvement or nodal disease will determine if they are candidates for resection; CT tends to be preferred in these patients. CT angiography (CTA) of the pancreas allows for more accurate and rapid determination of local invasion than does MR. MR may become the study of choice in a patient with renal insufficiency in whom contrast-induced nephropathy is of concern.

☐ Lesion characterization: Pancreatic lesions are often incidental findings on imaging studies performed for other indications. MRI may be useful in characterizing these lesions. However, MR may not be able to determine if a lesion is neoplastic, thus ERCP may be required.

☐ Preoperative planning: In patients with known pancreatic malignancy who are scheduled for surgical resection, MR may be performed to evaluate anatomy and vascular involvement preoperatively. CTA of the pancreas, however, is often the study of choice for this indication.

CONTRAINDICATIONS

☐ Patients with acute pancreatitis (by laboratory values and clinical presentation) may not be optimally evaluated with MR due to the active inflammation. It may be difficult to differentiate between acute mass-like inflammation and a focal pancreatic mass. It may be more appropriate to allow for subsidence of the acute event prior to imaging.

LIMITATIONS

☐ Patients unable to breath-hold or remain motionless during the study will produce degraded images, thus decreasing the quality of the study.

☐ As noted earlier, small pancreatic masses may be below the resolution of MRI. Thus, in a patient with a high clinical suspicion of pancreatic malignancy, additional imaging with CECT of the pancreas (pancreatic mass protocol CT) or endoscopic ultrasound may be required.

☐ Due to the long imaging times and inability to image very thin sections, CTA may be of greater usefulness than MR in assessing resectability of the tumor.

☐ Pancreatic lesions may be difficult to characterize as malignant or benign based upon MRI findings. For example, intraductal papillary mucinous neoplasms (IPMNs) may not be readily separable from benign processes such as pancreatic pseudocysts based upon their MRI characteristics. ERCP may thus be required in order to make the diagnosis (i.e. blue mucin arising from the duct on ERCP).

☐ Preoperative planning for resection of pancreatic neoplasms may be inadequate with MRI due to the spatial resolution; CTA may be of more benefit for this purpose.

☐ As with other imaging modalities, MR often cannot differentiate between focal pancreatitis and malignancy.

☐ Due to the long imaging times, young patients may require sedation or general anesthesia during the study. This limits the patient's ability to breath-hold and may degrade images.

☐ The small IVs used for pediatric patients do not allow power injectors to be used, which can affect the timing of the contrast bolus and limit the study.

MR of the Adrenal Glands

■ The study may or may not require the administration of IV contrast.

INDICATIONS

☐ Evaluation of adrenal masses in patients with neuroblastoma.

☐ Evaluation of adrenal masses incidentally identified at the time of imaging performed for an unrelated indication. This is the most common indication for dedicated adrenal imaging (i.e. the so-called adrenal incidentaloma). These are lesions, often seen at the time of abdominal CT imaging, which do not meet CT criteria for benign processes such as adrenal adenomas or myelolipomas. These patients are then referred for MR opposed phase imaging in order to determine if the lesion represents an adenoma. The vast majority of these lesions can be characterized as adenomas without the administration of IV contrast. If the mass is not an adenoma, IV contrast may be administered in order to determine if the mass represents a metastasis. Evaluation of suspected adrenal masses: In patients with symptoms suggestive of pheochromocytoma and elevated urinary catecholamines, MR of the adrenal glands may be performed in an attempt to identify a mass. If, however, the study is negative and there remains a high clinical suspicion for a pheochromocytoma, MRI of the abdomen/pelvis may be performed at another time to evaluate for possible masses along the sympathetic chain. Imaging of the neck also may be performed to evaluate for paragangliomas (extra-adrenal pheochromocytomas). Nuclear medicine imaging (iodine-131-metaiodobenzylguanidine [MIBG]) may be performed prior to imaging of the neck/chest/abdomen and pelvis as whole body imaging can be performed with a single injection of a radiotracer and may direct further MRI (see Chapter 11).

CONTRAINDICATIONS

☐ There is debate as to whether IV contrast material is contraindicated in patients with known or suspected pheochromocytomas. There is theoretic risk of precipitating an adrenergic storm. It is advisable to discuss these patients with the local radiology department prior to performance of the study.

LIMITATIONS

☐ Motion and respiratory artifact will degrade image quality and may render the study uninterpretable.

☐ Patients who have undergone prior adrenal/upper abdominal surgery (e.g. contralateral adrenal mass resection) will suffer image degradation due to the presence of surgical clips. This may render the MRIs uninterpretable.

☐ Although this is a relatively short examination, young patients may require sedation or general anesthesia.

MR of the Kidneys

■ The study requires non-contrast and contrast-enhanced imaging.

■ It requires the patient to breath-hold for 20–30 seconds.

■ It is often used to characterize lesions identified on other imaging studies (CT and ultrasound).

■ MR has better spatial resolution than CT, thus MR allows resolution of small lesions that are too small to be evaluated on CT imaging.

■ Multiplanar imaging capabilities of MR may be useful in evaluation of lesions.

INDICATIONS

☐ Evaluation of patients with nephroblastomatosis or known Wilms tumor to stage the disease, evaluate the extent of the tumor, and evaluate for contralateral or recurrent tumor.

☐ In patients with abdominal masses in whom it is unclear if the mass is of renal or adrenal origin, the multiplanar capabilities of MR may allow for determination of the site of origin of the tumor.

☐ MR is useful to evaluate for tumor or bland (i.e. non-tumorous thrombus) within the renal veins, inferior vena cava (IVC), and right atrium. This has clear implications for tumor staging and surgical planning (Wilms tumor).

☐ Identification of ectopic kidneys, which cannot be identified on ultrasound. It is preferred to CT in that no ionizing radiation is required.

☐ Characterization of lesions identified on alternate imaging modalities (e.g. CT or ultrasound). MR is the study of choice to evaluate cystic renal masses, which may represent cystic renal tumors.

☐ Follow-up of renal masses: Cystic renal lesions that are not clearly malignant but do not represent simple cysts (i.e. Bosniak IIf lesions) may be followed with MRI to assess for stability or progression to malignancy.

☐ Surveillance: In patients with prior partial or complete nephrectomy for renal malignancy (e.g. Wilms tumor), MR may be performed to evaluate for lesion recurrence or synchronous lesions. MR is preferable to CT in these patients as their renal function is often compromised due to prior renal resection, thus MR contrast (gadolinium) is preferred to the more nephrotoxic CT contrast.

☐ Staging: Patients with known or suspected renal neoplasms may be staged with contrast-enhanced MRI. This is particularly important for evaluation of tumor extension into the renal veins and IVC as this has obvious prognostic and surgical implications. MR has the ability to evaluate vascular involvement and to determine if vascular thrombus is bland (i.e. clot only) or tumor thrombus. It is also of paramount importance to evaluate for involvement of the IVC and right atrium by thrombus as this not only will change the patient's staging but also will determine the surgical approach. If there is thrombus within the IVC at or above the level of the hepatic veins, a cardiothoracic surgeon must be part of the surgical team in order to resect the thoracic extent of intravascular tumor thrombus.

CONTRAINDICATIONS

☐ Patients with renal compromise are at increased risk of developing NSF following IV contrast administration. If a patient has a low eGFR and cannot receive IV contrast, MR is of limited use. IV contrast is often required for evaluation of known or suspected renal masses.

LIMITATIONS

☐ Respiratory and motion artifact often will degrade image quality and render a study uninterpretable.

☐ Surgical clips in patients with prior partial nephrectomy or complete nephrectomy will produce artifacts that may degrade the image quality.

☐ Small lesions may be below the resolution of MRI for identification and characterization.

☐ MR may not enable assessment of the urothelium and ureters for synchronous or metachronous lesions. MR urography may be helpful, although it remains less useful than CT/CT-IVP examinations.

☐ Due to the long imaging times, young patients may require sedation or general anesthesia during the study. This limits the patient's ability to breath-hold and may degrade images.

☐ Respiratory motion causes artifacts, which may render the study uninterpretable.

MR Angiography of the Renal Arteries

▧ It is rapidly becoming a primary indication for MRI.

▧ The most common indication is refractory hypertension.

▧ It is performed without and with IV contrast.

▧ It requires the patient to be able to breath-hold for 20–30 seconds.

▧ MRA of renal arteries is optimal for proximal and ostial lesions. It is less sensitive for distal arterial stenoses (i.e. in the distal branch vessels of the renal vasculature).

■ It is often performed as part of an MRI of the kidneys; however, for billing purposes, it must be specifically requested in addition to MRI of the kidneys.

INDICATIONS

☐ Evaluation of renovascular hypertension

☐ Evaluation of renovascular anatomy

☐ Evaluation of venous thrombosis (tumor or bland thrombus) in patients with Wilms tumor

CONTRAINDICATIONS

☐ Renal artery stents may render the study suboptimal or may overestimate the degree of stenosis. An alternate study such as CTA, ultrasound, or conventional catheter angiography may be a more appropriate investigation for these patients.

LIMITATIONS

☐ Respiratory and motion artifact will often degrade image quality and render a study uninterpretable.

☐ Small accessory renal arteries may be out of the imaging plane or may be diminutive and thus not be recognized with MRA. These small accessory vessels may be stenotic and thus may be symptomatic.

☐ Distal and branch vessels of the renal arteries may not be adequately evaluated with MRA due to the limitations of spatial resolution. Thus, stenosis in these vessels as a cause of symptoms may be overlooked.

☐ Due to the long imaging times, patients may require sedation or anesthesia. This prevents the patient from cooperating with breath holding, which can degrade images and render the study uninterpetable.

☐ Young patients often cannot comply with breath holding, thus limiting the quality of the study.

☐ The small IVs used for pediatric patients do not allow power injectors to be used, which can affect the timing of the contrast bolus and limit the study.

Cardiac MR Imaging

■ It is increasingly used to evaluate cardiac abnormalities, particularly valvular disease and congenital heart disease.

■ The study is typically performed without IV contrast, although there are certain indications for the administration of IV contrast (including evaluation of cardiac masses, assessment of myocardial viability).

■ It requires the patient to be in normal sinus rhythm as the study is performed with cardiac gating (i.e. the scanner is triggered to start scanning based upon the peripheral cardiac tracing). Patients with arrythmias are poor candidates for cardiac MRI as the scanner is inconsistently triggered to start scanning.

■ The clinical question to be answered must be clearly communicated to the interpreting radiologist prior to the study so that the examination can be specifically tailored to provide the appropriate diagnostic information.

INDICATIONS

☐ Valvular: Echocardiography remains the gold standard for the evaluation of valvular cardiac disease (typically left heart valves). Cardiac MR, however, has emerged as a new modality to identify and quantify the amount of valvular disease present. There is good correlation of the quantification of disease with both modalities. Evaluation of valvular disease with MR is time-consuming and not routinely performed unless specifically requested. IV contrast is not administered for this indication.

☐ Vascular (pulmonary artery/aorta):
  • MR can evaluate the location of the main pulmonary artery and aorta and arterial-ventricular relationships in patients with suspected congenital cardiac anomalies. This does not require IV contrast administration.
  • Evaluation of the size of the main pulmonary artery and aorta may be performed in patients with suspected aneurysm. This may be performed without IV contrast; however, it is often performed as part of a contrast-enhanced examination.
  • Patients with suspected supracardiac congenital anomalies such as partial or total anomalous pulmonary venous return (PAPVR/TAPVR) are excellent candidates for evaluation with MRI. These patients require administration of IV contrast material.

☐ Evaluation of intra- and extracardiac shunts including surgical shunts/baffles:
  • Patients with suspected congenital intracardiac or extracardiac shunts (e.g. persistent ductus arteriosis) may be non-invasively evaluated with MRI. IV contrast is not required for this study; however, contrast may be helpful in certain instances (use is often determined at the time of the study by the monitoring radiologist).

- Patients with surgically placed conduits, baffles, and shunts may be monitored for stenosis and patency with MR. The degree of shunting can be assessed and monitored with MR. The study is often performed without and with IV contrast.

☐ Intracardiac (e.g. congenital anomalies): Patients (particularly infants) with suspected congenital cardiac disease may be non-invasively evaluated with MRI. The study is typically performed without IV contrast unless there is a question of an associated supracardiac vascular anomaly.

☐ Myocardial: This is one of the most important emerging applications for cardiac MRI. There are two main applications for myocardial imaging:

- Perfusion: This type of study is performed as a monitored examination as pharmacologic vasodilation (typically with adenosine) is performed. The study is performed as part of a complete cardiac imaging study. The perfusion portion of the examination allows for evaluation of myocardial blood flow. Areas with abnormal perfusion are interpreted as regions of ischemia.

- Diffusion (delayed myocardial enhancement): This type of study is performed in conjunction with a complete cardiac MR examination (often with perfusion). The study is performed following the administration of IV contrast such that approximately 8–10 minutes following contrast administration, images are obtained. Areas of myocardium that display late (delayed) enhancement are considered abnormal and represent areas of myocardial scar. There is typically a corresponding perfusion abnormality with regions of abnormal myocardial contraction.

☐ Epicardial (e.g. invasion): Mediastinal or pulmonary parenchymal disease may extend into the epicardial region. MR may be performed to evaluate the extent of local involvement.

☐ Pericardial:

- As just noted for epicardial disease, MR may be performed to evaluate for pericardial involvement by adjacent neoplastic or inflammatory disease. Malignant and benign pericardial effusions also may be identified.

- The primary role for MR in the evaluation of pericardial disease is in the differentiation of constrictive pericarditis from restrictive cardiomyopathy. Unlike restrictive cardiomyopathy, constrictive pericarditis is a treatable cause of heart failure. Constrictive pericarditis is well-evaluated by MR such that even small focal areas of pericardial thickening can be identified and the diagnosis made. The study is performed as part of a complete cardiac examination as other causes of heart failure may be identified. Additionally, secondary signs of constrictive pericarditis such as interventricular septal wall motion abnormalities may be identified and further confirm the diagnosis.

CONTRAINDICATIONS

☐ Patients not in sinus rhythm are not good candidates for cardiac MR as ECG gating cannot be adequately performed, thus the scanner cannot be triggered to scan.

☐ Patients with ECG changes or recent acute MI are not candidates for stress perfusion imaging due to the risks of pharmacologic stress.

☐ Patients with pacemakers and AICDs are not candidates for MR examinations.

☐ There is debate as to whether implanted epicardial pacer leads are contraindicated for cardiac MR examinations due to the risk of heating during the study. This should be discussed with the radiologist prior to the examination.

LIMITATIONS

☐ Patient factors:

• Patients with large body habitus may not be evaluable with MRI.

• Patients who cannot comply with multiple, repeated breath holding imaging sequences are poor candidates for cardiac MRI. Due to the exquisite sensitivity to motion and respiratory artifact, patients must remain motionless and suspend respiration in order for adequate images to be obtained. However, some scanners are able to image patients who are not able to breath-hold for the examination. These cases should be discussed with the radiologist prior to the study.

• Patients with arrhythmias are poor candidates for cardiac MRI as the scanner is triggered to scan based upon the R-R interval. Newer MR scanners may allow for limited studies in patients who are not in sinus rhythm.

☐ Technical factors:
  • Due to the mechanics of the MR scanner, the T wave
    may be enlarged and may mimic an R wave, thus inap-
    propriately triggering the scan and producing significant
    artifacts.

Vascular MRI

■ It is performed without and with IV contrast.
■ Patients must be clinically stable enough to undergo the exam-
  ination.
■ MR of the aorta is particularly useful in patients with suspected
  dissection who are unable to receive non-ionic IV contrast for
  CT imaging (based on poor renal function or documented con-
  trast allergy) or for assessing gradients across a stenosis (i.e. in
  children with coarctation of the aorta).
■ Peripheral vascular imaging:
  ☐ It is often used to evaluate peripheral vessels of the lower
    extremities in patients unable to undergo conventional
    angiography.
  ☐ It is performed without and with IV contrast.
  ☐ It requires the patient to lie supine and immobile for
    extended periods of time (the examination can require up
    to 1 hour of imaging time per extremity).
  ☐ Surgical clips can degrade the study. The artifact can be
    minimized by using different imaging techniques; however,
    it is helpful to be aware of the presence of clips prior to
    commencement of imaging.
  INDICATIONS
  ☐ Arterial:
    • Evaluation of patients with known or suspected aortic
      coarctation
    • Evaluation of patients with suspected vascular stenosis
      (e.g. patients with Williams syndrome)
    • Evaluation of vascular involvement by tumor to allow
      surgical planning
  ☐ Venous:
    • Evaluation of suspected DVT or thrombosis of the IVC
      and pelvic vessels in patients with negative or suboptimal
      lower extremity DVT ultrasound studies.

- Evaluation of suspected upper extremity or SVC thrombosis
- Evaluation of the presence and extent of tumor thrombus (e.g. into the renal veins/IVC in patients with renal cell carcinoma, or portal vein thrombus, in patients with hepatocellular carcinoma

CONTRAINDICATIONS

☐ Patients who cannot receive IV contrast are not candidates for MRA.

☐ Patients who cannot remain immobile are not candidates for the examination as it is essential that the patient be in exactly the same position for multiple image acquisitions in order to obtain diagnostic information.

☐ Patients who are unstable should not be placed in the magnet.

LIMITATIONS

☐ The small size of the vessels involved may lead to under- or overestimation of stenosis.

☐ Patient factors:

- Patients unable to remain motionless are poor candidates for the examination as motion artifact significantly degrades the images and can simulate or obscure areas of stenosis.
- Patients unable to breath-hold are poor candidates for studies such as evaluation of mesenteric or renal artery stenosis as respiratory motion may mask areas of stenosis.
- Patients in whom a large bore IV cannot be placed are not eligible for contrast administration by power injector. These patients are administered the contrast by hand injection, thus a tight bolus of contrast cannot be obtained and suboptimal imaging often occurs.
- Patients with IVC filters, renal artery stents, arterial stents, or metallic surgical clips are suboptimal candidates for MRA as these devices cause significant artifact and areas of disease may be obscured.
- Technical factors: Older MR scanners may not be able to adequately image the entire vascular system (e.g. the aorto-popliteal system) as the images cannot be acquired rapidly enough to prevent venous contamination. This renders areas of arterial disease difficult to identify.

Pelvic MR (for Gynecology)

■ The study may be performed without or with IV contrast, depending upon the study indication.

■ Patients may not eat 4–6 hours prior to the examination and they must avoid caffeine for 24 hours (to decrease bowel peristalsis and thus decrease artifacts).

INDICATIONS

☐ Uterine anomalies: MR may be definitive for the identification and characterization of congenital uterine anomalies. Limited renal imaging should be performed at the same time due to the associations of renal and genitourinary anomalies.

☐ Evaluation of cloacal abnormalities

☐ Ovarian: MR is very useful to evaluate known or suspected ovarian pathology.

• This is particularly true for known or suspected endometriosis. IV contrast is not required for the imaging of endometriosis.

• MR is a valuable study for ovarian masses that do not demonstrate characteristics of endometriosis. A diagnosis may be suggested or confirmed with MR. IV contrast may be required, depending upon the imaging appearance of the ovarian mass; however, this is often not predictable until the study is performed. Therefore, it is suggested that the study be requested with IV contrast. If the contrast is not required, it will not be administered.

• MR may be useful in the diagnosis of suspected ovarian torsion. Ultrasound (with pulsed Doppler) is the imaging modality of choice for the diagnosis of ovarian torsion. If there is high clinical suspicion of ovarian torsion in the setting of a negative or inconclusive ultrasound, however, MR may be helpful to identify ovarian edema and enlargement, which would suggest the diagnosis.

LIMITATIONS

☐ Due to the small size of the patients and gynecologic organs, resolution may be limited.

☐ The lack of pelvic fat may limit evaluation of pelvic abnormalities.

MRI of the Brain

■ It may be performed as a contrast-enhanced or non-contrast study depending upon the indication for the examination. Due to increasingly stringent insurance precertification requirements, it is essential to be aware of the type of study being requested prior to scheduling so that the examination is not cancelled due to billing errors. If a question arises as to whether or not IV contrast may be required, it is advisable to contact the imaging center prior to scheduling so that the appropriate examination may be scheduled and conducted.

Non-Contrast MR of the Brain

■ It is performed as a routine without IV contrast unless an abnormality requiring contrast administration is identified while the examination is in progress.

■ All non-contrast examinations may be ordered in the same manner, regardless of the indication (including evaluation of seizures). The protocol prescribed by the radiologist will be dependent upon the indication for the examination. For the most part, routine sequences are performed for all of the above listed indications, with the exception of patients with seizures. In these patients, high-resolution images are obtained with a surface coil.

INDICATIONS

☐ Evaluation of headaches (in children and adults)

☐ Evaluation of patients with a history of trauma. MR is not indicated in the evaluation of patients with suspected subarachnoid hemorrhage as it is often not detectable with MRI unless it is recurrent, chronic, or long-standing. MRI may be helpful in dating the age of subdural/epidural hemorrhage, although this is less clear-cut than dating parenchymal hemorrhage. The main advantage of MRI in sub/epidural collections is determination of acute or chronic hemorrhage, which may be of value in suspected non-accidental trauma in children.

☐ Follow-up of ventricular size in patients with known hydrocephalus

☐ Evaluation of patients with seizures

☐ Evaluation of patients with known or suspected cardiovascular accident (CVA).

CONTRAINDICATIONS

☐ Patients who are actively seizing should not be placed in the magnet due to the inability to fully monitor the patient's clinical status.

☐ General contraindications for MRI

LIMITATIONS

☐ Areas of abnormal diffusion will normalize over time, thus yielding false negatives for areas of subacute ischemia.

☐ Small or subtle masses or areas of infection may not be identifiable on non-contrast imaging unless there is surrounding parenchymal edema; IV contrast should be administered if there is concern for intracranial infection or mass.

☐ Small areas such as the internal auditory canal or pituitary are not adequately imaged with routine brain protocols; if there is concern for pathology in these regions, dedicated imaging should be performed.

☐ If patients are unable to hold still, imaging may be uninterpretable. Unlike CT imaging in which only a portion of the study is affected if a patient moves, in MRI, patient motion for even a portion of the image acquisition will affect the whole sequence. This is due to the manner in which data are acquired and processed in MRI.

☐ Small lesions may be below the resolution of MRI.

☐ It may be difficult to differentiate between infection and tumor.

Contrast-Enhanced MR of the Brain

■ The study is performed as routine non-contrast images followed by contrast-enhanced images.

■ Although non-contrast images are obtained in addition to contrast-enhanced images, the study is ordered as a contrast-enhanced MR of the brain (not as a without/with contrast study).

INDICATIONS

☐ Evaluation of patients with altered mental status to evaluate for underlying structural or mass lesion

☐ Evaluation of patients with known or suspected metastatic disease. MR has a higher sensitivity for detection of parenchymal and leptomeningeal metastatic disease; however, CT is superior to MR for identification of osseous metastatic disease.

☐ Characterization of masses identified with CT
☐ Follow-up of known primary CNS neoplasms
☐ Evaluation of intracranial infection. It is most useful for parenchymal lesions (i.e. abscess) or epidural collections. Meningeal enhancement may be seen in cases of meningitis (particularly tuberculous, fungal, or aseptic); however, meningeal enhancement may be seen following lumbar puncture, thus leading to false-positive results. It is advisable to defer lumbar puncture if MRI is planned for the evaluation of suspected meningitis or leptomeningeal spread of tumor.
☐ Evaluation of demyelinating disease (e.g. multiple sclerosis). Although the majority of evaluations may be performed without IV contrast to confirm a suspected diagnosis of demyelinating disease, IV contrast is helpful in the identification of active foci of demyelination as these tend to demonstrate peripheral enhancement.

CONTRAINDICATIONS
☐ Patients who are actively seizing should not be placed in the magnet due to the inability to fully monitor the patient's clinical status.
☐ General contraindications for MRI

LIMITATIONS
☐ It may not be possible to differentiate between infection and tumor.
☐ It may not be possible to differentiate between postsurgical changes, radiation-induced changes, and recurrent tumor. MR spectroscopy and diffusion imaging may be useful to provide additional information in these cases.
☐ Areas of subacute ischemia can be mass-like and will demonstrate enhancement in this phase; this may make it difficult to differentiate from tumor or infection.
☐ Small areas such as the internal auditory canal or pituitary are not adequately imaged with routine brain protocols; if there is concern for pathology in these regions, dedicated imaging should be performed.
☐ If patients are unable to hold still, imaging may be uninterpretable. Unlike CT imaging, in which only a portion of the

study is affected if a patient moves, in MRI, patient motion for even a portion of the image acquisition will affect the whole sequence. This is due to the manner in which data are acquired and processed in MRI.

☐ Small lesions may be below the resolution of MRI.

MR of the Nasopharynx

■ It is performed as a routine with IV contrast.

■ It does not image the brain parenchyma; dedicated images of the nasopharynx are obtained. Imaging does include sequences to evaluate for the presence of lymphadenopathy within the neck.

INDICATIONS

☐ Identification of suspected nasopharyngeal mass

☐ Restaging of known nasopharyngeal malignancy

☐ Evaluation of aggressive sinus infection in the setting of immunocompromise

CONTRAINDICATIONS

☐ Patients with known or suspected gas-forming organisms are better imaged with CT. This is due to the poor imaging capabilities of MR in the presence of air.

☐ General contraindications for MRI

LIMITATIONS

☐ Air within the sinuses creates artifact that makes it difficult to image the region.

☐ A primary head and neck malignancy may be occult on imaging; only metastatic disease may be identifiable.

☐ Subtle areas of vascular involvement may be below the resolution of MRI; CT may be useful for this purpose.

☐ Artifacts from surgical clips may make image acquisition and interpretation difficult.

MR of the Orbits

■ It is performed as a routine with IV contrast.

■ It does image the brain parenchyma as it is often performed for evaluation of demyelinating disease.

INDICATIONS

☐ Evaluation of involvement of the orbits in demyelinating disease

☐ Evaluation of suspected ophthalmopathy (particularly Graves)

☐ Evaluation of nerve entrapment or involvement by masses

☐ Evaluation of metastatic disease (particularly melanoma and breast)

☐ Evaluation of primary intraocular tumors (e.g. retinoblastoma, ocular melanoma) and inflammatory lesions (e.g. orbital pseudotumor)

CONTRAINDICATIONS

☐ Surgical clips or metal within the eye may move in the magnetic field. The type of clip should be cleared with a physicist for safety prior to imaging.

☐ General contraindications to MRI

LIMITATIONS

☐ Ocular movement or patient movement may render images uninterpretable.

☐ It may be difficult to differentiate tumor from infection or demyelination.

☐ If masses are large, it may be difficult to determine if they arise from the intraconal or extraconal space. This has implications on determining what is the likeliest (e.g. tumor or infection) to cause the abnormality.

☐ Artifacts from surgical clips may make image acquisition and interpretation difficult.

MR of the Pituitary

▪ It is performed as a routine with IV contrast.

▪ It includes evaluation of the brain parenchyma as well as high-resolution images of the sella turcica with dynamic contrast enhancement.

▪ The indication for the study and the patient's symptoms are critical pieces of information prior to performing the examination as the study is performed in a different manner depending upon the indication (i.e. pituitary microadenoma versus macroadenoma).

INDICATIONS

☐ Evaluation of patients with suspected pituitary macroadenoma (mass effect/visual changes)

☐ Evaluation of suspected microadenoma (hormonal stimulation)

☐ Evaluation of suspected mass in the sella turcica

☐ Evaluation of absent or ectopic pituitary

☐ Evaluation of suspected pituitary infundibular lesion (e.g. diabetes insipidus) such as sarcoid, eosinophilic granuloma

☐ Evaluation of pituitary hemorrhage (e.g. postpartum, Sheehan's syndrome)

☐ Evaluation of hypothalamic dysfunction

☐ Evaluation of hypothalamic masses (e.g. hypothalamic hamartomas [patients with gelastic seizures], optic gliomas)

CONTRAINDICATIONS

☐ General contraindications to MRI

LIMITATIONS

☐ Small masses may be below the resolution of MR.

☐ Subtle areas of enhancement may be difficult to recognize, which may make diagnosis of an abnormality difficult.

☐ It may be difficult to differentiate tumor from demyelination and granulomatous disease.

☐ Artifacts from the adjacent paranasal sinuses and surgical clips may render image acquisition and interpretation difficult.

☐ Areas of hemorrhage may complicate interpretation as it may be difficult to differentiate hemorrhage from a mass unless blood products and enhancement characteristics are considered.

MR of the Neck

■ It may be performed without or with IV contrast, depending upon the indication for the study.

■ If the study is performed for evaluation of lymphadenopathy or for localization of parathyroid adenomas, no IV contrast is required.

■ If the study is performed as an MRA for the purposes of evaluation of carotid or basivertebral disease, IV contrast is required.

Non-Contrast MR of the Neck

INDICATIONS

☐ Evaluation of suspected lymphadenopathy in patients with a history of head and neck malignancy. This is of particular importance in patients with a history of thyroid malignancy as CT of the neck requires the administration of IV contrast to identify lymphadenopathy. This is disadvantageous in patients with thyroid neoplasms as the iodine-containing contrast may interfere with other imaging modalities or even with planned therapy.

☐ Evaluation of orthotopic or ectopic parathyroid adenomas

Contrast-Enhanced MR of the Neck (MRA)

INDICATIONS

☐ Evaluation of suspected extracranial carotid/basivertebral disease including stenosis and dissection

☐ Preoperative evaluation of vessel involvement by tumor

CONTRAINDICATIONS

☐ General contraindications to MRI

LIMITATIONS

☐ Small masses may be below the resolution of MRI

☐ Ectopic thyroid or parathyroid glands may be located within the mediastinum. This region is generally not imaged at the time the neck is imaged.

☐ Lymphadenopathy is deemed pathologic on the basis of size criteria only (short axis >1.5 cm). However, microscopic disease that does not enlarge the lymph node is not recognized on routine MR of the neck.

☐ Motion artifact will limit image interpretation.

☐ Subtle areas of vascular involvement by tumor may be below the resolution of MRI.

MR Angiography/MR Venography

▓ It is performed as a routine with IV contrast.

▓ It is typically performed in conjunction with complete imaging of the brain parenchyma.

▓ It must be ordered as a separate study from MRI (for billing/insurance purposes).

INDICATIONS

☐ Evaluation of known or suspected CVA to evaluate vessel occlusion or stenosis

☐ Evaluation of known or suspected aneurysms of the Circle of Willis

☐ Evaluation of suspected or known vascular malformations

☐ Evaluation of suspected venous occlusion (MR venography [MRV]). It must be specifically requested as it is not performed routinely with MRA imaging. The indication for

MRV should be clearly stated at the time of the request for the examination. It is often requested in patients with mastoiditis, patients who are pregnant, and patients in hypercoagulable states.

CONTRAINDICATIONS
☐ General contraindications to MRI

LIMITATIONS
☐ Very slowly flowing blood can mimic thrombus and vessel occlusion.
☐ Slow flow in vascular malformations may make it difficult to determine what type of malformation the lesion represents.
☐ Motion artifact can limit the examination.

MR Spectroscopy

▪ It is performed as a routine without IV contrast.
▪ It is typically performed in conjunction with complete MRI of the brain.
▪ It must be requested as a separate study in conjunction with a routine MR examination.
▪ It is not performed routinely due to the length of the imaging sequence as well as due to the fact that it remains a research tool to some extent with limited application in clinical settings.

INDICATIONS
☐ Evaluation of mass lesions in the brain to help differentiate neoplastic from non-neoplastic conditions
☐ Evaluation of suspected toxic/metabolic conditions (e.g. Leigh's disease)

CONTRAINDICATIONS
☐ General contraindications to MRI

LIMITATIONS
☐ The lesion must be large enough for an adequate amount of the lesion to be sampled with spectroscopy.
☐ MR spectroscopy is not sensitive; it may remain difficult to differentiate between tumor and other processes such as radiation change.
☐ It is a relatively time-consuming sequence during which patients must lie still. Due to the length of the image acquisition, it is not routinely used.

MR of the Spine

▪ It may be performed as a non-contrast or a contrast-enhanced study, depending on the indication for the study.

Pediatric MRI

- As with MRI of the brain, it is essential to request the appropriate study at the time of scheduling so that insurance precertification may be obtained appropriately.

Non-Contrast MR of the Spine

- It is performed as a routine without IV contrast unless an abnormality requiring contrast administration is identified while the examination is in progress.
- It requires prolonged immobility and supine positioning. For patients with significant pain in these settings, some degree of sedation or pain relief may be required.

INDICATIONS
- ☐ Evaluation of disc disease
- ☐ Evaluation of acute spine trauma (particularly the cervical spine)
- ☐ Evaluation of demyelinating disease, although contrast may be required to evaluate the extent of active disease (see section, Non-Contrast MR of the Brain)
- ☐ Evaluation of cord pathology due to disc disease, trauma, XRT, congenital malformations (e.g. tethered cord, Chiari malformation, meningomyelocele), cord compression from disc disease

CONTRAINDICATIONS
- ☐ General contraindications to MRI

LIMITATIONS
- ☐ Surgical hardware may cause artifact that will render image acquisition and interpretation difficult.
- ☐ Motion artifact can significantly limit interpretation.
- ☐ It may be difficult to differentiate cord pathology due to ischemia, infection, and infarction.

Contrast-Enhanced MR of the Spine

- It is performed as a routine with IV contrast.
- It requires prolonged immobility and supine positioning. For patients with significant pain in these settings, some degree of sedation or pain relief may be required.

INDICATIONS
- ☐ Evaluation of suspected osteomyelitis/discitis
- ☐ Evaluation of suspected arachnoiditis
- ☐ Evaluation of suspected epidural abscess (surgical emergency)

- [ ] Evaluation of neoplasm including vertebral body metastases (although CT and nuclear medicine bone scan are the studies of choice), drop metastases, leptomeningeal spread of tumor
- [ ] Evaluation of cord compression from neoplasm/osseous metastatic disease
- [ ] Evaluation of primary tumors of the spinal cord

CONTRAINDICATIONS

- [ ] General contraindications to MRI

LIMITATIONS

- [ ] Patient motion may limit the examination.
- [ ] It may not be possible to differentiate among infection, inflammation, and tumor.
- [ ] It may not be possible to differentiate between recurrent disc disease and scar tissue in the postoperative patient.

APPENDIX I

Common Clinical Questions and Key Studies to Order

Right Upper Quadrant Pain

Study	Information obtained	Significant limitation
KUB	▪ ± Gallstones ▪ Pneumobilia ▪ Pneumoperitoneum ▪ Emphysematous cholecystitis	▪ Not specific or sensitive for visceral abnormalities
Ultrasound	▪ Cholelithiasis ▪ Acute cholecystitis ▪ Intra/extrahepatic biliary ductal dilation ▪ Choledocholithiasis ▪ Pancreatitis (in thin patients) ▪ Right renal obstruction	▪ False negatives for cholecystitis can occur, especially if early or acalculous ▪ Poor sensitivity for choledocholithiasis ▪ Recent meal or morphine administration can lead to gallbladder contraction, limiting evaluation
CT	▪ Pancreatitis ▪ Biliary obstruction from masses ▪ Obstructing renal calculus ▪ Bowel pathology (e.g. ascending colon, small bowel abnormality) ▪ ± Cholecystitis	▪ Early/mild pancreatitis may be occult on CT ▪ Mild biliary obstruction may be occult ▪ Cholecystitis not well-evaluated on CT; cholelithiasis may be occult on CT

329

Study	Information obtained	Significant limitation
MR/MRCP	■ Intra/extrahepatic biliary dilation ■ Choledocholithiasis ■ Acute cholecystitis	■ Artifacts such as biliary air (e.g. prior papillotomy) may mimic stones ■ Small stones may not be identified
HIDA	■ Acute cholecystitis ■ Chronic cholecystitis ■ Biliary atresia	■ Recent meal ■ Recent morphine administration

Evaluation of Liver Function Test Abnormalities

Study	Information obtained	Significant limitation
Ultrasound	■ Intra/extrahepatic biliary ductal dilation ■ Choledocholithiasis ■ Fatty liver ■ Cirrhosis/portal hypertension ■ Liver metastases	■ Limited sensitivity for metastases/HCC
CT	■ Intra/extrahepatic biliary ductal dilation ■ Choledocholithiasis ■ Fatty liver ■ Cirrhosis/portal hypertension ■ Liver metastases	■ Limited sensitivity for minimal ductal dilation
MR	■ Intra/extrahepatic biliary ductal dilation ■ Choledocholithiasis ■ Fatty liver ■ Cirrhosis/portal hypertension ■ Liver metastases	■ Biliary air can cause artifacts that can mimic stones
Sulfur colloid study	■ Evaluation of portal hypertension	■ Minimal degrees of hepatocellular dysfunction may not be detectable

Evaluation of Gallbladder Disease

Study	Information obtained	Significant limitation
KUB	▪ Radiodense gallstones ▪ Emphysematous cholecystitis	▪ Not all gallstones are radiodense
Ultrasound	▪ Evaluation of cholelithiasis ▪ Evaluation of acute cholecystitis ▪ Evaluation of choledocholithiasis ▪ Evaluation of biliary obstruction	▪ Ultrasound may be negative or equivocal for early cholecystitis ▪ Low sensitivity for choledocholithiasis
CT	▪ Evaluation of choledocholithiasis ▪ Evaluation of biliary obstruction	▪ Low sensitivity for choledocholithiasis ▪ Low sensitivity for minimal biliary ductal dilation
MR	▪ Evaluation of cholelithiasis ▪ Evaluation of acute cholecystitis ▪ Evaluation of choledocholithiasis ▪ Evaluation of biliary obstruction ▪ Evaluation of choledocholithiasis ▪ Evaluation of biliary obstruction	▪ Biliary air can mimic stones
HIDA	▪ Evaluation of acute cholecystitis ▪ Evaluation of chronic cholecystitis ▪ Evaluation of biliary atresia	▪ False-negative studies can occur

Evaluation of Biliary Obstruction

Study	Information obtained	Significant limitation
Ultrasound	■ Presence of intra/extrahepatic biliary dilation ■ Presence of choledocholithiasis ■ Presence of obstructing mass	■ Low sensitivity for choledocholithiasis ■ Low sensitivity for hepatic masses
CT	■ Presence of intra/extrahepatic biliary dilation ■ Presence of choledocholithiasis ■ Presence of obstructing mass	■ Limited evaluation of subtle biliary dilation ■ Non-contrast CT poor for the evaluation of liver masses; CECT is the study of choice
MR	■ Presence of intra/extrahepatic biliary dilation ■ Presence of biliary stricture (MRCP) ■ Presence of choledocholithiasis ■ Presence of obstructing mass	■ Biliary air can mimic stones ■ Cholangiocarcinoma may not be identified unless delayed imaging following IV contrast administration is performed
HIDA	■ Evaluation of cholecystitis ■ Evaluation of CBD obstruction ■ Evaluation of biliary atresia	■ In patients with very poor liver function or very elevated bilirubins, the tracer may not be taken up by the liver or concentrated, rendering the examination uninterpretable

Evaluation of Bile Leaks

Study	Information obtained	Significant limitation
Ultrasound	▪ Presence of perihepatic/gallbladder fossa fluid	▪ Ultrasound cannot differentiate normal postoperative fluid from bile
CT	▪ Presence of perihepatic/gallbladder fossa fluid	▪ CT cannot differentiate normal postoperative fluid from bile
MR	▪ Presence of perihepatic/gallbladder fossa fluid	▪ MR cannot differentiate normal postoperative fluid from bile unless a biliary specific/excreted contrast agent is given. This is not routinely available in most clinical practices.
HIDA	▪ Presence of activity in the gallbladder fossa in cholecystectomy patients ▪ Delayed (at 24 hours) accumulation of activity in the peritoneal cavity	▪ In patients with poor liver function, tracer may not be taken up or excreted from the liver

Evaluation of Liver Masses

Study	Information obtained	Significant limitation
Ultrasound	▪ Presence of mass	▪ Poor sensitivity for masses, particularly in heterogeneous/fatty livers
CT	▪ Presence of mass ▪ Enhancement pattern of mass ▪ Other sites of abdominal tumor	▪ Phase of contrast enhancement affects sensitivity ▪ Small masses may be below the resolution of CT

Study	Information obtained	Significant limitation
MR	■ Presence of mass ■ Characterization of mass for diagnosis ■ Other sites of abdominal tumor	■ Phase of contrast enhancement affects sensitivity ■ Small masses may be below the resolution of MR ■ It may not be possible to characterize the mass; may require biopsy for diagnosis
Nuclear imaging	■ Differentiation of FNH from adenoma (HIDA) ■ Identification of hepatoma (HIDA) ■ Confirmation of hemangioma (RBC study)	■ Small masses may be below the resolution of nuclear imaging

Evaluation of Flank Pain

Study	Information obtained	Significant limitation
KUB	■ Presence of renal stone	■ Not all stones are dense on x-ray
Ultrasound	■ Presence of renal stone ■ Presence of obstruction (hydronephrosis)	■ Ureteral stones may be difficult to visualize due to shadowing from adjacent bowel air
CT	■ Presence of renal/ureteral stone ■ Presence of renal/ureteral obstruction	■ In thin patients without retroperitoneal fat, it may be difficult to visualize small ureteral stones or separate them from phleboliths (venous calcifications)
MR	■ Presence of hydronephrosis/level of obstruction	■ Patient motion can obscure small stones

Evaluation of Renal Infection

Study	Information obtained	Significant limitation
Ultrasound	▪ Renal abscess ▪ Hydronephrosis ▪ Obstructing stone as nidus of infection	▪ Renal abscess may be occult on ultrasound
CT (contrast-enhanced)	▪ Striated nephrogram suggesting pyelonephritis ▪ Renal abscess ▪ Obstructing stone acting as nidus of infection ▪ Bladder wall thickening suggesting cystitis	▪ CT may be normal in pyelonephritis
MR	▪ Renal abscess ▪ Hydronephrosis	▪ MR may be normal in pyelonephritis

Evaluation of Renal Mass

Study	Information obtained	Significant limitation
Ultrasound	▪ Simple vs. complex cyst ▪ Solid vs. cystic mass	▪ In obese patients, it may not be possible to identify a mass or characterize it as a simple cyst
CT (with/without contrast)	▪ Cyst vs. cystic renal neoplasm ▪ Enhancing renal mass ▪ Staging of known or suspicious renal cell carcinoma ▪ Evaluation of local extension/vascular invasion of renal cell carcinoma ▪ Preoperative planning partial nephrectomy for neoplasm	▪ Poor contrast bolus may limit the examination ▪ In obese patients, it may be difficult to evaluate for enhancement based on streak artifact ▪ If patients have poor renal function, they may not concentrate contrast, therefore, enhancement of renal lesions may not be demonstrated

Study	Information obtained	Significant limitation
MR (with/ without contrast)	■ Cyst vs. cystic renal neoplasm ■ Enhancing renal mass ■ Staging of known or suspected renal cell carcinoma ■ Evaluation of local extension/vascular invasion of renal cell carcinoma ■ Preoperative planning partial nephrectomy for neoplasm ■ Surveillance for tumor recurrence, contralateral renal cell carcinoma	■ If patients are unable to hold their breath the same way for the contrast-enhanced portion of the examination, it may be impossible to determine if contrast enhancement is present ■ Motion artifact may significantly limit the examination

Evaluation of Hypertension/Renal Artery Stenosis

Study	Information obtained	Significant limitation
Ultrasound	■ Elevation of velocities in the renal artery suggesting stenosis ■ Indication of renal parenchymal disease ■ Evaluation of renal size	■ Relatively poor sensitivity and specificity ■ Limited in obese patients ■ Limited in noncompliant patients unable to comply with breath holding instructions ■ Cannot be performed on ventilated patients due to inability to suspend respiration
CTA	■ Direct evaluation of renal artery lumen for stenosis ■ Evaluation of renal size	■ Patients with renal impairment are not candidates for the study ■ Arterial calcification can cause artifact, limiting evaluation of renal artery stenosis

Study	Information obtained	Significant limitation
MRA	■ Direct evaluation of renal artery lumen for stenosis ■ Evaluation of renal size	■ Patients with renal impairment are not candidates for the study ■ Arterial calcification/stents cause artifacts that can overestimate stenosis
Nuclear medicine	■ Identification of renal artery stenosis	■ If bilateral renal artery stenosis is present, it can lead to false-negative results
Angiography	■ Direct evaluation of renal artery lumen for stenosis	■ Invasive ■ Risk of contrast nephropathy

Evaluation of Acute Renal Failure

Study	Information obtained	Significant limitation
Ultrasound	■ Hydronephrosis ■ Intrinsic renal disease	■ In obese patients, it may be difficult to visualize the kidneys

Evaluation of Renal Function

Study	Information obtained	Significant limitation
CT (contrast-enhanced)	■ Gross estimation of renal enhancement ■ Identification of renal excretion ■ Identification of renal artery stenosis (CTA)	■ Patients with significantly impaired renal function (Cr >1.5 mg/dL) are not candidates for the study due to the risk of contrast-induced nephropathy ■ Patients with poor unilateral renal function may not demonstrate enhancement unless significantly delayed images are obtained; this leads to increased radiation exposure

Study	Information obtained	Significant limitation
		▪ Patients with heavy arterial calcification may not be eligible for CTA for RAS due to the artifact from the calcium
MR	▪ Gross estimation of renal enhancement ▪ Identification of renal excretion ▪ Identification of renal artery stenosis (MRA)	▪ Patients with markedly impaired renal function (eGFR <30) are not candidates for the study due to the risk of NSF ▪ Patients with heavily calcified arteries or renal artery stents cannot be well-assessed for stenosis due to artifact
Nuclear medicine	▪ Quantification of renal function ▪ Determination of renal excretion, delayed excretion ▪ Identification of UPJ obstruction ▪ Identification of renal artery stenosis	▪ Patients with very delayed renal function may require significantly prolonged imaging times

Evaluation of Hematuria

Study	Information obtained	Significant limitation
Ultrasound	▪ Renal stones ▪ Renal mass ▪ Bladder wall thickening ▪ Bladder debris ▪ Bladder mass ▪ Bladder stone	▪ Transitional cell carcinoma in the ureter is typically not seen with ultrasound

Study	Information obtained	Significant limitation
CT (with/ without contrast)	<ul><li>Renal stones</li><li>Renal mass</li><li>Ureteral mass (CT urogram)</li><li>Bladder wall thickening</li><li>Bladder debris</li><li>Bladder mass</li><li>Bladder stone</li></ul>	<ul><li>Small bladder masses may be occult on CT</li><li>In patients with poor renal function, the kidneys may not concentrate contrast; enhancement cannot be assessed</li></ul>
MR (with/ without contrast)	<ul><li>Renal stones</li><li>Renal mass</li><li>Ureteral mass (MR urogram)</li><li>Bladder wall thickening</li><li>Bladder debris</li><li>Bladder mass</li><li>Bladder stone</li></ul>	<ul><li>If there is poor excretion into the collecting systems, transitional cell carcinomas may be occult</li></ul>
Cystogram	<ul><li>Filling defects from clot, infection, tumor</li><li>Bladder trabeculation, diverticula from chronic outlet obstruction</li><li>Invasion of the bladder from adjacent tumor (e.g. prostate)</li></ul>	<ul><li>Small filling defects may be obscured</li></ul>

Evaluation of Chronic Bladder Abnormality

Study	Information obtained	Significant limitation
Ultrasound	<ul><li>Bladder wall thickening</li><li>Bladder diverticula</li><li>Bladder stones</li><li>Bladder outlet obstruction</li></ul>	<ul><li>If underdistended, the bladder cannot be well evaluated</li></ul>

Common Clinical Questions and Key Studies to Order

Study	Information obtained	Significant limitation
CT	■ Bladder wall thickening ■ Bladder diverticula ■ Bladder outlet obstruction ■ Bladder fistulas ■ Bladder stones	■ If underdistended, the bladder cannot be well evaluated ■ Small fistulas may not be readily identified
MR	■ Bladder wall thickening ■ Bladder diverticula ■ Bladder outlet obstruction ■ Bladder fistulas ■ Bladder stones	■ If underdistended, the bladder cannot be well evaluated ■ Small fistulas may not be readily identified
Cystogram	■ Bladder outlet obstruction ■ Bladder trabeculation/diverticula ■ Bladder fistula ■ Bladder erosion from adjacent mass	■ Small fistulas may be difficult to identify

Evaluation of Adrenal Abnormality

Study	Information obtained	Significant limitation
CT (non-contrast/ CECT with washout)	■ Identification of adrenal mass ■ Characterization of adrenal mass ■ Identification of adrenal hemorrhage	■ Lipid-poor adenomas may be difficult to characterize with CT
MRI	■ Identification of adrenal mass ■ Identification of adrenal hemorrhage ■ Characterization of adrenal mass	■ Small masses may be difficult to characterize ■ Lipid-poor adenomas may be difficult to characterize ■ Respiratory motion can render the study uninterpretable

Study	Information obtained	Significant limitation
Nuclear Imaging	▓ Identification of primary and metastatic adrenal neoplasms (e.g. neuroblastoma)	▓ Small sites of disease may be below the resolution of nuclear imaging
Angiography	▓ Adrenal vein sampling for elevated rennin levels	▓ Invasive ▓ Time-consuming

Evaluation of Splenic Abnormality

Study	Information obtained	Significant limitation
Conventional radiographs	▓ Splenomegaly	▓ Low sensitivity
Ultrasound	▓ Splenomegaly ▓ Asplenia/polysplenia ▓ Splenic laceration ▓ Splenic infarction ▓ Splenic abscess ▓ Splenic mass	▓ Difficult to characterize splenic masses
CT	▓ Splenomegaly ▓ Asplenia/polysplenia ▓ Splenic laceration ▓ Splenic infarction ▓ Splenic abscess ▓ Splenic mass	▓ Difficult to characterize splenic masses
MR	▓ Splenomegaly ▓ Asplenia/polysplenia ▓ Splenic laceration ▓ Splenic infarction ▓ Splenic abscess ▓ Splenic mass	▓ Difficult to characterize splenic masses
Nuclear medicine	▓ Presence and location of residual splenic tissue in ITP	▓ Small deposits of splenic tissue may be below the resolution of nuclear imaging

Common Clinical Questions and Key Studies to Order

Study	Information obtained	Significant limitation
	■ Colloid shift to spleen in portal hypertension ■ Identification of splenosis	
Angiography	■ Diagnosis and treatment of traumatic splenic injury	■ Patients may be hemodynamically unstable ■ Invasive

Evaluation of Bowel Abnormality

Study	Information obtained	Significant limitation
Conventional radiographs	■ Pneumoperitoneum ■ Portal venous air ■ Pneumatosis ■ Bowel obstruction ■ Ileus ■ Constipation	■ Non-specific ■ Cannot evaluate for intra-abdominal abscesses
Ultrasound	■ Appendicitis ■ Intussusception	■ The appendix is difficult to identify, particularly if normal
CT	■ Bowel obstruction ■ Bowel infection ■ Bowel ischemia ■ Bowel inflammation (e.g. appendicitis, diverticulitis) ■ Intra-abdominal abscess	■ Bowel ischemia is very difficult to identify without IV contrast ■ Inadequate distension with oral contrast may make it difficult to identify bowel wall thickening ■ Lack of IV contrast severely limits ability to identify abscess
MR	■ Appendicitis in pregnancy ■ Bowel fistulas	■ Small fistula may be difficult to identify ■ Bowel motion may limit evaluation of the bowel

Study	Information obtained	Significant limitation
Nuclear medicine	▪ Meckel's scan ▪ GI bleeding site (GI bleeding study)	▪ If the Meckel's does not contain gastric mucosa, there will be a false-negative result
Angiography	▪ Diagnosis and treatment of GI bleeding	▪ It may be difficult to localize the site of GI bleed ▪ Bleeding has often stopped by the time angiography is performed ▪ It may not be possible to treat the site of bleeding percutaneously; surgery may be required

Evaluation of the Acute Abdomen

Study	Information obtained	Significant limitation
Conventional radiographs	▪ Pneumoperitoneum ▪ Pneumatosis	▪ Low sensitivity
Ultrasound	▪ Appendicitis ▪ Intussusception ▪ Ascites for spontaneous bacterial peritonitis	▪ The appendix may be difficult to identify, particularly if normal
CT	▪ Pneumoperitoneum ▪ Bowel obstruction ▪ Bowel ischemia/ infection/infarction ▪ Bowel perforation ▪ Bowel volvulus ▪ Appendicitis ▪ Diverticulitis	▪ The study may be limited if inadequate bowel distension with oral contrast
MRI	▪ Appendicitis in pregnancy	▪ The appendix is often difficult to visualize

Evaluation of Pancreatitis

Study	Information obtained	Significant limitation
KUB	■ Radiodense gallstones	■ Not all gallstones are dense on x-ray
Ultrasound	■ Presence of cholelithiasis as etiology of pancreatitis ■ Presence of choledocholithiasis ■ Edematous pancreas ■ Pancreatic duct dilation	■ Low sensitivity for choledocholithiasis ■ Pancreas is often poorly visualized, particularly in obese patients
CT	■ Presence of choledocholithiasis ■ Pancreatic duct dilation/edema ■ Presence of complications of pancreatitis (e.g. pseudocyst formation, necrosis, vascular aneurysms, hemorrhagic pancreatitis) ■ Presence of pancreatic mass	■ Complications of pancreatitis and pancreatic mass are not routinely identified without IV contrast; CECT is the diagnostic study of choice ■ Low sensitivity for choledocholithiasis
MR	■ Presence of choledocholithiasis ■ Pancreatic duct dilation/edema ■ Presence of complications of pancreatitis (e.g. pseudocyst formation, necrosis, vascular aneurysms, hemorrhagic pancreatitis) ■ Presence of pancreatic mass	■ Biliary air may mimic stones

Evaluation of Pregnancy

Study	Information obtained	Significant limitation
Ultrasound	▪ Presence of intrauterine gestation ▪ Dating of pregnancy ▪ Presence of ectopic gestation ▪ Risk stratification/fetal anatomic survey for fetal anomalies ▪ Evaluation of bleeding	▪ Early gestations may not be identified ▪ Fetal anomalies may be difficult to identify, particularly in early gestation (anatomic surveys should be performed at 18–20 weeks' gestation) ▪ Early ectopic gestations may not be visible; if there is no gestational sac in the uterus and no adnexal mass, ectopic cannot be excluded and follow-up ultrasound is necessary
MR	▪ Fetal anomalies ▪ Placenta acreta, percreta, increta	▪ Motion of the fetus can limit the study ▪ Placental abnormalities are very difficult to identify with MR; percreta is typically the only placental invasion possible to identify with MR

Evaluation of Pregnancy Complications

Study	Information obtained	Significant limitation
Ultrasound	▪ Evaluation of fetal demise ▪ Evaluation of ectopic gestation ▪ Placenta previa, acreta, increta, percreta	▪ Early ectopic gestations may not be visible; if there is no gestational sac in the uterus and no adnexal mass, ectopic gestation cannot be excluded and follow-up ultrasound is necessary

Study	Information obtained	Significant limitation
	■ Evaluation of twin-twin transfusion syndrome ■ Evaluation of bleeding ■ Retained products of conception ■ Endometritis	■ Retained products of conception cannot be fully excluded even in the setting of a negative ultrasound ■ It may be difficult to differentiate retained products from endometritis with ultrasound
CT (contrast-enhanced)	■ Post-delivery pelvic infection	■ Endometritis cannot be demonstrated on CT
MR (non-contrast)	■ Appendicitis in pregnancy ■ Placenta acreta/percreta/increta ■ Ureteral stones/renal obstruction	■ Patient and fetal motion may limit the examination ■ Bowel motion may limit evaluation of the appendix
Angiography	■ Uterine artery embolization in emergency C-section	■ The procedure is invasive

Evaluation of the Acute Abdomen in Pregnancy

Study	Information obtained	Significant limitation
Ultrasound	■ Evaluation of appendicitis ■ Evaluation of renal obstruction ■ Evaluation of placental abruption	■ The appendix is very difficult to visualize due to bowel displacement by the gravid uterus ■ Placental abruption is typically a clinical diagnosis/emergency. Fetal compromise can be identified with ultrasound.

Study	Information obtained	Significant limitation
MR (non-contrast)	▪ Evaluation of appendicitis ▪ Evaluation of renal obstruction	▪ Patient and fetal motion may limit the examination ▪ Bowel motion may limit evaluation of the appendix

Evaluation Pelvic Pain (non-pregnant)

Study	Information obtained	Significant limitation
Ultrasound	▪ Ovarian torsion ▪ Ovarian mass ▪ Fibroids ▪ Tubo-ovarian abscess ▪ Ovarian cyst rupture, hemorrhagic cyst	▪ The ovaries have a dual arterial supply; therefore, arterial flow can be present even in acute torsion. This can lead to false-negative study. ▪ It may be difficult to differentiate a complicated ovarian cyst from a cystic neoplasm; these patients require follow-up ultrasound or MR
CT	▪ Gonadal vein thrombosis ▪ Ovarian mass ▪ Ovarian cyst ▪ Fibroids	▪ CT does not have good contrast resolution for gynecologic pathology and is of limited value unless the mass is calcified or has fat (dermoid)
MR	▪ Gonadal vein thrombosis ▪ Ovarian mass ▪ Ovarian torsion ▪ Ovarian cyst ▪ Endometriosis ▪ Fibroids	▪ Ovarian torsion is difficult to identify on MR

Study	Information obtained	Significant limitation
Angiography	■ Fibroid treatment (embolization)	■ Invasive procedure ■ Risk of procedure failure ■ Fibroids can regrow despite embolization

Evaluation of Pelvic Infection and Fistula

Study	Information obtained	Significant limitation
Ultrasound	■ Endometritis ■ Tubo-ovarian abscess ■ Pyosalpinx	■ It may not be possible to differentiate pyosalpinx from hematosalpinx on ultrasound
CT	■ Tubo-ovarian abscess ■ Presence of pelvic bowel, bladder, uterine fistula	■ It may be difficult to differentiate tubo-ovarian abscess from other pelvic sources of abscess ■ Small fistulas may be difficult to visualize
MR	■ Tubo-ovarian abscess ■ Pyosalpinx ■ Presence of pelvic bowel, bladder, uterine fistula	■ Small fistulas or air-containing fistulas may be difficult to visualize
Fluoroscopy (fistulogram)	■ Evaluation of cutaneous fistulas from bowel, bladder	■ If the cutaneous fistula cannot be cannulated with a catheter, it cannot be evaluated

Evaluation Pelvic Malignancy

Study	Information obtained	Significant limitation
Ultrasound	■ Evaluation of suspected ovarian masses ■ Evaluation of suspected uterine malignancy (i.e. abnormal vaginal bleeding)	■ It may not be possible to differentiate benign from malignant ovarian masses

Study	Information obtained	Significant limitation
	■ Evaluation of complications of disease (e.g. hydronephrosis)	
CT (contrast-enhanced)	■ Staging of disease ■ Complications of malignancy (e.g. renal obstruction, typhlitis)	■ Mesenteric implants may be difficult to visualize without oral contrast or if patients are thin without mesenteric fat
MR	■ Staging of disease ■ Complications of malignancy	■ Implants may be difficult to visualize if patients lack intra-abdominal fat

Evaluation of Infertility and Recurrent Pregnancy Loss

Study	Information obtained	Significant limitation
Ultrasound	■ Presence and location of fibroids ■ Presence of uterine anomaly ■ Presence of endometrial mass ■ Dilated fallopian tubes ■ Ovarian cysts, masses, endometriomas	■ Uterine anomalies may be difficult to identify and characterize on ultrasound due to difficulty visualizing the uterine fundus ■ Dilated fallopian tubes may simulate ovarian cysts
Hysterosonogram	■ Evaluation of endometrial abnormalities (e.g. fibroids, polyps) ■ Patency of fallopian tubes ■ Evaluation of ovarian masses, cysts, endometriomas ■ Evaluation of uterine anomalies	■ Uterine anomalies may be difficult to identify and characterize on ultrasound due to difficulty visualizing the uterine fundus ■ Dilated fallopian tubes may simulate ovarian cysts

Study	Information obtained	Significant limitation
Hysterosalpin-gography (HSG)	■ Evaluation of endometrial synechiae ■ Evaluation of fibroids ■ Evaluation of uterine anomaly ■ Patency of fallopian tubes	■ Fibroids are difficult to visualize with this technique ■ Uterine anomalies are often not recognized with this technique and the uterine contour is not evaluated
MR	■ Evaluation of uterine anomaly ■ Evaluation of fibroids, adenomyosis ■ Evaluation of endometriosis	■ Endometrial abnormalities are not well evaluated with MR

Evaluation of Acute Osseous Trauma

Study	Information obtained	Significant limitation
Conventional radiographs	■ Presence and characterization of fracture ■ Presence of pathologic fracture ■ Presence of soft tissue swelling, laceration ■ Postreduction alignment of fracture fragments ■ Evaluation of ORIF hardware positioning and complication	■ Non-displaced fractures may be radiographically occult ■ If adequate positioning for films is not obtained, fractures may not be identified
CT	■ Characterization of known fracture for preoperative planning ■ Identification of radiographically occult fracture	■ If patients cannot be appropriately positioned, it may be difficult to obtain images that allow adequate evaluation of the fracture

Study	Information obtained	Significant limitation
MR	▨ Identification of radiographically occult fracture ▨ Evaluation of acute osteochondral defect	▨ There are many contraindications to MR imaging (see box below), including external fixators
Nuclear medicine (bone scan)	▨ Identification of shin splints ▨ Identification of stress fractures ▨ Identification of pathologic fractures ▨ Identification of post-traumatic reflex sympathetic dystrophy	▨ Nuclear imaging is not specific for the disease process (e.g. arthritis and acute fracture may both show uptake of radiotracer) ▨ Precise localization of the uptake may be difficult due to the poor spatial resolution of nuclear imaging

Evaluation of Musculoskeletal Tumors

Study	Information obtained	Significant limitation
Conventional radiographs	▨ Presence and characterization of bone lesion ▨ Presence of soft tissue component ▨ Follow-up of benign bone tumors ▨ Follow-up of malignant tumors after treatment ▨ Identification of pathologic fracture	▨ Soft tissue masses are not well visualized on conventional radiographs ▨ Recurrence of tumor may not be visible on conventional radiographs, particularly if it is a soft tissue recurrence ▨ Radiation changes may be difficult to differentiate from recurrence
CT	▨ Presence and characterization of bone lesion ▨ Presence of soft tissue component	▨ Soft tissue extension of tumor may be difficult to determine on CT ▨ It may be difficult to differentiate recurrence from radiation change

Study	Information obtained	Significant limitation
	▪ Follow-up of benign bone tumors ▪ Follow-up of malignant tumors after treatment ▪ Identification of pathologic fracture	▪ Metallic fixation hardware can significantly limit the examination due to artifact
MR	▪ Presence and characterization of bone lesion ▪ Presence of soft tissue component ▪ Follow-up of benign bone tumors ▪ Follow-up of malignant tumors after treatment ▪ Identification of pathologic fracture	▪ It may be difficult to differentiate recurrence from radiation change ▪ Metallic surgical hardware can produce artifacts, which limit the study
Nuclear medicine (bone scan)	▪ Identification of primary bone lesion ▪ Identification of sites of metachronous or metastatic disease	▪ Nuclear imaging has a limited role in the follow-up of local recurrence as it may not be possible to differentiate postsurgical activity from tumor ▪ Precise localization of the extent of disease is difficult to determine with nuclear imaging

Evaluation of Osseous Metastases

Study	Information obtained	Significant limitation
Conventional radiographs	▪ Presence and location of osseous metastases ▪ Complications of metastases (i.e. pathologic fractures)	▪ Low sensitivity, particularly in obese patients

Study	Information obtained	Significant limitation
CT	▣ Presence and location of osseous metastases ▣ Complications of metastases (i.e. pathologic fractures) ▣ Soft tissue masses associated with osseous metastases	▣ Some metastases are occult on CT or are in the plane of the images and therefore not visible ▣ Soft tissue masses may be difficult to visualize on CT
MR	▣ Presence and location of osseous metastases ▣ Complications of metastases (i.e. pathologic fractures) ▣ Early metastatic disease without cortical abnormality ▣ Soft tissue masses associated with osseous metastases ▣ Cord compression for spinal metastases	▣ Motion can limit the examination
Nuclear medicine (bone scan)	▣ Evaluation of presence and extent of osseous metastatic disease	▣ False negatives can occur in multiple myeloma and eosinophilic granulomatosis ▣ False-positive results can occur within 6 weeks following chemotherapy; the reparative phase of bone turnover occurs and the metastatic disease may falsely appear worse

Evaluation of Soft Tissue Tumors

Study	Information obtained	Significant limitation
Conventional radiographs	■ Presence of soft tissue mass ± bone destruction ■ Presence of calcification within soft tissue mass, which can aid in diagnosis	■ Soft tissue masses may not be visible, particularly in obese patients
CT	■ Presence of soft tissue mass ± bone destruction ■ Presence of calcification within soft tissue mass, which can aid in diagnosis ■ Presence of multiple sites of disease	■ Extent of soft tissue masses may be difficult to visualize on CT
MR	■ Presence of soft tissue mass ■ Assessment of enhancement patterns of mass ■ Bony change associated with soft tissue mass ■ Presence of multiple sites of disease	■ The entire body is not typically imaged; therefore, distant sites of disease will not be evaluated

Evaluation of Primary Bone Tumors

Study	Information obtained	Significant limitation
Conventional radiographs	■ Presence and extent of lesion ■ Characterization of lesion ■ Identification of pathologic fracture	■ Lesions in certain locations (e.g. the sacrum may not be visible if there is significant stool or bowel air obscuring the region)
CT	■ Presence and extent of lesion ■ Characterization of lesion	■ The soft tissue mass may not be well evaluated with CT

Study	Information obtained	Significant limitation
	▪ Presence of soft tissue mass ▪ Identification of pathologic fracture	▪ Non-displaced fractures may not be visible if in the plane of the scan; reconstructed images in different planes are required for complete evaluation
MR	▪ Presence and extent of lesion ▪ Characterization of lesion ▪ Presence and extent of soft tissue mass ▪ Identification of pathologic fracture	▪ It may not be possible to characterize a bone tumor with MR; biopsy is often required
Nuclear medicine	▪ Identification of primary bone lesion ▪ Identification of sites of metachronous or metastatic disease	▪ Precise localization of the extent of tumor is difficult with nuclear imaging due to the poor spatial resolution

Evaluation of Arthritis

Study	Information obtained	Significant limitation
Conventional radiographs	▪ Presence and location of erosions ▪ Soft tissue changes and calcifications	▪ It may be difficult to identify early changes of arthritis
CT	▪ Presence of erosions ▪ Pathologic fractures	▪ Limited use in the evaluation of small body parts for arthritis (e.g. hands)
MR	▪ Presence of erosions ▪ Presence of inflammatory tissue ▪ Ligamentous and muscle rupture that can be seen in inflammatory arthritis	▪ Motion artifact can limit the examination

Evaluation of Tendon and Ligament Injury

Study	Information obtained	Significant limitation
MR	■ Evaluation of presence and extent of ligament tears ■ Presence and extent of tendon tears ■ Associated bone changes ■ Associated cartilage changes ■ Presence and extent of tendonitis	■ Motion artifact can severely limit interpretation ■ In patients with suspected rotator cuff or labral injury, MR arthrography is the study of choice ■ Postoperative joints should be imaged with MR arthrography to allow identification of reinjury

Evaluation of the Postoperative Joint (e.g. arthrography)

Study	Information obtained	Significant limitation
Conventional arthrography	■ Presence of ligament disruption ■ Presence of tendon tears ■ Presence of disruption of surgical repair	■ Limited evaluation of partial thickness tears ■ Does not adequately evaluate cartilage
CT arthrography	■ Presence of ligament disruption ■ Presence of tendon tears ■ Presence of disruption of surgical repair ■ Presence of cartilage abnormality	■ Motion artifact can limit the examination
MR arthrography	■ Presence of ligament disruption ■ Presence of tendon tears ■ Presence of disruption of surgical repair ■ Presence of cartilage abnormality ■ Presence of associated bone edema	■ Motion artifact can limit the examination

Evaluation Acute Stroke: CT, MR with Diffusion, Carotid Ultrasound, Echo

Study	Information obtained	Significant limitation
CT (non-contrast)	▪ Ischemic stroke ▪ Embolic stroke ▪ Hemorrhagic conversion of stroke ▪ Intravascular thrombus (e.g. dense MCA sign) ▪ Cerebral edema ▪ Mass effect	▪ Early ischemic infarction may be occult < 6 hours
MR (non-contrast)	▪ Early ischemic stroke ▪ Embolic stroke ▪ Hemorrhagic conversion of stroke ▪ Intravascular thrombus (e.g. dense MCA sign) ▪ Cerebral edema ▪ Mass effect	▪ Motion artifact can limit the study
Ultrasound (carotid)	▪ Carotid occlusion ▪ Critical carotid stenosis ▪ Plaque burden in carotid arteries ▪ Friable plaque at risk of embolization ▪ Vertebral artery occlusion ▪ Subclavian steal	▪ Very slow flow in the carotid artery may not be detectable and can mimic carotid occlusion
Echocardiography	▪ Intracardiac source of thromboembolic disease ▪ Poor cardiac output	▪ May be limited by patient body habitus ▪ Poor imaging windows can limit the examination ▪ TEE is invasive

Common Clinical Questions and Key Studies to Order

Evaluation of Intracranial Tumor

Study	Information obtained	Significant limitation
CT (contrast-enhanced)	■ Presence of mass ■ Extent of mass ■ Multifocal disease ■ Mass effect ■ Herniation ■ Hemorrhagic conversion of mass	■ It may be difficult to differentiate between infection and tumor ■ Small masses may be below the resolution of CT
MR (contrast-enhanced)	■ Presence of mass ■ Extent of mass ■ Multifocal disease ■ Mass effect ■ Herniation ■ Hemorrhagic conversion of mass ■ Leptomeningeal metastatic disease or primary malignancy (e.g. lymphoma)	■ It may be difficult to differentiate between infection and tumor

Evaluation of Infection

Study	Information obtained	Significant limitation
CT (contrast-enhanced)	■ Presence of abscess ■ Extent of abscess ■ Multifocal disease ■ Mass effect ■ Herniation ■ Hemorrhagic conversion of lesion	■ It may be difficult to differentiate between infection and tumor ■ Leptomeningeal infection may be difficult to identify on CT
MR (contrast-enhanced)	■ Presence of abscess ■ Extent of abscess ■ Multifocal disease ■ Mass effect ■ Herniation	■ It may be difficult to differentiate between infection and tumor

Study	Information obtained	Significant limitation
	■ Hemorrhagic conversion of lesion ■ Leptomeningeal infection (e.g. viral or tuberculous meningitis)	

Evaluation of Intracranial Trauma

Study	Information obtained	Significant limitation
CT (non-contrast)	■ Parenchymal hemorrhage ■ Subdural, epidural hematoma ■ Subarachnoid hemorrhage ■ Mass effect ■ Herniation ■ Calvarial fractures	■ Diffuse axonal injury is typically occult on CT ■ Subtle hemorrhage may be difficult to identify, particularly if there is patient motion
MR (non-contrast)	■ Parenchymal hemorrhage ■ Subdural, epidural hematoma ■ Subarachnoid hemorrhage ■ Mass effect ■ Herniation ■ Diffuse axonal injury	■ Subarachnoid hemorrhage is difficult to identify on MR unless chronic (hemosiderin can be seen on MR)
Nuclear medicine (brain death study)	■ Brain perfusion ■ Lack of brain perfusion in brain death	■ May need to be repeated if minimal blood flow remains present

Evaluation of Carotid Trauma

Study	Information obtained	Significant limitation
Ultrasound (carotid)	■ Carotid dissection flap ■ Carotid occlusion	■ Dissection flaps may not be readily identifiable on ultrasound ■ Very slow flow may not be detectable and can mimic complete carotid occlusion

Study	Information obtained	Significant limitation
CTA (carotid CTA)	■ Carotid dissection ■ Carotid occlusion	■ Very slow flow can mimic occlusion
MRA (carotid MRA)	■ Carotid dissection ■ Carotid occlusion	■ Artifacts such as calcification can mimic segments of occlusion or high grade stenosis

Evaluation of Mental Status Change

Study	Information obtained	Significant limitation
CT (non-contrast)	■ Traumatic injury; subdural, epidural, subarachnoid hemorrhage ■ Stroke ■ Diffuse brain edema	■ Early stroke may not be detectable on CT; MR is more sensitive
CT (contrast-enhanced)	■ Intracranial mass ■ Intracranial infection	■ Small lesions may be below the resolution of CT ■ It may be difficult to differentiate between infection and tumor
MR (non-contrast)	■ Traumatic injury; subdural, epidural, subarachnoid hemorrhage ■ Diffuse axonal injury ■ Stroke ■ Diffuse brain edema	■ Motion can limit the examination
MR (contrast-enhanced)	■ Intracranial mass ■ Intracranial infection	■ It may be difficult to differentiate between infection and tumor

Evaluation of Vascular Anomalies/Subarachnoid Hemorrhage with CT Angiography

Study	Information obtained	Significant limitation
CT (non-contrast)	▪ Parenchymal hemorrhage ▪ Subarachnoid hemorrhage	▪ Subtle subarachnoid hemorrhage may be difficult to identify
CTA (contrast-enhanced)	▪ Identification of aneurysms, venous malformations, vascular malformations	▪ If the timing bolus of IV contrast material is inadequate, vascular lesions may not be identified or appropriately characterized
MRA (contrast-enhanced)	▪ Identification of aneurysms, venous malformations, vascular malformations	▪ If the timing bolus of IV contrast material is inadequate, vascular lesions may not be identified or appropriately characterized ▪ Partially thrombosed or calcified lesions may be difficult to evaluate on MR

Sinus Disease

Study	Information obtained	Significant limitation
Conventional radiographs	▪ Evaluation of acute sinusitis	▪ Low sensitivity
CT (non-contrast)	▪ Presence and location of acute sinus disease ▪ Presence and location of chronic sinus disease	▪ High radiation dose to lens of eye

Study	Information obtained	Significant limitation
CT (contrast-enhanced)	■ Presence and extent of acute fungal sinusitis in immunosuppressed patients ■ Extension of sinus disease into the brain (epidural abscess)	■ High radiation dose to lens of eye
MR (contrast-enhanced)	■ Presence and extent of acute fungal sinusitis in immunosuppressed patients ■ Extension of sinus disease into the brain (epidural abscess)	■ Air within the sinuses may cause artifact that can limit the examination

Facial Trauma

Study	Information obtained	Significant limitation
Conventional radiographs	■ Displaced facial bone fractures	■ Low sensitivity
CT of the facial bones (non-contrast)	■ Displaced and non-displaced facial bone fractures	■ Fractures in the plane of the scan may not be visible without reconstruction into other planes
CT of the orbits (non-contrast)	■ Displaced and non-displaced fractures of the orbits	■ Fractures in the plane of the scan may not be visible without reconstruction into other planes

Cervical Spine Trauma

Study	Information obtained	Significant limitation
Conventional radiographs	▪ Cervical spine fracture ▪ Malalignment suggesting ligamentous injury	▪ Low sensitivity for non-displaced and subtle fractures compared with CT ▪ Disc abnormalities cannot be visualized
CT (non-contrast)	▪ Cervical spine fracture ▪ Malalignment suggesting ligamentous injury ▪ Traumatic disc herniation/ protrusion	▪ Ligaments are not directly visualized; therefore, ligamentous injury cannot be excluded ▪ Spinal cord trauma cannot be evaluated
MR (non-contrast)	▪ Cervical spine fracture ▪ Malalignment suggesting ligamentous injury ▪ Traumatic disc herniation/protrusion ▪ Spinal cord injury	▪ Motion artifact can limit the examination

Disc Disease

Study	Information obtained	Significant limitation
CT (non-contrast)	▪ Disc herniation/protrusion ▪ Narrowing of the spinal canal, lateral recesses	▪ Cord contusion or edema due to disc disease is not visible on CT
CT (contrast-enhanced)	▪ Disc infection (discitis)	▪ Does not allow evaluation of the adjacent bone for early osteomyelitis
MR (non-contrast)	▪ Disc herniation/protrusion ▪ Narrowing of the spinal canal, lateral recesses ▪ Edema in muscles supplied by the affected nerves	▪ Motion can limit the examination

Study	Information obtained	Significant limitation
	▪ Spinal cord signal abnormality from compression	
MR (contrast-enhanced)	▪ Discitis/osteomyelitis	▪ If patients cannot receive IV contrast, evaluation of osteomyelitis is limited as degenerative disease can have a similar non-contrast appearance

Spinal Cord Injury, Demyelination, Cord Compression

Study	Information obtained	Significant limitation
CT (non-contrast)	▪ Identification of osseous injury to spinal column ▪ Evaluation of disc extrusion/bony encroachment of spinal cord	▪ The spinal cord cannot be evaluated with CT
MR (non-contrast)	▪ Identification of osseous injury to spinal column ▪ Evaluation of disc extrusion/bony encroachment of spinal cord ▪ Evaluation of spinal cord edema, contusion, hemorrhage, transsection demyelination	▪ Motion artifact can limit the study
MR (contrast-enhanced)	▪ Allows for determination of sites of active demyelination (enhancement) ▪ Allows evaluation of enhancing spinal metastases	▪ Small masses may be below the resolution of MR

Central or Peripheral Neuropathy

Study	Information obtained	Significant limitation
CT (non-contrast)	▪ Spinal canal or lateral recess narrowing ▪ Masses related to the spinal canal or brachial plexus	▪ The nerves and muscle edema cannot be evaluated with CT
MR (non-contrast)	▪ Spinal canal or lateral recess narrowing ▪ Masses related to the spinal canal or brachial plexus ▪ Abnormal signal in the nerves or muscles	▪ Masses related to the nerves are not fully evaluated without IV contrast
MR (contrast-enhanced)	▪ Spinal canal or lateral recess narrowing ▪ Masses related to the spinal canal or brachial plexus ▪ Abnormal signal in the nerves or muscles ▪ Enhancing masses related to the nerves	▪ Motion limits the examination

Evaluation of Metastatic Disease

Study	Information obtained	Significant limitation
CT (contrast-enhanced)	▪ Presence of intracranial or spinal metastasis ▪ Multifocal lesions ▪ Extent of disease ▪ Brain edema/herniation	▪ It may be difficult to differentiate residual tumor from radiation change or infection
MR (contrast-enhanced)	▪ Presence of intracranial or spinal metastasis ▪ Multifocal lesions ▪ Extent of disease ▪ Brain edema/herniation	▪ It may be difficult to differentiate residual tumor from radiation change or infection

Study	Information obtained	Significant limitation
PET CT	■ Presence of intracranial or spinal metastasis ■ Multifocal lesions ■ Extent of disease	■ Small lesions may be below the resolution of PET CT

Evaluation of Infection in the Head and Neck

Study	Information obtained	Significant limitation
Conventional radiographs	■ Bone destruction	■ Low sensitivity
CT (contrast-enhanced)	■ Bone destruction ■ Soft tissue mass ■ Presence, location, and extent of enhancing abscess collection	■ Soft tissue masses may be difficult to identify
MR (contrast-enhanced)	■ Bone destruction ■ Soft tissue mass ■ Presence, location, and extent of enhancing abscess collection	■ Motion may limit the examination
Nuclear medicine (bone scan)	■ Abnormal radiotracer activity in area of osteomyelitis	■ The findings are non-specific and can be seen in other bone abnormalities (e.g. degenerative disease)

Evaluation of Aortic Disease

Study	Information obtained	Significant limitation
Conventional radiographs	■ Displaced aortic calcification in aortic dissection ■ Aneurysmal dilation of the aorta	■ Low sensitivity for displaced calcification

Study	Information obtained	Significant limitation
Ultrasound	▪ Evaluation of thoracic/abdominal aortic aneurysm ▪ Evaluation of aortic dissection	▪ Poor evaluation of thoracic aorta with TTE; TEE required
CT	▪ Evaluation of presence and size of aortic aneurysm (non-contrast) ▪ Evaluation of aortic dissection (CECT) ▪ Evaluation of aortic pseudoaneurysm/ mycotic aneurysm ▪ Evaluation of vasculitis/aortitis (CECT) ▪ Evaluation of acute aortic traumatic injury (CECT) ▪ Evaluation of atherosclerotic disease ▪ Evaluation of aortic coarctation	▪ Patients who cannot receive IV contrast cannot be evaluated with CT for an aortic dissection; MR or TEE should be considered in these patients
MR	▪ Evaluation of presence and size of aortic aneurysm (non-contrast) ▪ Evaluation of aortic dissection (contrast-enhanced) ▪ Evaluation of aortic pseudoaneurysm/ mycotic aneurysm ▪ Evaluation of vasculitis/aortitis (contrast-enhanced)	▪ Limited evaluation for aortic dissection if patients cannot receive IV contrast

Study	Information obtained	Significant limitation
	▪ Evaluation of acute aortic traumatic injury (contrast-enhanced) ▪ Evaluation of atherosclerotic disease ▪ Evaluation of aortic coarctation	
Angiography	▪ Evaluation of atherosclerotic disease ▪ Evaluation and treatment (stenting) of acute aortic trauma ▪ Evaluation of aortic dissection ▪ Evaluation of aortic coarctation	▪ Aortic dissection may not be identified on catheter angiography if the true lumen is not significantly narrowed by the false lumen
Nuclear medicine (FDG PET CT)	▪ Inflammation of the aortic wall in vasculitis, infection	▪ False negatives may occur if inflammation is mild

Evaluation of Peripheral Vascular Disease

Study	Information obtained	Significant limitation
Ultrasound	▪ Evaluation of vascular grafts	▪ Slow flow may not be detected and can mimic occlusion
CTA (contrast-enhanced)	▪ Evaluation of known or suspected peripheral vascular disease ▪ Evaluation of acute vascular injury (e.g. trauma)	▪ Heavily calcified vessels may be difficult to evaluate ▪ Patients who cannot be appropriately positioned may have suboptimal studies

Study	Information obtained	Significant limitation
MRA (contrast-enhanced)	▨ Evaluation of known or suspected peripheral vascular disease	▨ Heavily calcified vessels may be difficult to evaluate ▨ Patients who cannot be appropriately positioned may have suboptimal studies ▨ Motion artifacts may render a study uninterpretable
Angiography	▨ Evaluation of presence and extent of suspected peripheral vascular disease ▨ Treatment of peripheral vascular disease	▨ Some lesions are not amenable to percutaneous treatment and may require surgical management

Evaluation of Deep Venous Thrombosis

Study	Information obtained	Significant limitation
Ultrasound	▨ Presence and extent of occlusive and non-occlusive thrombus ▨ Follow-up of known thrombus	▨ Limited evaluation of pelvic and IVC clot ▨ Limited study in obese patients
CT (contrast-enhanced)	▨ Evaluation of pelvic and thigh clot	▨ If timing of the bolus is inaccurate, false results may occur
MR (contrast-enhanced)	▨ Evaluation of deep pelvic thrombus	▨ If timing of the bolus is inaccurate, false results may occur ▨ Artifacts can occur, which can lead to false results

Common Clinical Questions and Key Studies to Order

Study	Information obtained	Significant limitation
Venography	■ Evaluation of lower or upper extremity thrombus in patients with high clinical suspicion of deep venous thrombosis with negative workup	■ There may be significant collateral vessel formation, which can limit evaluation of the main vessels

Acute Chest Pain

Study	Information obtained	Significant limitation
Conventional radiographs	■ Non-cardiac causes of chest pain ■ Findings of heart failure in the setting of MR ■ Aortic abnormalities (e.g. aortic dissection)	■ Low sensitivity for aortic dissection
CT (contrast-enhanced)	■ Aortic dissection ■ PE ■ Acute coronary occlusion (coronary CT angiography)	■ If contrast bolus timing is incorrect, pathology may not be identified (e.g. PE may not be identified if the bolus is timed to the aorta and not the pulmonary arteries)
MR (contrast-enhanced)	■ Aortic dissection ■ Acute cardiac abnormality (e.g. myocardial ischemia, infarction)	■ Patients may be too unstable to undergo the relatively long imaging time required for MR
Angiography	■ Aortic dissection ■ Acute coronary artery occlusion ■ Coronary artery stenosis ■ PE	■ Invasive
Nuclear medicine (cardiac)	■ Acute myocardial ischemia	■ False negatives may occur if three-vessel balanced disease is present

Stable Angina

Study	Information obtained	Significant limitation
Conventional radiographs	▪ Cardiomegaly ▪ Coronary artery stents ▪ Pacemaker/AICD ▪ Pulmonary edema	▪ Does not provide functional information
CTA (contrast-enhanced)	▪ Presence and extent of coronary atheroma ▪ Degree of luminal narrowing from plaque ▪ Cardiac wall motion abnormalities ▪ Assessment of ejection fraction	▪ Elevated heart rates cause significant artifact that can render the study uninterpretable ▪ Heavily calcified vessels create artifact that can render regions of the vessels uninterpretable
MR (contrast-enhanced)	▪ Presence of stress perfusion abnormalities ▪ Areas of scar and ischemia ▪ Cardiac wall motion abnormalities ▪ Assessment of ejection fraction	▪ Patients who cannot receive IV contrast are not candidates for the evaluation of perfusion abnormalities and scar; wall motion abnormalities can be assessed without IV contrast
Nuclear imaging	▪ Presence and extent of ischemia ▪ Presence and extent of scar ▪ Cardiac wall motion abnormalities ▪ Assessment of ejection fraction	▪ Balanced disease (i.e. flow limiting stenosis in all three vessels can lead to false-negative studies) ▪ Studies can be limited by patient obesity and motion

Common Clinical Questions and Key Studies to Order

Study	Information obtained	Significant limitation
Angiography	■ Presence and degree of coronary artery luminal compromise by atheroma	■ Early or subclinical (< 50% narrowing) disease may be missed by this technique as it affects the wall of the coronary artery and only the lumen is evaluated with conventional catheter angiography (IV ultrasound can evaluate the wall)

Unstable Angina

Study	Information obtained	Significant limitation
Angiography	■ Coronary artery spasm ■ Coronary artery critical stenosis ■ Coronary artery occlusion	■ Invasive ■ Lesions may not be amenable to percutaneous treatment; may require surgical treatment

Cardiac Viability

Study	Information obtained	Significant limitation
Echocardio-graphy	■ Global and regional wall motion abnormalities ■ Evaluation of ejection fraction	■ May be limited by large patient body habitus ■ Poor imaging windows can limit the examination ■ TEE is invasive
MR (contrast-enhanced)	■ Stress perfusion abnormalities suggest ischemia/scar ■ Delayed hyperenhancement characterizes regions of scar and allows prediction of long-term outcome ■ Evaluation of global and regional wall motion abnormalities	■ Patients who cannot receive IV contrast are not candidates for the evaluation of perfusion abnormalities and scar; wall motion abnormalities can be assessed without IV contrast

Study	Information obtained	Significant limitation
Nuclear medicine	▦ Perfusion abnormalities can be determined with SPECT or Rb-82 PET CT ▦ FDG PET CT in combination with Rb-82 PET CT can determine areas that have decreased perfusion with viable myocardium ▦ Evaluation of global and regional wall motion abnormalities	▦ Balanced disease (i.e. flow limiting stenosis in all three vessels can lead to false-negative studies) ▦ Studies can be limited by patient obesity and motion

Coronary Disease

Study	Information obtained	Significant limitation
Conventional radiographs	▦ Cardiomegaly ▦ Coronary artery stents ▦ Pacemaker/AICD ▦ Pulmonary edema	▦ Does not provide functional information
Coronary calcium scoring	▦ Presence and extent of calcified atheroma ▦ Follow-up of coronary artery disease (calcified plaque)	▦ Non-calcified plaque cannot be identified with this technique, resulting in false negatives
CTA (contrast-enhanced)	▦ Presence and extent of coronary atheroma ▦ Degree of luminal narrowing from plaque ▦ Cardiac wall motion abnormalities ▦ Assessment of ejection fraction	▦ Elevated heart rates cause significant artifact that can render the study uninterpretable ▦ Heavily calcified vessels create artifact that can render regions of the vessels uninterpretable

Study	Information obtained	Significant limitation
MR (contrast-enhanced)	■ Presence of stress perfusion abnormalities ■ Areas of scar and ischemia ■ Cardiac wall motion abnormalities ■ Assessment of ejection fraction	■ Patients who cannot receive IV contrast are not candidates for the evaluation of perfusion abnormalities and scar; wall motion abnormalities can be assessed without IV contrast
Echocardiography	■ Global and regional wall motion abnormalities ■ Evaluation of ejection fraction	■ May be limited by large patient body habitus ■ Poor imaging windows can limit the examination ■ TEE is invasive
Nuclear medicine	■ Presence and extent of ischemia ■ Presence and extent of scar ■ Cardiac wall motion abnormalities ■ Assessment of ejection fraction	■ Balanced disease (i.e. flow limiting stenosis in all three vessels can lead to false-negative studies) ■ Studies can be limited by patient obesity and motion
Angiography	■ Presence and degree of coronary artery luminal compromise by atheroma ■ Coronary artery spasm ■ Coronary artery critical stenosis ■ Coronary artery occlusion	■ Early or subclinical ($< 50\%$ narrowing) disease may be missed by this technique as it affects the wall of the coronary artery, and only the lumen is evaluated with conventional catheter angiography (intravascular ultrasound can evaluate the wall)

Estimation of Cardiac Function

Study	Information obtained	Significant limitation
Echocardiography	■ Evaluation of regional and global wall motion abnormalities ■ Estimation of ejection fraction ■ Evaluation of valve function	■ May be limited by large patient body habitus ■ Poor imaging windows can limit the examination ■ TEE is invasive
CTA (contrast-enhanced)	■ Evaluation of regional and global wall motion abnormalities ■ Estimation of ejection fraction ■ Evaluation of valve function	■ Elevated heart rates cause significant artifact that can render the study uninterpretable ■ Heavily calcified vessels create artifact that can render regions of the vessels uninterpretable
MR (non-contrast)	■ Evaluation of regional and global wall motion abnormalities ■ Estimation of ejection fraction ■ Evaluation of valve function	■ If patients are unable to breath-hold, the study will be limited due to motion artifact
Nuclear medicine	■ Evaluation of regional and global wall motion abnormalities ■ Estimation of ejection fraction	■ Balanced disease (i.e. flow limiting stenosis in all three vessels can lead to false-negative studies) ■ Studies can be limited by patient obesity and motion
Angiography	■ Left ventriculography	■ Invasive

Evaluation of Pulmonary Embolism

Study	Information obtained	Significant limitation
Conventional radiograph	■ Pulmonary disease that may explain patient's symptoms (e.g. pneumonia)	■ Limited use for diagnosis of PE
CTPA (contrast-enhanced)	■ Acute pulmonary thromboemboli ■ Subacute/chronic pulmonary thromboemboli ■ Pulmonary artery enlargement ■ Right heart strain	■ Poor contrast bolus timing may render the study non-diagnostic ■ High radiation dose to the breast in young women ■ In obese patients, streak artifact may significantly limit the study
Nuclear medicine (V/Q)	■ Acute pulmonary thromboemboli ■ Right to left shunts	■ If patients are intubated, the ventilation component of the examination cannot be performed. Thus, only a likelihood and not a probability of PE can be assigned ■ In patients with abnormal chest radiographs (e.g. pneumonia, the results may be equivocal for the presence of PE)
Ultrasound (DVT)	■ Presence and extent of deep venous thrombosis in patients with known or suspected PE	■ Obese patients are difficult to evaluate due to poor visualization of the vessels and inability to compress the vessels

Study	Information obtained	Significant limitation
Angiography (PAgram)	▪ Acute pulmonary thromboemboli ▪ Subacute/chronic thromboemboli ▪ Pulmonary artery pressures; pulmonary arterial hypertension	▪ Invasive

Pediatrics

Evaluation of Vomiting

Study	Information obtained	Significant limitation
Conventional radiographs	▪ Distended stomach suggesting outlet obstruction (e.g. pyloric stenosis) ▪ Small bowel obstruction ▪ Necrotizing enterocolitis	▪ Low sensitivity ▪ Often non-specific bowel gas pattern
Ultrasound	▪ Presence of pyloric stenosis	▪ Early pyloric stenosis may have false-negative ultrasound results
Fluoroscopy	▪ Presence of malrotation and midgut volvulus ▪ Presence of gastroesophageal reflux ▪ Presence and location of small bowel obstruction ▪ Colonic obstruction with resultant small bowel obstruction	▪ Failure to demonstrate gastroesophageal reflux does not exclude it; it is an intermittent process
CT (contrast-enhanced)	▪ Presence and location of small bowel obstruction ▪ Presence of acute abdomen (e.g. appendicitis with perforation)	▪ The appendix may be difficult to identify, particularly in thin patients with no intra-abdominal fat

Evaluation of Acute Abdominal Pain

Study	Information obtained	Significant limitation
Conventional radiographs	▪ Free intraperitoneal air ▪ Bowel obstruction ▪ Renal calculi ▪ Pneumobilia	▪ Many renal stones are radiolucent ▪ Renal obstruction cannot be determined on conventional radiographs
Ultrasound	▪ Intussusception ▪ Appendicitis	▪ The appendix may not be identified with ultrasound, particularly if normal
CT (contrast-enhanced)	▪ Free intraperitoneal air ▪ Bowel obstruction ▪ Obstructing renal calculi ▪ Appendicitis ▪ Infectious bowel pathology ▪ Sequela of trauma (e.g. liver/spleen laceration) ▪ Pancreatitis ▪ Adrenal hemorrhage ▪ Abscess formation	▪ Subtle traumatic injury may be difficult to identify ▪ It may be difficult to differentiate bowel from abscess cavities, particularly if the bowel is not adequately distended with oral contrast

Evaluation of Chronic Abdominal Pain with Weight Loss

Study	Information obtained	Significant limitation
Conventional radiographs	▪ Abnormal bowel gas pattern (e.g. obstruction, bowel wall thickening) ▪ Abnormal calcifications (e.g. in the liver in metastatic neuroblastoma) ▪ Organomegaly (e.g. splenomegaly, hepatomegaly)	▪ Bowel gas pattern is often non-specific ▪ Low sensitivity for organomegaly

Study	Information obtained	Significant limitation
Ultrasound	■ Solid organ masses (e.g. liver mass, splenomegaly in Epstein-Barr virus, etc.)	■ If the liver is heterogeneous, cirrhotic or fatty infiltrated, masses may not be visible by ultrasound
CT (contrast-enhanced)	■ Abdominal masses ■ Bowel thickening/ stricture (e.g. Crohn's disease) ■ Abdominal infection	■ Small masses or implants may not be visible ■ It may be difficult to differentiate tumor from infection
MR (contrast-enhanced)	■ Abdominal masses ■ Bowel thickening/ stricture (e.g. Crohn's disease) ■ Abdominal infection	■ Small masses or implants may not be visible ■ It may be difficult to differentiate tumor from infection

Evaluation of Palpable Abdominal Mass

Study	Information obtained	Significant limitation
Conventional radiograph	■ Presence of formed stool, which can present as a palpable mass ■ Organomegaly ■ Calcifications suggesting mass	■ Low sensitivity for organomegaly ■ Calcifications may be difficult to visualize
Ultrasound	■ Organomegaly ■ Solid organ mass	■ If the liver is heterogeneous, cirrhotic, or fatty infiltrated, masses may not be visible by ultrasound
CT (contrast-enhanced)	■ Organomegaly ■ Solid organ mass ■ Bowel mass ■ Mesenteric mass	■ Bowel masses (particularly if mucosal) may be difficult to visualize

Common Clinical Questions and Key Studies to Order

Study	Information obtained	Significant limitation
	■ Osseous mass with soft tissue component ■ Sites of metastatic disease from primary tumor	
MR (contrast-enhanced)	■ Organomegaly ■ Solid organ mass ■ Bowel mass ■ Mesenteric mass ■ Osseous mass with soft tissue component ■ Sites of metastatic disease from primary tumor	■ Bowel masses (particularly if mucosal) may be difficult to visualize

Evaluation of Vesicoureteral Reflux

Study	Information obtained	Significant limitation
Ultrasound	■ Presence of parenchymal scar ■ Presence of duplicated collecting system ■ Presence and degree of renal obstruction ■ Presence of collecting system dilation with full bladder, suggesting reflux	■ It does not provide information on renal function ■ A capacious, non-obstructed system may be difficult to differentiate from an obstructed system with ultrasound
CT (contrast-enhanced)	■ Presence of renal scar	■ Routine CECT does not assess renal function
MR (contrast-enhanced)	■ Presence of renal scar ■ Evaluation of renal function (contrast enhancement and excretion)	■ Renal function cannot be quantitated on MR, unlike nuclear medicine studies

Study	Information obtained	Significant limitation
VCUG	■ Presence and degree of vesicoureteral reflux ■ Presence of ureterocele ■ Presence of posterior urethral valves	■ False negatives may occur; if reflux is not demonstrated, it does not exclude its presence
Nuclear medicine	■ Presence of renal scar (DMSA) ■ Evaluation of renal function (DTPA, MAG-3) ■ Indirect evaluation of vesicoureteral reflux ■ Direct evaluation of vesicoureteral reflux (nuclear VCUG)	■ High radiation dose

Evaluation of Hydronephrosis

Study	Information obtained	Significant limitation
Ultrasound	■ Presence and degree of collecting system dilation ■ Changes of UPJ obstruction ■ Follow-up of degree of renal obstruction ■ Presence of obstructing mass/stone ■ Associated cortical thinning in long-standing obstruction	■ Dilation of the collecting system/capacious systems cannot always be differentiated from obstructed systems as ultrasound is an anatomic study, not a dynamic or functional study
CT	■ Presence and degree of renal obstruction ■ Presence of obstructing mass/calculus	■ Small masses may be difficult to visualize
MR	■ Presence and degree of renal obstruction	■ Motion may limit the examination

Study	Information obtained	Significant limitation
	■ Presence of obstructing mass/calculus ■ Relative function of the obstructed kidney (i.e. contrast enhancement and excretion relative to the normal kidney)	
Nuclear imaging	■ Presence of renal obstruction vs. dilated, functional system (functional study) ■ Differentiation of obstruction from dilated, non-obstructed system ■ Evaluation of renal artery stenosis	■ If bilateral renal artery stenosis is present, a false-negative result may occur

Evaluation of Intracranial Bleed

Study	Information obtained	Significant limitation
Ultrasound	■ Neonatal head ultrasound can evaluate for the presence and grade of germinal matrix hemorrhage ■ Evaluation of parenchymal hemorrhage ■ Evaluation of extra-axial fluid collection (e.g. epidural, subdural)	■ The study can be performed only if the fontanelle is open to allow the ultrasound beam to penetrate ■ Ultrasound is limited for the evaluation of extra-axial fluid, cerebral edema, and subarachnoid hemorrhage
CT (non-contrast)	■ Presence and location of intraparenchymal hemorrhage, subdural, epidural, subarachnoid hemorrhage ■ Presence of diffuse cerebral edema	■ Limited for the evaluation of subtle or early diffuse cerebral edema

Study	Information obtained	Significant limitation
MR (non-contrast)	▪ Presence and location of intraparenchymal hemorrhage, subdural, epidural, subarachnoid hemorrhage ▪ MR can date the hemorrhage ▪ Presence of diffuse cerebral edema	▪ Very susceptible to motion artifact, particularly given relatively long imaging time required compared with CT or ultrasound

Evaluation of Fever of Unknown Origin

Study	Information obtained	Significant limitation
Conventional radiographs (CXR)	▪ Pneumonia is one of the most common causes of fever of unknown origin	▪ Early pneumonia, atypical or viral pneumonia may be radiographically occult
CT (contrast-enhanced)	▪ Abscess ▪ Malignancy ▪ Solid organ or visceral abnormality	▪ Poor contrast bolus can limit evaluation ▪ It may be difficult to differentiate infection from necrotic tumor (e.g. ring-enhancing hepatic mass)
MR (contrast-enhanced)	▪ Abscess ▪ Malignancy ▪ Solid organ or visceral abnormality	▪ Poor contrast bolus can limit evaluation ▪ It may be difficult to differentiate infection from necrotic tumor (e.g. ring-enhancing hepatic mass)

Study	Information obtained	Significant limitation
Nuclear medicine (gallium, WBC, PET CT)	▪ Abscess ▪ Malignancy	▪ Poor resolution for determination of precise location of abnormality ▪ May be difficult to differentiate infection from malignancy; often requires confirmatory study (e.g. CECT)

Contrast Premedication Protocol

Regimen 1
▪ Medication: Prednisone
▪ Route: Oral
▪ Dose: 50 mg
▪ Schedule: 13, 7, and 1 hour prior to CECT
▪ Benadryl 50 mg oral or IV is also administered 1 hour prior to CECT.
▪ Cimetidine also may be administered for its H_2 antagonist effects

Regimen 2
▪ Medication: Solu-Medrol
▪ Route: IV
▪ Dose: 125 mg
▪ Schedule: 6 and 1 hour prior to CECT
▪ Benadryl 50 mg oral or IV also is administered 1 hour prior to CECT.
▪ IV cimetidine may also be administered for its H_2 antagonist effects.

Contraindications to MR Imaging

Absolute contraindications
▪ Cardiac valves (now only St. Jude valve)
▪ Metallic foreign bodies within the orbits (patients with exposure history should be screened for metal with orbital radiographs prior to the MR examination)
▪ Patients with ferromagnetic surgical clips (e.g. cerebral aneurysm clips)
▪ Patients with pacemakers or AICDs cannot be imaged with MR due to the effect of the magnetic field upon the devices.

Relative contraindications

- Recently placed cardiac stents (within 1–2 days)
- Obesity: The majority of MR scanners have a table limit of 350 lbs. Patients exceeding this limit cannot be imaged on conventional MR scanners. Patient girth is also a limitation; if patients exceed a certain circumference, they will not fit into the bore of the magnet.
- Claustrophobia: Many patients are unable to tolerate a complete MR examination based on claustrophobia. If there is a preexisting history of claustrophobia, the patient may be booked for the examination with sedation or may require anesthesia if sedation is inadequate to allow completion of the study.
- Inability to lie supine: Patients who are unable to lie completely flat are often poor candidates for MRI. Images may be suboptimal due to patient positioning. Additionally, if patients are unable to be appropriately positioned based upon respiratory compromise when in a supine position, they are often unable to tolerate the examination. MRI of solid organs such as the liver and kidneys often requires the patient to breath-hold for 20–30 seconds. If patients are unable to do so, the images may be degraded to the degree of being uninterpretable.

Common Clinical Questions and Key Studies to Order

APPENDIX II

Recommended Studies by Clinical Indication

★ = Recommended studies are listed below each clinical indication.

Acute cholecystitis
- ★ Ultrasound
- MR
- ★ HIDA

Biliary obstruction
- ★ Ultrasound
- ★ ERCP
- PTC
- CT
- ★ MRCP

Choledocholithiasis
- Ultrasound
- ★ MRCP
- CT
- ★ ERCP

Liver mass
- Ultrasound
- ★ MR (enhanced)
- ★ CT (enhanced)
- Nuclear imaging

Hepatic vessel occlusion
- ★ Ultrasound (Doppler)
- MR (enhanced)
- CT (enhanced)
- Angiography

Portal hypertension
- ★ Ultrasound (Doppler)
- MR (enhanced)
- Angiography
- CT (enhanced)
- ★ Nuclear imaging

Pancreatitis
- ⋆ Ultrasound (gallstones)
- MR (enhanced)
- ⋆ CT (enhanced)

Renal colic
- Conventional x-ray
- ⋆ CT (non-contrast)
- ⋆ Ultrasound

Renal mass
- Ultrasound
- ⋆ MR
- ⋆ CT

Hematuria
- KUB (stones)
- ⋆ CT (enhanced)
- Cystogram
- Ultrasound
- ⋆ MR (enhanced)

Bowel obstruction
- Conventional x-ray
- Fluoroscopy
- ⋆ CT (enhanced)

Bowel perforation
- Conventional x-ray
- ⋆ CT (enhanced)

Ischemic bowel
- Conventional x-ray
- ⋆ CT (enhanced)

Colitis/inflammatory bowel disease
- Conventional x-ray
- CT enterography
- Fluoroscopy
- ⋆ CT (enhanced)
- MR enterography

Appendicitis
- Ultrasound
- MR (non-contrast)
- ⋆ CT (enhanced)

Diverticulitis
- ⋆ CT (enhanced)

GI bleed
- ⋆ CT (enhanced)
- ⋆ Angiography
- ⋆ Nuclear Imaging

Recommended Studies by Clinical Indication

Abdominal trauma
Ultrasound   ★ CT (enhanced)

Acute abdomen
Conventional x-ray   ★ CT (enhanced)

Pelvic pain (non-pregnant)
★ Ultrasound (transvaginal)   CT (enhanced)
★ MR   Angiography (fibroids)

Pelvic pain (pregnant)
★ Ultrasound   ★ MR (non-contrast)

Ectopic
★ Ultrasound

Recurrent pregnancy loss
Ultrasound   HSG
★ Hysterosonography   ★ MR

Infertility
Ultrasound   ★ HSG
★ Hysterosonography   ★ MR

Pelvic infection
Ultrasound   ★ CT (enhanced)
★ MR (enhanced)

Pelvic mass
★ Ultrasound   CT (enhanced)
★ MR (enhanced)

Malignancy staging
★ CT (enhanced)   ★ MR (enhanced)
★ PET CT

Fever of unknown origin
Conventional x-ray   Ultrasound
★ CT (enhanced)   MR (enhanced)
★ Nuclear imaging

Pulmonary nodule
Conventional x-ray   ★ CT (non-contrast)
PET CT

Interstitial lung disease
    Conventional x-ray
    Nuclear imaging

★ CT (high resolution)

Chest pain
★ Conventional x-ray
    Echocardiography
    Nuclear imaging

★ CT (enhanced)
    ETT
    Angiography

Stable angina
★ Coronary CTA
★ Nuclear imaging

★ ETT
    Angiography

Unstable angina
★ Angiography

Pulmonary embolism
    Conventional x-ray
★ CTPA (enhanced)
    Angiography

★ Ultrasound (DVT)
★ Nuclear imaging (V/Q)

Leg Swelling/DVT
★ Ultrasound
    MR venography

    CT venography (enhanced)
    Angiography

Peripheral vascular disease
    Ultrasound
★ MRA (enhanced)

★ CTA (enhanced)
★ Angiography

Hypertension
★ Ultrasound (Doppler RAS)
★ MRA (enhanced)
    Angiography

★ CTA (enhanced)
    Nuclear imaging

Aortic dissection
    Conventional x-ray
    MR (enhanced)
    Angiography

★ CT (enhanced)
    TEE

Carotid disease
★ Ultrasound
★ MRA (enhanced)

★ CTA (enhanced)
    Angiography

Acute bone trauma
★ Conventional x-rays
★ MR (non-contrast)

★ CT (non-contrast)
Nuclear imaging

Soft tissue/muscle/ligament/tendon injury
★ MR (non-contrast)

Osteomyelitis
Conventional x-rays
★ MR (enhanced)

CT
★ Nuclear imaging

Primary bone tumor
★ Conventional x-rays
MR (enhanced)

★ CT (non-contrast)
Nuclear imaging

Bone metastases
Conventional x-rays
MR (enhanced)

★ CT (non-contrast)
★ Nuclear imaging

Headache
★ CT (non-contrast)

MR (non-contrast)

Altered mental status
★ CT (non-contrast)

MR

Acute head trauma
★ CT (non-contrast)

MR (non-contrast)

Seizure
★ CT (non-contrast)

★ MR (contrast)

Brain tumor/infection
★ CT (enhanced)
Nuclear imaging

★ MR (enhanced)

Cervical spine injury
★ Conventional x-rays
MR (non-contrast)

★ CT (non-contrast)

Cord compression/injury
CT

★ MR

Disc disease
CT (non-contrast)

★ MR (non-contrast)

Back pain
- ★ Conventional x-rays
- ★ MR (non-contrast)

CT (non-contrast)
Nuclear imaging

Pediatric imaging

Vomiting
- Conventional x-rays
- ★ Ultrasound

- ★ Upper GI
- CT

Acute abdominal pain
- ★ Conventional x-rays
- ★ CT

- ★ Ultrasound

Failure to pass meconium
- Conventional x-rays

- ★ Hypaque enema

Hip pain
- Conventional x-rays

- ★ Ultrasound

Urinary tract infection
- ★ Ultrasound
- MR (enhanced)
- Nuclear imaging

CT (enhanced)
- ★ VCUG

Index